Prostaglandins and Leukotrienes

HEMATOLOGY

Series Editor

Kenneth M. Brinkhous, M.D.
Department of Pathology
University of North Carolina
School of Medicine
Chapel Hill, North Carolina

Volume 1 Prostaglandins and Leukotrienes: Blood and Vascular Cell Function, *Jonathan M. Gerrard*

Other Volumes in Preparation

Hematopoietic Stem Cells, *edited by David W. Golde and Fumimaro Takaku*

Bone Marrow Transplantation, *edited by Dirk W. van Bekkum*

Prostaglandins and Leukotrienes

Blood and Vascular Cell Function

Jonathan M. Gerrard
Department of Pediatrics
University of Manitoba
Manitoba Institute of Cell Biology
Winnipeg, Canada

MARCEL DEKKER, INC. New York and Basel

Library of Congress Cataloging in Publication Data

Gerrard, Jonathan M., date
Prostaglandins and leukotrienes.

(Hematology; v. 1)
Includes index.
1. Blood cells. 2. Blood platelets. 3. Prostaglandins –Physiological effect. 4. Leukotrienes–Physiological effect. I. Title. II. Series: Hematology (New York, N.Y.) ; v. 1. [DNLM: 1. Blood Cells–physiology. 2. Prostaglandins–blood. 3. Prostaglandins–physiology. 4. SRS-A–blood. 5. SRS-A–physiology.
W1 HE873 v. 1 / QU 90 G378p]
QP94.G47 1984 599'.0113 84-19969
ISBN 0-8247-7259-8

Marcel Dekker, Inc.
270 Madison Avenue, New York, New York 10016

Current printing (last digit):
10 9 8 7 6 5 4 3 2 1

Printed in the United States of America

Introduction to the Series

This book represents the first volume in the new Hematology Series from Marcel Dekker, Inc. This series is designed to provide up-to-date and authoritative presentations on current topics in hematology, with emphasis on new knowledge and its clinical significance. In perspective, hematology as a field has followed a pattern for many years of major scientific advances, improved understanding of disease, and rapid applications in the clinic. Looking back, this pattern was set in the first half of this century. A gauge of major advances of that period is provided by physicians and scientists working in hematology who became Nobel Laureates in Physiology and Medicine. This list includes Karl Landsteiner for discovery of blood groups, 1930; George Whipple, George Minot, and William Murphy for discoveries on liver therapy for anemia, 1934; and Henrik Dam and Edward Doisy for the discovery of vitamin K and its chemical nature, 1944. The pace of advance continues and seems to be accelerating, hence the perceived need for this new series in hematology. It is anticipated that succeeding volumes in the series will deal with a wide scope of subjects in hematology regarding which a new body of significant knowledge has developed. It is hoped that these collected works become important volumes for general reading, for updating one's information, and for reference.

It is appropriate that the first volume of the series should be devoted to the role of prostaglandins and related compounds on blood cell function and to the implications of this important regulatory system for prevention and management of disease. The word "prostaglandin" was coined 50 years ago by von Euler, one of the discoverers of this new class of bioactive compounds. He originally but erroneously thought them to be of prostatic gland origin. The name, in spite of its wrong connotation, has become deeply embedded in the language. The biologic importance of these compounds is attested to by an ever enlarging literature. It was not until the last decade, however, that the importance of the prostaglandin-based regulatory system in hematology was appreciated. This was marked by the first international symposium on prostaglandins and hematology, held in 1976. The leadoff paper was co-authored by Jonathan M. Gerrard, the author of this volume. During the late 1970s there were many significant developments in this field. In rapid order, several groups of compounds with potent biological effects on blood cells and blood-vascular function were recognized. These included prostacyclin, the thromboxanes and the leukotrienes. The latter two, like the prostaglandins, are metabolically derived from essential fatty acids, notably arachidonic acid, through a number of enzymatic pathways with many cofactors. The names, thromboxane and leukotriene, are derived in part from the blood cell from which they were isolated, thrombocyte and leukocyte, respectively. A marvel of modern science is the rapidity with which the structures of these compounds were established and with which many analogues were synthesized. Since the discovery in 1971 that aspirin limited prostaglandin production by inhibiting cyclooxygenase, many other inhibitors with different modes of action have been identified. The potential for development of drugs which would precisely modulate in a specific way cell metabolism and cellular responses has become widely appreciated. Dr. Gerrard, a physician and a productive investigator in this field, provides the reader with a well-organized and clearly illustrated presentation regarding the nature and significance of prostaglandins and related compounds in blood, vascular, and inflammatory diseases.

Kenneth M. Brinkhous
Series Editor

Preface

The award of the Nobel Prize to Dr. Sune Bergstrom, Dr. Bengt Samuelsson, and Dr. John Vane in 1982 highlighted the importance of prostaglandins and related chemicals in biological processes. It has taken a long time from the original discovery of a smooth muscle-contracting activity in semen in 1930 by Kurzrok and Lieb to the widespread study of these active chemicals. Research on blood cells has been at the forefront of this research area. Thromboxane A_2 made in platelets was first identified by Mats Hamberg and others working with Bengt Samuelsson. Prostacyclin made in vascular tissue was next discovered by Salvador Moncada and others working with John Vane. Most recently, leukotrienes, produced by white blood cells, have been structurally characterized and studied by several groups.

The general importance of understanding something of this area of research to modern medical care is emphasized by the widespread use of inhibitors of prostaglandin and thromboxane production including aspirin, indomethacin, ibuprofen, and many others. Steroids, like prednisone, also widely used, also interfere with prostaglandin formation, but act at a more basic level—inhibition of release of the precursor fatty acids from phospholipids. There is currently a considerable gap between those who do research in this area, and those who are trying to use these drugs in a meaningful way clinically. Part of the reason for this gap is that most medical doctors lack much of the fundamental knowledge of lipids essential to understanding how they work. This book is written as an attempt to bridge this gap. At the same time, individuals working with blood cells often find that they know their own cell type intimately, but lack basic knowledge of similar cell types important to their research. This book, in combining the essential details of each cell type and the relevant interactions of prostaglandins and related chemicals, can be a useful reference tool.

The book is written as a single-authored book to allow uniform treatment of the various prostaglandins and related chemicals in their interactions with each blood cell type. In the early chapters, I have followed the guiding principle that complex biological interactions can be best understood in terms of simpler fundamental processes common to a wide variety of cell types. In some instances, our knowledge of such basic processes is still sketchy. In others, we can now begin to comprehend at a molecular level the reason behind the specific mechanism and its evolution. Chapters 1-5 therefore look at the nature of the lipids of interest and the common threads in the dynamic interactions of these lipids in various cell types.

In Chapters 6-14, each individual blood cell type is discussed in sequence. This approach was essential since the pattern of synthesis and effect of prostaglandins and related lipids appears to have evolved uniquely in each cell type to match cellular functional requirements. In each chapter there is first a brief overview of cell structure and function. This is then followed by a discussion of our current knowledge of the cellular synthesis of these lipids and the effects of endogenously and exogenously produced compounds on cell function. A short overview at the end of each of these chapters summarizes what now appear to be the most salient features. For the researcher, important species differences are covered in an appendix.

In Chapters 15-19, the stage moves to address in vivo interactions of blood cells. Specific problems are associated with this more complex world. Measuring in vivo production of prostaglandins and related chemicals has been frustrating because of their rapid metabolism. It is difficult enough to assess simultaneously all the relevant metabolites of a single cell type without having to be concerned with the even broader range of production possible in the mixed cell systems in the body. Nevertheless, emerging concepts of the role of blood cells and their lipid metabolites in hemostasis and thrombosis, in inflammation and host defense, in hypersensitivity reactions, and in blood cell production are discussed.

The final chapter provides in summary form an overview of the concepts presented in this book. It is written to give a concise perspective on the role of prostaglandins, thromboxanes, hydroxy fatty acids, and leukotrienes in blood cell biology, and the current and future application of this knowledge to understanding and treating human diseases.

A glossary at the end of the book provides a ready reference for those unfamiliar with the terminology in this rapidly expanding area of medical science.

Jonathan M. Gerrard

Acknowledgments

I am indebted to Jim White for encouraging my interest in research, for his tutelage during the years we spent together in Minneapolis, and for his support and advice at several points during the writing of this book. There are many individuals who taught me various facets of what I know about prostaglandins. These include Bill Krivit, who initially invited me to do a fellowship in pediatric hematology working on prostaglandins; Mel Silver and Bryan Smith, with whom I spent a critical 3 days early in my training; and Bill Sweeney, who showed me how to use the gas chromatograph-mass spectrometer to analyze prostaglandins. From those with whom I have collaborated, including Gundu Rao, Doug Peterson, Dewayne Townsend, Gustav Graff, Nelson Goldberg, David Glass, David Brown, Marie Stuart, Carl Witkop, Jr., Ian Dresner, Roger Carroll, and Fletcher Taylor, I have had many fruitful discussions. Students and technicians who have worked with me, including Beatrice Heagan, Marcy Krumwiede, Janet Peller, Steve Stoddard, Ralph Shapiro, Doug Tate, Steve Kindom, Katie Krantz, Ailie Butler, Anna Schorer, Shiela Glover, Ann Benton, Jan McCrea, Jeanine Savard, Kathi Fast, Pauline Robinson, Gillian Woodfield, and Laura Friesen, have provided careful and often painstaking effort to produce the experimental data to try to answer many questions. During the preparation of this book, Drs. L. A.

Boxer, Kenneth M. Brinkhous, J. W. Gerrard, A. H. Greenberg, S. J. Israels, N. L. Kobrinsky, D. A. Peterson, D. M. Smith, and N. L. Stephens provided helpful comments after reading drafts of one or more chapters. I am indebted to Lori Devlin for typing this book and to the staff of Marcel Dekker for their assistance and support.

I owe much to my wife and family for their support and their understanding when I am off traveling or busy writing.

Contents

PART II: SPECIFIC BLOOD CELL TYPES

PART III: THE ROLE OF PROSTAGLANDINS AND RELATED CHEMICALS IN VIVO IN CELL-CELL INTERACTIONS INVOLVING BLOOD CELLS

Prostaglandins and Leukotrienes

I

GENERAL CONCEPTS

1
An Introduction to Prostaglandins

Within and adjacent to the bloodstream are a wide variety of cell types. Modulation of the function of blood cells by prostaglandins and related chemicals now occurs in a bewildering variety of ways. Essential to an appreciation of the reason for the importance of these chemicals is some understanding of their nature and their chemical properties. These compounds act as local "hormones" or autocoids. Knowledge of their origin, their structure, their solubility, and their instability shows why they have a wide variety of effects on cells.

I. THE PROSTAGLANDINS AND CELL INJURY: AN APPRECIATION OF WHY THESE COMPOUNDS ARE IMPORTANT

Prostaglandins and related chemicals are derived from polyunsaturated fatty acids such as arachidonic acid (Fig. 1-1). Arachidonic acid is a basic constituent of cells, but in normal circumstances it is bound as an integral part of phospholipids, triglycerides, or cholesterol esters. Under conditions of cellular damage or cellular stimulation arachidonic acid is released from these essential

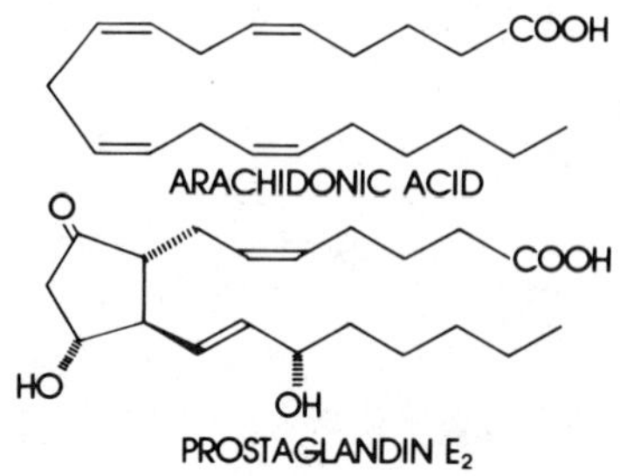

Fig. 1-1 Conversion of arachidonic acid to prostaglandin E_2 produces a compound with a rigid 5-carbon ring, with a ketone (=0), and with two hydroxyls (OH) added in a stereospecific fashion (≡ indicates below the plane of the carbons). The ketone on the top right of PGE_2 is called a β-hydroxy ketone as an OH group is attached two carbons distant. The OH in the middle center is referred to as an allylic hydroxy because there is a double bone on the other side of the carbon, one removed from the carbon where the OH is attached.

cellular components and is rapidly oxidized to prostaglandins and similar compounds. The rapid formation of these compounds under conditions of cellular stimulation or cellular damage and their nature (with many functional groups, and intermediate lipid:water solubility) allow them to interact with a wide variety of other chemicals (ions and proteins in particular) to modulate cellular functions. The *rapid formation* and the *reactive nature* of these compounds are keys to their understanding.

II. UNDERSTANDING THE ACTIVITY AND REACTIVITY OF PROSTAGLANDINS AND RELATED CHEMICALS

The oxidation of polyunsaturated fatty acids like arachidonic acid (Fig. 1-1) produces chemicals with a wide variety of functional groups. For instance, prostaglandin E_2 (PGE_2) (Fig. 1-1) has (a) a carboxyl, (b) a labile β-hydroxy ketone, (c) a secondary allylic alcohol, and (d) two double bonds. The variety of transformations possible (see Ch. 2) enables a wide variety of different chemical structures to be formed. The oxygen atoms added (as hydroxyls, ketones, and so on) during these oxygenation reactions vastly improve the ability of the compounds to attach to metals or proteins and thus to modulate cell function. Also, the addition of these oxygen-containing substituent groups transforms arachidonic acid (a highly lipophilic or membrane-soluble compound) into compounds of intermediate lipid:water solubility. This change in solubility properties allows the prostaglandins and related chemicals better diffusion through water phases and better access to cytoplasmic constituents. The conversion of arachidonic acid also creates a compound with a five-membered ring that makes part of the molecule considerably more rigid than the free fatty acid. This aspect may be important to fitting of these chemicals to receptors.

III. RAPID RELEASE OF ARACHIDONIC ACID FROM CELLS BY INJURY OR SPECIFIC STIMULUS

Synthesis of prostaglandins and related chemicals is usually activated within cells by release of the precursor fatty acid—and most frequently arachidonic acid. The release of arachidonic acid from cellular membranes where it is bound within phospholipids depends in all cells which have been well studied on a mechanism of hair-trigger sensitivity. Even very mild nonspecific cellular perturbations can lead to some synthesis of prostaglandins. The degree to which prostaglandins and related chemicals are formed depends in this nonspecific circumstance on the degree of cell injury as well as on the amount of cellular synthetic enzyme. However, for most cells, there is a specific pathway or pathways for arachidonic acid liberation, triggered by specific cellular interactions with stimulatory chemicals. Such pathways are evaluated in detail in Ch. 4.

IV. THE EVOLUTION OF PROSTAGLANDINS

Cellular components which are fundamental and necessary to life such as cytochrome C and actin have changed little through long periods of time and are practically identical from one mammalian cell to the next. In contrast to this, the pattern of production and effect of prostaglandins and related chemicals sometimes varies in a major way even from one mammalian species to another. Prostaglandins and related chemicals are formed for the most part in mammalian cells as a response to injury or stimulus. The wide variety of metabolic products of arachidonic acid and the variation from animal to animal suggest that this group of compounds has probably evolved its current complexity relatively recently on an evolutionary time frame and has retained an adaptability to the specific requirements of each species.

BIBLIOGRAPHY

U. S. von Euler and R. Eliasson. *Prostaglandins.* Academic Press, New York (1967).

S. M. M. Karim and K. Hillier. *The Prostaglandins.* Wiley-Interscience, New York (1967).

M. F. Cuthbert (ed.). *The Prostaglandins, Pharmacological and Therapeutic Advances.* J. B. Lippincott, Philadelphia (1973).

P. W. Ramwell (ed.). *The Prostaglandins*, Volume 1. Plenum Press, New York (1973).

S. M. M. Karim (ed.). *Prostaglandins: Chemical and Biochemical Aspects.* University Park Press, Baltimore (1976).

P. B. Curtis-Prior. *Prostaglandins.* Elsevier/North-Holland, Amsterdam (1976).

S. M. M. Karim. *Practical Applications of Prostaglandins and Their Synthesis Inhibitors.* University Park Press, Baltimore (1979).

S. Greenberg, P. J. Kadowitz, and T. F. Burks. *Prostaglandins, Organ and Tissue-Specific Actions.* Marcel Dekker, New York (1982).

2

The Structures and General Functional Properties of Prostaglandins and Related Chemicals

This chapter will introduce the compounds of interest, their precursors, their metabolites, and related active substances.

I. CELL MEMBRANES AND PHOSPHOLIPIDS

Fundamental to an understanding of mammalian cells is a knowledge of phospholipids and their organization into a lipid bilayer. Most phospholipids are characterized by a glycerol backbone (Fig. 2-1) with a polar phosphate attached on the third carbon and two nonpolar fatty acid chains attached to carbons 1 and 2. To the phosphate group on carbon 3 there is usually a further polar constituent (choline, ethanolamine, inositol, or serine) (Fig. 2-2). The result of this structure is a molecule with a polar (head) end, which prefers to exist in a water environment, and a hydrophobic tail, which prefers to exist in a lipid environment. One conformation in which groups of these molecules exist together is a bilayer with one layer of phospholipids associated tail to tail with another layer of phospholipids (Fig. 2-3). In such a bilayer, the hydrocarbon of the acyl (derived from fatty acids) tails of these molecules associates in the middle to give a central lipid layer. The polar head ends associate with

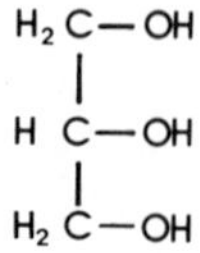

Fig. 2-1 Glycerol is the starting material from which phospholipids are synthesized.

the outside water phases. It is this structure which forms the basis for cell membranes. The central lipid domain (back-to-back fatty acid chains) is relatively impermeable to most polar water-soluble constituents, including ions such as Na^+, K^+, Ca^{2+}, and Mg^{2+}, proteins, and carbohydrates. This enables the cell to maintain an intracellular microenvironment very different from the extracellular milieu. Maintenance of the integrity of this lipid bilayer is of fundamental importance to cells, and any influence which affects the bilayer integrity must be responded to by the cell.

In addition to phospholipids, within the bilayer are several other lipids and many proteins. Bilayer membranes must have a certain stiffness and a certain fluidity. Individual cellular membranes may vary somewhat in the relative degree of fluidity. The fluidity of a membrane depends on the lipid constituents and on the associated proteins, with the nature of the acyl (fatty acid) chains of the phospholipids being one important factor (see Sec. II).

The polar head group of the phospholipid has important interactions with components of the water phase. Phosphatidylcholine, which has no net charge over a wide range of pH, has less interaction with the cations (Na^+, K^+, Ca^{2+}, and so on) and positively charged groups on proteins than phosphatidylinositol, phosphatidylserine, phosphatidylethanolamine and phosphatidic acid, all of which carry a net negative charge at physiologic pH. Sphingomyelin, a sphingolipid that can function in a lipid bilayer similar to the above phospholipids has a slight net positive charge on the surface due to the presence of the free hydroxy group of the 4-sphingosine, which lessens the acidity of the phosphate group by ion-dipole interaction.

The phospholipids and sphingolipids are not uniformly distributed in cell membranes. Red blood cells and platelet plasma membranes are enriched in phosphatidylcholine and sphingomyelin on their outer leaflet and in phosphatidylethanolamine, phosphatidylserine, and phosphatidylinositol on their inner leaflet (Fig. 2-4).

PHOSPHATIDYLCHOLINE

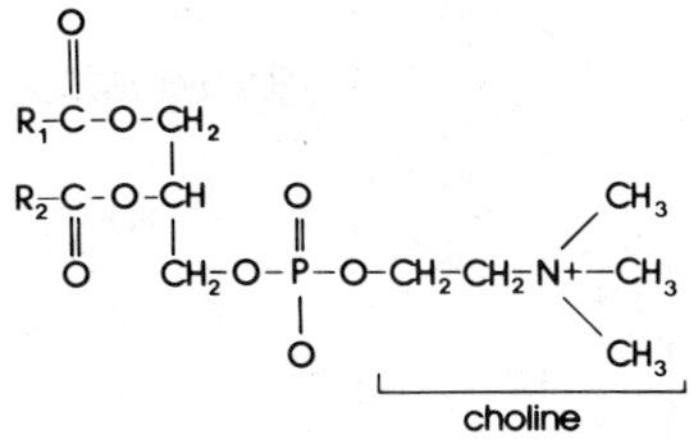

PHOSPHATIDYLETHANOLAMINE

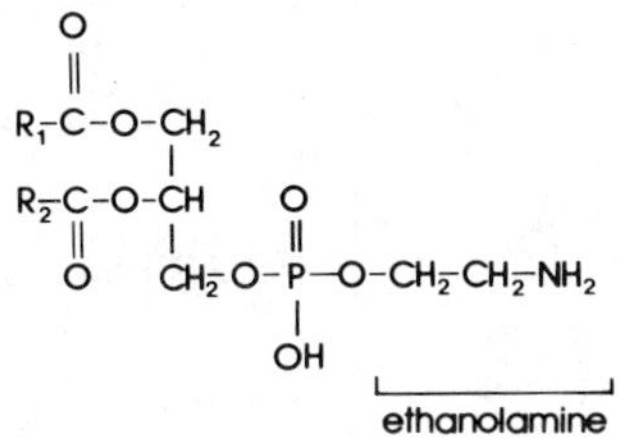

PHOSPHATIDYLINOSITOL

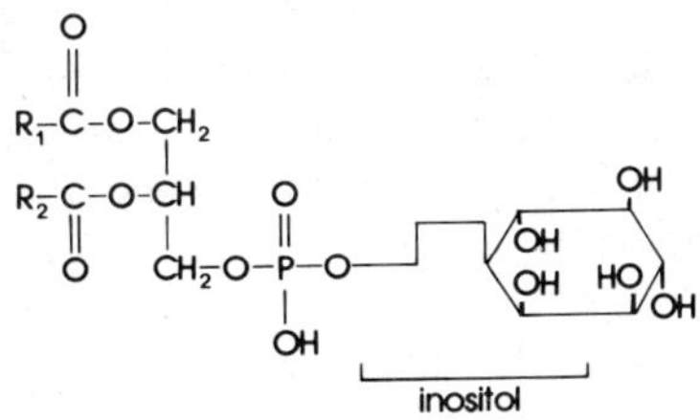

PHOSPHATIDYLSERINE

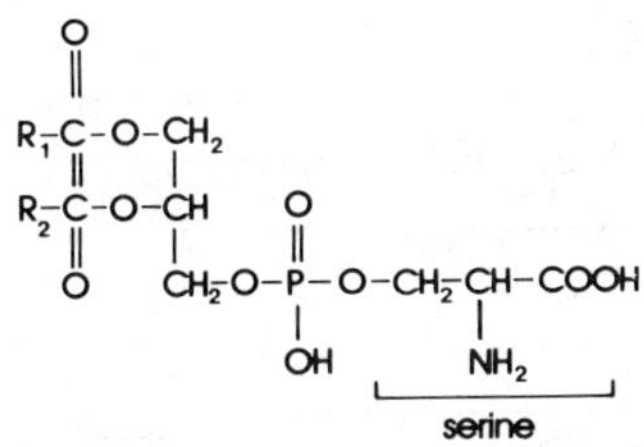

Fig. 2-2 The principal phospholipid types in biological membranes are phosphatidylcholine, phosphatidylethanolamine, phosphatidylinositol, and phosphatidylserine. A related sphingolipid, sphingomyelin (not shown), is also an important species in many biological membranes. R_1 and R_2 indicate the hydrocarbon chains of the fatty acids. In biological membranes the fatty acid in the 1-position is usually a saturated fatty acid while the fatty acid in the 2-position is usually an unsaturated one. Deviating from the usual form for drawing these phospholids, the two fatty acid chains are drawn on the same side of the glycerol backbone, and the phosphate and base on the other, as this is the way these groups will orient in a bilayer membrane. (See Fig. 2-3.)

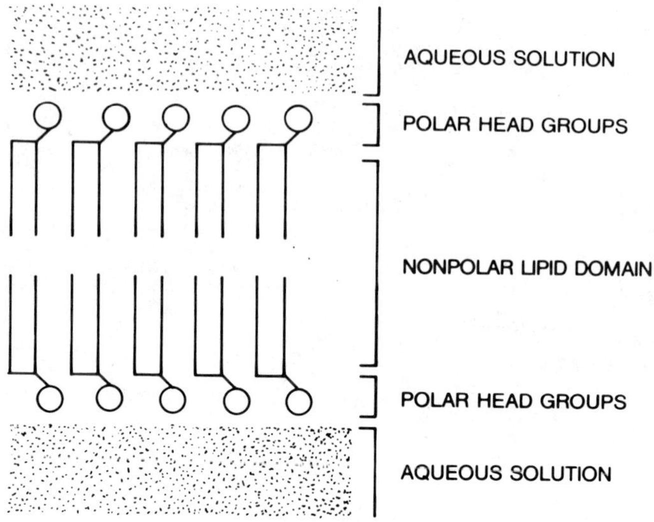

Fig. 2-3 The basic structure of cell membranes is two layers of phospholipids. The central lipid zone containing the fatty acid chains is relatively impermeable to water and polar or ionized species allowing the cell to maintain its own internal microenvironment.

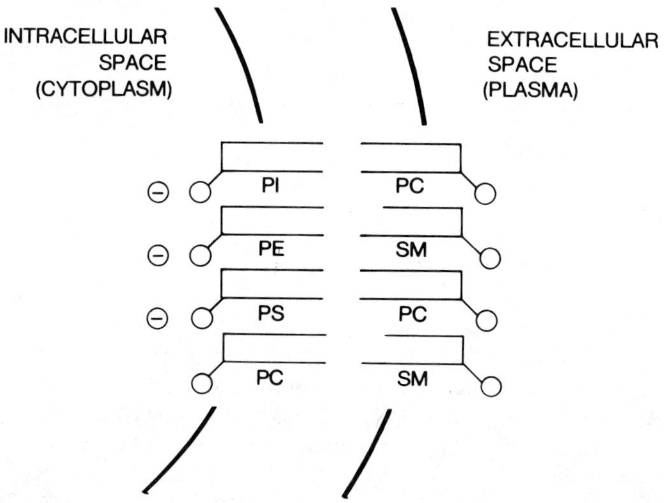

Fig. 2-4 In red blood cells and platelets, and probably in other blood cells as well, the outer plasma membrane is asymmetrical. Phosphatidylcholine (PC) and sphingomyelin (SM) are the major constituents of the outer bilayer. Phosphatidylethanolamine (PE), phosphatidylcholine (PC), phosphatidylserine (PS), and phosphatidylinositol (PI) are the major phospholipids of the inner bilayer. ⊖ indicates a negative charge on the polar "head" end of the phospholipid.

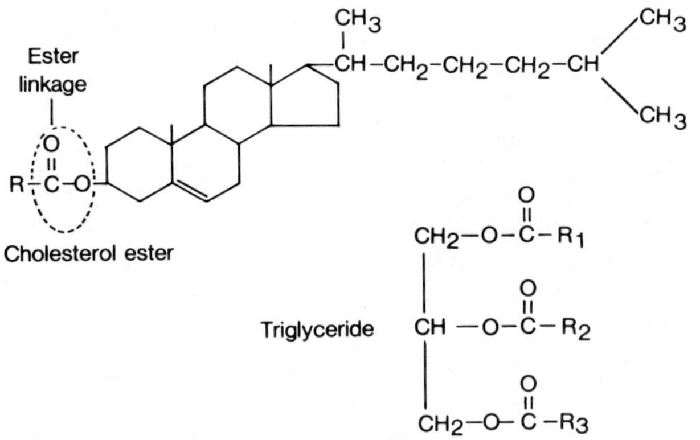

Fig. 2-5 In addition to phospholipids, fatty acid (acyl) chains are found on cholesterol and triglycerides, and in some cells these could be important reservoirs for the fatty acid precursors needed for synthesis of prostaglandins and related chemicals. In the cholesterol ester the fatty acid species is attached through an ester linkage to cholesterol. As in Fig. 2-2, R is used to designate the hydrocarbon chain of the fatty acid.

Two other lipids which may contain arachidonic acid which could be released to make this fatty acid available for prostaglandin synthesis are *cholesterol esters* and *triglycerides* (Fig. 2-5). To date, evidence points to the phospholipids as the major sources in most cell types for arachidonic acid, but these two compounds are mentioned briefly as they may, at some future time, also turn out to have a role.

II. FATTY ACIDS: THE SUBSTRATES FOR SYNTHESIS OF PROSTAGLANDINS AND SIMILAR CHEMICALS

Fatty acids are a component of the phospholipid in cell membranes, and the substrate for the formation of prostaglandins. Fatty acids esterified at the 1- and 2-carbon positions form the acyl chains of the phospholipids described above. When the ester bond joining the fatty acid to the glycerol backbone of the phospholipid is hydrolyzed, free fatty acid is made available. The mechanisms for this hydrolysis will be discussed in Ch. 4. Here, we are concerned with the nature of the fatty acids. Most naturally occurring fatty acids are essentially long hydrocarbon chains with a carboxylic acid group at one end. The fatty acids are characterized by the length of the chain of carbon atoms,

STRUCTURE

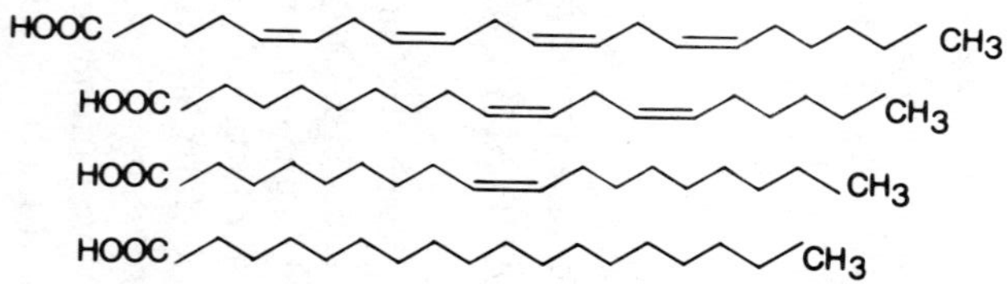

NAME	SYMBOLIC REPRESENTATION
ARACHIDONIC ACID	5,8,11,14,-20:4 or 20:4 ω 6
LINOLEIC ACID	9,12-18:2 or 18:2 ω 6
OLEIC ACID	9-18:1 or 18:1 ω 9
STEARIC ACID	18:0

Fig. 2-6 Examples of the principal fatty acids of mammalian membranes include stearic acid, oleic acid, linoleic acid, and arachidonic acid. In the nomenclature on the far right, ω-9 indicates the distance of the double bond from the ω terminal CH_3 group is nine carbons.

the number of double bonds, and the position and orientation of the double bonds. Four examples are shown in Fig. 2-6. Saturated (with no double bond) fatty acids in mammalian tissues are predominantly palmitic (16 carbons) and stearic (18 carbons). The principal unsaturated (with double bonds) fatty acids of most human tissues are oleic acid (18 carbons: 1 double bond), linoleic acid (18 carbons: 2 double bonds), and arachidonic acid (20 carbons: 4 double bonds). In selected tissues, other polyunsaturated fatty acids are important constituents. For example, adrenal gland cholesterol esters contain large amounts of 7,10,13,16-docosatetraenoic acid (22:4 w 6) (1).

A. Fatty Acids and Membrane Fluidity

Because fatty acids have a polar group (the carboxyl) and a nonpolar tail (the hydrocarbon chain), fatty acids can be aligned in a monolayer on a water surface with a carboxyl group in the water and the fatty acid chain extending above the surface. This property has been useful for studying the packing of fatty acids. It has been found that saturated fatty acids can pack more closely together in monolayers. Correspondingly, within a bilayer, phospholipids with predominantly saturated acyl chains form more densely packed and more rigid membranes. Monolayers of unsaturated fatty acids are less densely packed, and bilayer membranes with a higher proportion of unsaturated fatty acids are more fluid. The relative effect of various fatty acids on membrane fluidity can also be appreciated from an evaluation of their relative melting points (Table 2-1).

The effect of the nature of fatty acids on the liquid crystal-gel transition temperature is critical. It appears to be important that the transition temperature be below but quite close to the ambient operating temperature of the biomembrane. In this regard, it is of interest that fish (for instance the guppy) respond to a decrease in water temperature by changing their

Table 2-1 Melting Points of Several Fatty Acids

Fatty acid	Melting point (°C)
Stearic acid (18:0)	70
Oleic acid (18:1w9)	11
Linoleic acid (18:2w6)	- 5
Arachidonic acid (20:4w6)	–50
Eicosapentaenoic acid (20:5w2)	-54

phospholipids so that they have a higher proportion of polyunsaturated fatty acids. If the fish did not so alter their lipids, their cell membranes likely would be too stiff to function effectively. Diet also influences the nature of cell membrane fatty acids, an important consideration for those interested in prostaglandins. For instance, Greenland Eskimos eating a high-fish or fish-based diet (i.e., seals which eat fish) (note: the fish are from cold northern waters) have a high level of eicosapentaenoic acid (with five double bonds) in their cellular phospholipids, whereas most North Americans have a low level of eicosapentaenoic acid and a high level of arachidonic acid (2).

B. Oxidation of Fatty Acids

Unsaturated fatty acids oxidize relatively easily. Avoiding this oxidation has been a major problem in regard to the storage and shipment of cooking oils, where rancid or oxidized oils are of poor quality. Oxidation of unsaturated fatty acids occurs because they have one or more double bonds (C=C) where oxygen can attach with relative ease under the appropriate circumstances. The addition of oxygen usually creates a radical, probably initially (C-C=C-C + O^2 → C-C(O-O•)-C•-C), but further oxidation will create a wide variety of products (Fig. 2-7). The initial radical formed is unstable. Depending on the particular circumstance,

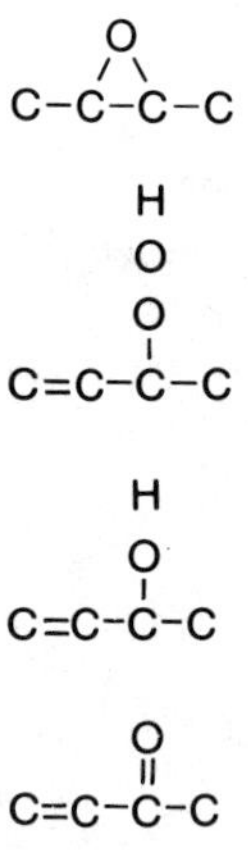

epoxide

hydroperoxide

hydroxyl

ketone

Fig. 2-7 Various oxidized products results from addition of oxygen at the site of a double bond in a fatty acid.

this unstable radical (a) may break up leaving the original reactants, (b) may lead to stable oxidized products, or (c) may lead to the generation of a wide variety of secondary oxygen radicals (3-5). In this third circumstance, there may be a variety of secondary reactions or even something akin to a chain reaction leading to further and more extensive fatty acid oxidation.

Metals are crucial to the oxidation of fatty acids, in part because the positive charge on metals such as Fe^{2+} or Zn^{2+} will associate with the negative carboxyl group of the fatty acid, and with the slight negative charge (due to charge dissociation) on the oxygen. Oxygen itself, when associated with a metal (so that the charge is dissociated), will now tend to associate with a double bond. The result is illustrated in Fig. 2-8 (3). Because iron is a transition metal and will readily undergo a change from the Fe^{2+} form to Fe^{3+}, it will readily donate an electron. The result of a donated electron will be breakdown of the unstable complex to give either production of an oxygen radical, that is, superoxide [Fe^{2+} + fatty acid + $O_2 \rightarrow Fe^{3+} + O_2^-$ + fatty acid (4)] or production of a fatty acid hydroperoxide (Fe^{2+} + fatty acid + $O_2 \rightarrow Fe^{3+}$ + fatty acid $-O-O^- + \dot{H}$). This is probably the first step in the oxidation of fatty acids by Fe^{2+}. Beyond this, because of the variety of oxygen radicals possible and the variety of fatty acid oxidation steps, the situation may be very variable.

This, in a very simplified fashion, is why most enzymes responsible for metabolizing fatty acids to stable oxidized products contain iron or heme. This may be why nontransition metals like Zn^{2+} are found in enzymes which are desaturases (i.e., add double bonds without producing oxidized fatty acid products). For example, zinc, which exists only as Zn^{2+}, and not as Zn^{3+}, can

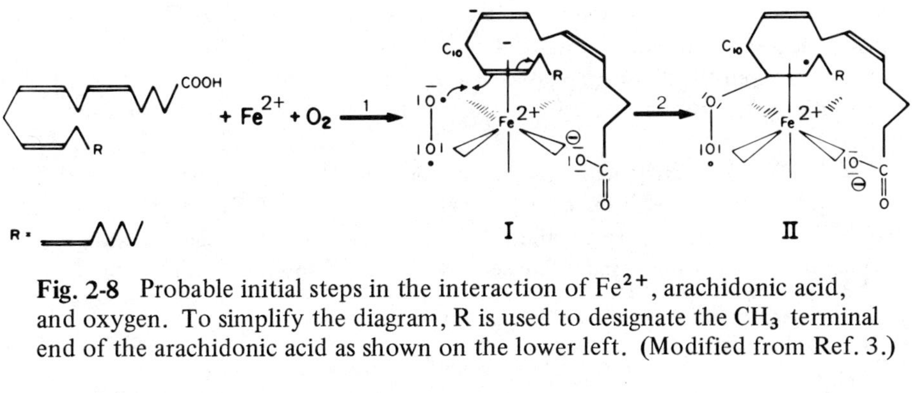

Fig. 2-8 Probable initial steps in the interaction of Fe^{2+}, arachidonic acid, and oxygen. To simplify the diagram, R is used to designate the CH_3 terminal end of the arachidonic acid as shown on the lower left. (Modified from Ref. 3.)

form the initial radical, probably as ($\dot{C}$–C–O–$\mathring{O}$:Zn^{2+}). However, since zinc cannot donate an electron in the simple situation of fatty acid-zinc interaction, the complex will readily fall apart giving the initial reactants (5). Extension of this result, suggests that new double bonds could be formed by Zn^{2+} interactions together with other components of the desaturase enzyme at a site where there was no double bond to create this radical which could then fall apart to give an unoxidized, unsaturated bond.

C. Protein Binding of Fatty Acids

In the blood plasma, fatty acids are largely bound to albumin, with very little fatty acid existing unbound. The albumin concentration of the medium used for suspension of blood cells can therefore have a considerable effect on the nature of fatty acid interaction with cells.

D. Fatty Acids as Precursors for the Synthesis of Prostaglandins and Related Chemicals

1. Synthesis of Prostaglandins

The three principal precursor fatty acids for prostaglandin synthesis are shown in Fig. 2-9. The first, 8,11,14-eicosatrienoic acid or dihomo-γ-linolenic acid, has three double bonds and is the precursor for PGE_1 and $PGF_{1\alpha}$. It is found in only very small quantities in most mammalian cells. Even when the diet contains much of this fatty acid, as with diets supplemented with evening primrose oil, the increase in its cellular content is relatively small, in part because many cells rapidly convert it to arachidonic acid.

The second fatty acid, arachidonic acid, has four double bonds and is the precursor for two-series prostaglandins, including PGE_2, $PGF_{2\alpha}$, and PGI_2. Arachidonic acid is present in considerable amounts in tissue from most mammals when the diet is vegetable or meat based. This fatty acid and its metabolic products are therefore, under most circumstances, the major ones to be considered.

The third fatty acid, eicosapentaenoic acid, has five double bonds. It is the precursor of the three-series prostaglandins PGE_3, $PGF_{3\alpha}$, and PGI_3. Whereas it is found in only small quantities in most diets, fish diets or diets which have fish-eating animals like seals as a major component will be enriched in this fatty acid.

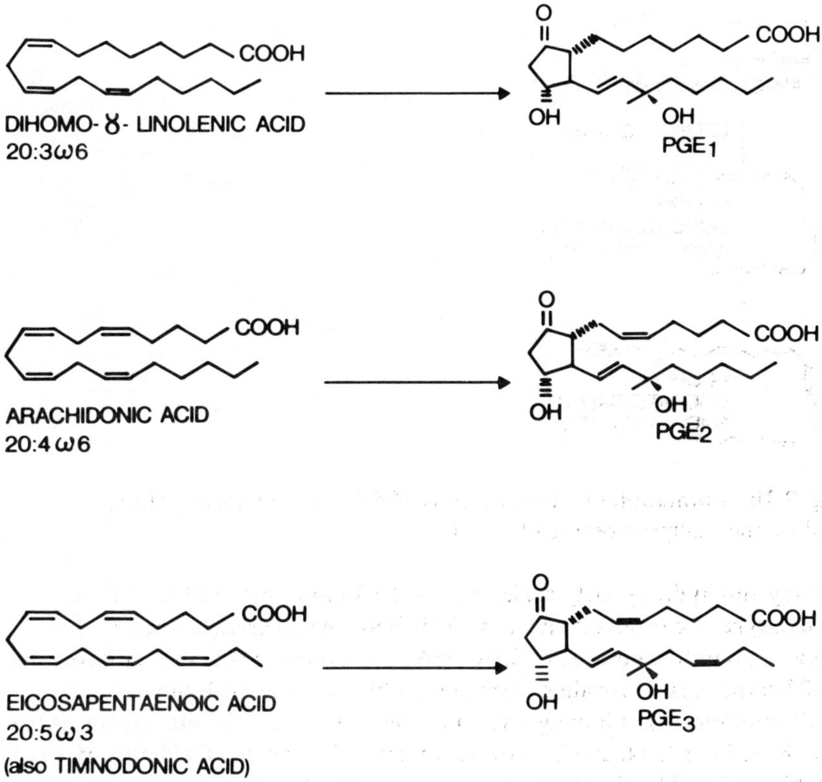

Fig. 2-9 Production of one-series prostaglandins (PGE_1, shown) two-series prostaglandins, and three-series prostaglandins from their respective fatty acid precursors.

2. Fatty Acids as Precursors for Formation of Other Oxygenated Products

It is often forgotten that acids such as linoleic acid, while not substrates for the synthesis of prostaglandins, can nevertheless be converted to other oxygenated products by the prostaglandin synthase enzyme (6). The role of such products is not known. However, more important, at least at our current state of knowledge, is the conversion of fatty acids by lipoxygenase enzymes. Lipoxygenase enzymes add oxygen to unsaturated fatty acids to form hydro-

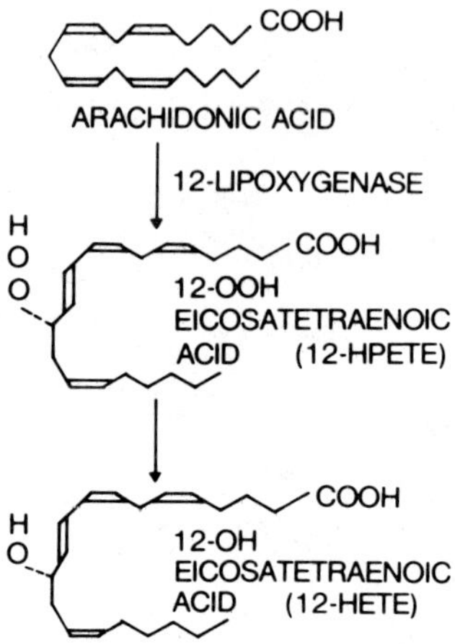

Fig. 2-10 Formation of a hydroperoxy (OOH) and a hydroxy (OH) fatty acid by the 12-lipoxygenase of platelets.

peroxy and hydroxy fatty acids. Figure 2-10 shows the products of the 12-lipoxygenase of blood platelets. This lipoxygenase reaction will add an oxygen group to a number of fatty acids, providing the overall chain length is 18-22 carbons and providing there are double bonds at both the ω-9 and ω-12 positions (7). Lipoxygenase enzymes can potentially add oxygen at the 5, 6, 8, 9, 11, 12, 14, and 15 carbons of arachidonic acid. Oxidation of arachidonic acid by lipoxygenase enzymes is the first step in the formation of leukotrienes.

III. PROSTAGLANDINS AND SIMILAR CHEMICALS INVOLVED IN CELL ACTIVATION

Appendix 2-1 contains a catalog of prostaglandins and related chemicals, their structure, and some of their activities. Appendix 2-2 gives a summary of the production and effects of these lipids as they relate to blood cells. This section provides a general introduction to the structures.

A. Prostaglandins

The basic prostanoic acid structure is shown in Fig. 2-11. All prostaglandins have a cyclopentane ring, two aliphatic side chains, and a terminal carboxylic

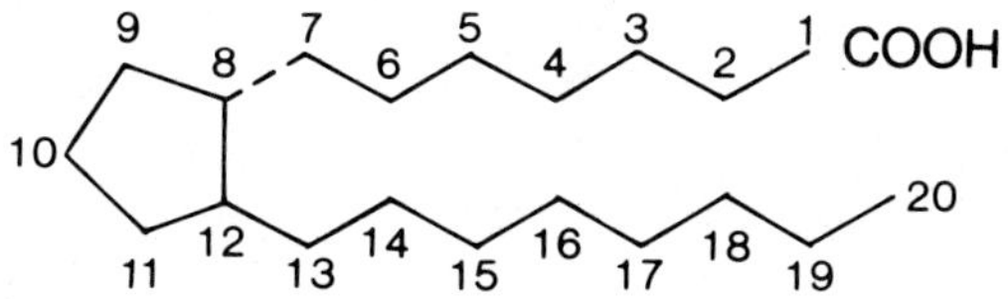

Fig. 2-11 The basic prostanoic acid structure. Carbons are numbered from 1 to 20 with the first carbon—the carboxy terminal carbon. The five-membered (cyclopentane) ring involves carbons 8-12.

acid as shown. In addition, all prostaglandins have a C-13:14 double bond and a 15-hydroxyl (or hydroperoxy) function which are important for prostaglandin biological activity. The precise solution conformation of the prostaglandins is unknown, and indeed there is likely to be some flexibility in the exact position of the aliphatic side chains; however, the conformation of PGE_2 and other prostaglandins when crystallized has been determined (8).

During the synthesis of prostaglandins (Fig. 2-12), the first stable intermediates formed by the prostaglandin synthase enzyme from arachidonic acid are the endoperoxides, PGG_2, and PGH_2 (9). Many nonsteroidal anti-inflammatory agents, including aspirin and indomethacin, have as a major effect the inhibition of prostaglandin synthase. Further details of the various synthetic enzymes and their inhibitors are in Ch. 5. PGG_2 and PGH_2 are very unstable with a half-life of about 5 min in water. Further enzymes are involved in the metabolism of these endoperoxides to other prostaglandins. Specific isomerases convert PGH_2 to PGD_2 and PGE_2. A reductase converts PGH_2 to PGF_2. Prostacyclin synthase converts PGH_2 to PGI_2. PGI_2 is relatively stable in basic solutions but is unstable under neutral or acidic conditions, with a half-life of about 6 min in blood at pH 7.4. Various prostaglandins with details of their structure are listed in App. 2-1.

B. The Thromboxanes

The basic structure of thrombanoic acid is shown in Fig. 2-13. Thrombanoic acid has a six-membered ring instead of the five-membered ring structure of prostaglandins. In the ring, between carbons 11 and 12 is an oxygen. The aliphatic chains attached to the ring are similar to those found in prostaglandins. Thromboxane A_2 is produced from PGH_2 by the enzyme thromboxane synthetase (Fig. 2-12). Thromboxane A_2, an unstable compound with a half-life of 30 sec in water at 37°C, is a potent platelet-aggregating and vasoconstrictor agent.

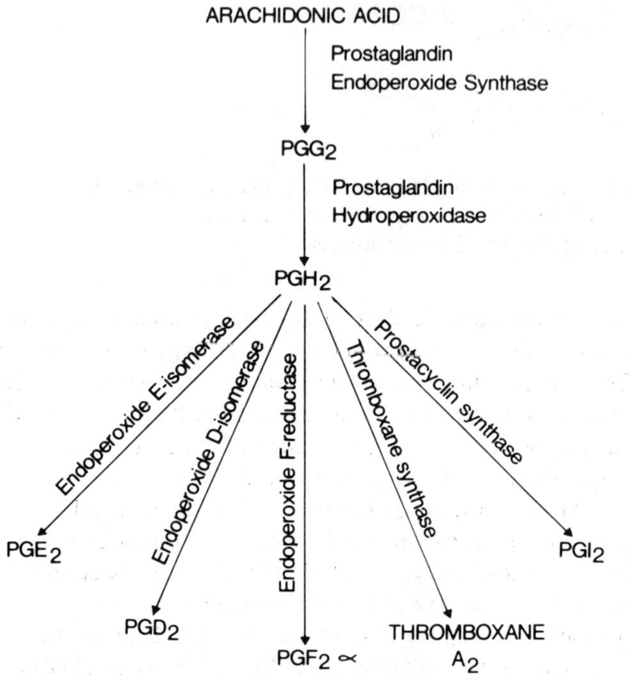

Fig. 2-12 The principal active biological products of the prostaglandin synthase or cyclooxygenase enzyme.

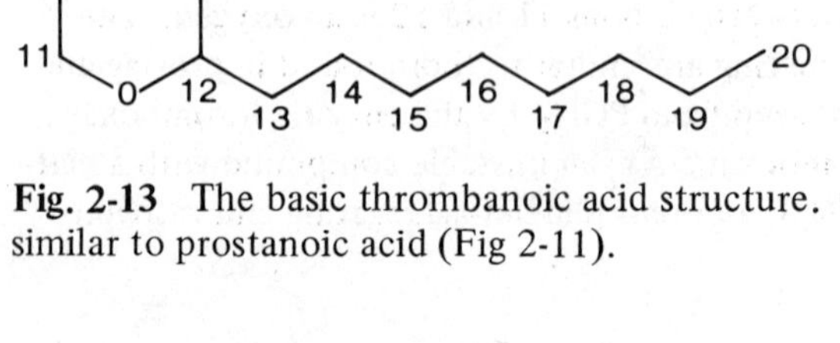

Fig. 2-13 The basic thrombanoic acid structure. Carbons are numbered similar to prostanoic acid (Fig 2-11).

C. The Hydroxy Fatty Acids

Lipoxygenase enzymes can convert arachidonic acid to a variety of hydroxy or hydroperoxy fatty acids. One of these, 12-hydroxyeicosatetraenoic acid (12-HETE), the primary product of the platelet lipoxygenase, is shown in Fig. 2-10. Hydroperoxy fatty acids are unstable intermediates. Hydroxy fatty acis are relatively stable compounds and are biologically active (i.e., 5-HETE and 12-HETE cause neutrophil chemotaxis).

D. The Leukotrienes and Slow-Reacting Substance of Anaphylaxis

Leukotrienes are synthesized through a route which begins with the 5-lipoxygenase pathway (10) (Fig. 2-14). Leukotrienes produced via the 15-lipoxygenase also exist, but their biological importance is not yet established. The first leukotriene formed is an unstable epoxide, leukotriene A_4 (LTA_4). LTA_4 can then be acted on by a hydrolase to give leukotriene B_4 (LTB_4) or by glutathione-S-transferease and gamma-glutamyl transpeptidase to form the peptolipids LTC_4, LTD_4, and LTE_4. Slow-reacting substance of anaphylaxis (SRS-A) from guinea pig lungs has been identified as LTD_4 (10) as has SRS from rat basophilic leukemia cells (10). SRS from murine mastocytoma cells has been identified as LTC_4 (11,12). The leukotrienes received their name since they are formed by leukocytes and contain a conjugated triene structure. Leukotrienes have significant biological effects on white blood cells and on smooth muscle cells.

E. Platelet-Activating Factor or Acetyl Glyceryl Ether Phosphorylcholine (AGEPC)

Platelet-activating factor is an unusual phospholipid with an ether instead of an ester linkage to the acyl chain in position 1 and a very short chain (only two carbons–the acetyl group) in position 2 (Fig. 2-15) (14). Platelet-activating factor is synthesized by several different cell types, with mast cells, monocytes, and neutrophils appearing to be most important.

F. Diglyceride, Phosphatidic Acid, and Lysophosphatidic Acid

Stimulation of a variety of different cell types results in the breakdown of phosphatidylinositols and the formation of diglyceride and phosphatidic

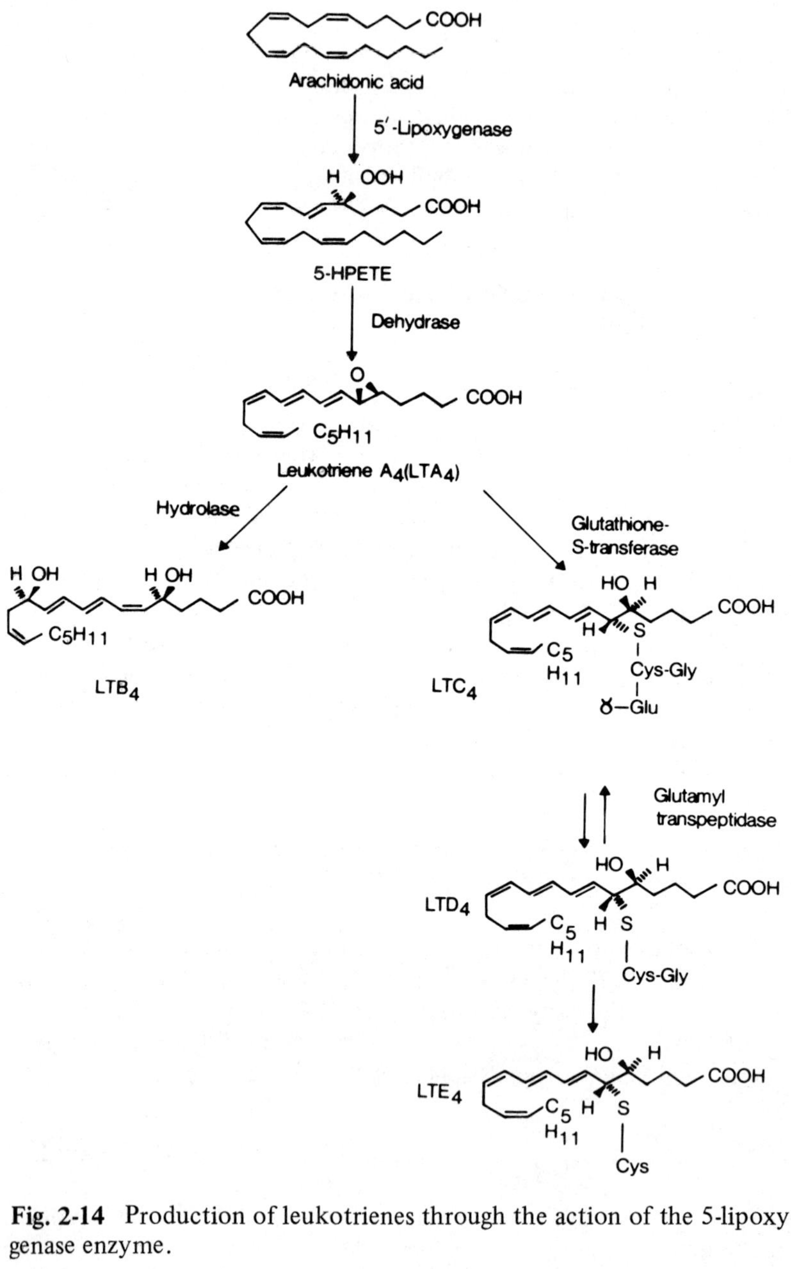

Fig. 2-14 Production of leukotrienes through the action of the 5-lipoxygenase enzyme.

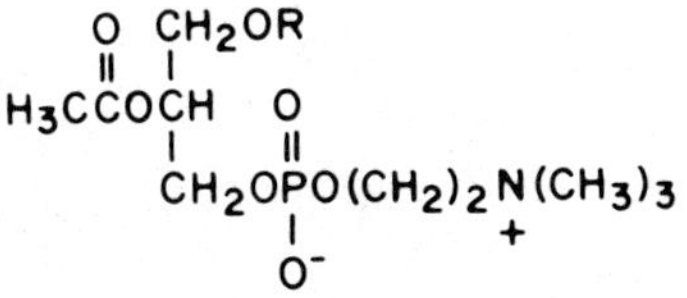

Fig. 2-15 The structure of platelet-activating factor, or, -0-alkyl-2-acetyl-sn-glyceryl-3-phosphoryl choline. Note the ether linkage (COR) to carbon 1 of the glycerol backbone, the acetyl group on carbon 2, and the phosphoryl choline attached to carbon 3.

acid (Fig. 2-16) (15). Lysophosphatidic acid has also been shown to be formed in platelets (16). Diglyceride promotes membrane fusion and activates a protein kinase C (17,18). Phosphatidic acid and lysophosphatidic acid can both function, under some circumstances, as calcium ionophores (19,20). All three lipids may be involved in cellular activation processes.

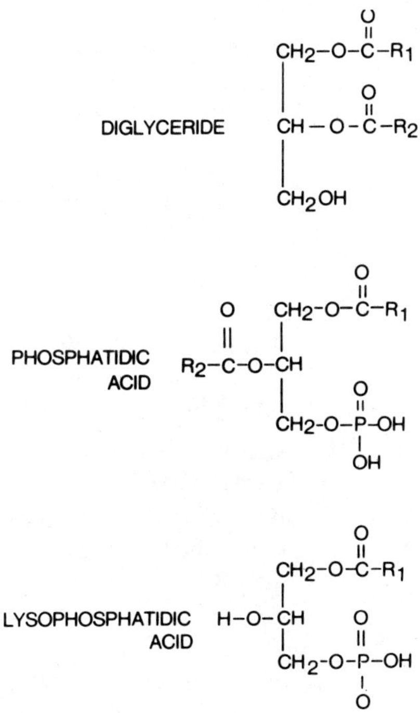

Fig. 2-16 Additional active lipids which are produced following breakdown of phosphatidylinositols.

APPENDIX 2-1

Various Prostaglandins

Prostaglandins	Substituent groups C9	C11	C15	Double bonds	Comments
PGA_2	=O	H	OH	C5, C10 C13	A derivative of PGE_2 which forms under acidic conditions. It has not yet been found to occur in mammalian species in vivo (21). It has biological effects including antihypertensive and antiviral actions.
PGB_2	=O	H	OH	C5, C8-12, C13	A derivative of PGE_2 which forms under basic conditions. It has not been demonstrated to occur in vivo in mammals.
PGC_2	=O	H	OH	C5,C11, C13	PGA_2 can be isomerized in plasma of certain species to give PGC_2 (22-24).
PGD_2	OH	=O	OH	C5,C13	PGD_2 is formed in vivo particulary by mast cells and in the brain. In some cells (i.e., platelets) it is effective at raising cellular cyclic adenosine monophosphate (cAMP) (25). In the brain, it may have a role in inducing sleep (26).
PGE_2	=O	OH	OH	C5, C13	PGE_2 is synthesized in a variety of tissues with the kidney and seminal vesicles being important ones. In blood cells, monocytes are a major source. PGE_2 has a wide spectrum of biological activity. In some cells, for example lymphocytes, PGE_2 activates cellular adenylate cyclase to raise the level of cAMP and inhibit cell function.

Various Prostaglandins (continued)

Prostaglandins	Substituent groups C9	C11	C15	Double bonds	Comments
$PGF_{2\alpha}$	OH	OH	OH	C5,C13	$PGF_{2\alpha}$ is produced by a variety of biological tissues. A significant role for $PGF_{2\alpha}$ in blood cell function, if it exists, has yet to be defined. $PGF_{2\alpha}$ does affect blood cell production (see Ch. 19) increasing colony-forming units-granulocyte macrophage (CFU-GM) and decreasing burst-forming units-erythrocytes (BFU-E).
PGG_2	O - - - -O (endoperoxide)		OOH	C5,C13	PGG_2 and PGH_2 are unstable endoperoxides which are intermediates in the formation of other naturally occurring prostaglandins and thromboxanes. Both have potent platelet-aggregating activity.
PGH_2	O - - - -O (endoperoxide)		OOH	C5, C13	
PGI_2	C_6–O–C_9	OH	OH	C5, C13	PGI_2 is produced in a variety of cells. From the point of view of blood cells, endothelial cells are the most important. PGI_2 in some cells (i.e., platelet and neutrophil) is a potent inhibitor of cell function acting by raising cell cAMP.

APPENDIX 2-2

Summary of the Production and Effects of Prostaglandins and Related Chemicals on Human Blood Cells[a]

Blood cell type	Arachidonic acid metabolite produced: Prostaglandin and thromboxanes	Arachidonic acid metabolite produced: Hydroxy fatty acids and leukotrienes
Red blood cells	None	15-HETE (reticulocytes only)
Platelets	Thromboxane A_2 (smaller amounts of PGD_2, PGE_2 & $PGF_{2\alpha}$)	HHT 12-HETE
Neutrophils	(Small amounts of PGE_2 $PGF_{2\alpha}$ & thromboxane A_2)	5-HETE, LTB_4, 15-HETE(?), (12, 20 DiHETE in mixtures of platelets and neutrophils only)
Basophils	PGD_2 (mast cells only) (small amounts of thromboxane A_2)	LTC_4, LTD_4 (5-HETE, LTB_4 - mast cells definitely, basophils ?)
Eosinophils	PGE_2 – ?	15-HETE, LTB_4, LTC_4
Lymphocytes		
T Lymphocytes	Probably none	15-HETE, 11-HETE, 5-HETE (small amounts LTB_4)
B Lymphocytes	Probably none	?
NK Cells	?	?
Monocytes	Thromboxane A_2, PGE_2, (small amounts of $PGF_{2\alpha}$ and PGI_2 ?)	5-HETE, LTB_4, LTC_4
Endothelial cells	PGI_2, PGE_2 (smaller amounts of thromboxane A_2)	15-HETE, 11-HETE
Vascular[d] Smooth muscle	PGI_2 (smaller amounts of PGE_2, $PGF_{2\alpha}$ and thromboxane A_2)	?

[a]The principal arachidonate species made by each blood cell types are listed. Under effects of the metabolites, only those metabolites which have been shown to have significant and consistent effects are listed. For additional details on each type the reader is referred to the individual cell chapters.

Effects of arachidonic acid metabolites	
Stimulatory substances	Inhibitory substances
—	—
PGG_2, PGH_2, Thromboxane A_2	PGD_2, PGH_2, PGI_2
LTB_4, 5-HETE, other HETEs, (thromboxane A_2 - ?)	PGE_2, PGI_2, PGE_1
5-HETE, 5-HPETE (LTB_4 - effective only with cyto chalasin B)	PGE_2, PGE_1, PGI_2 - ?
LTB_4, various HETEs, PGD_2	PGE_2, PGE_1
? (LTB_4 may enhance suppressor T cell activity)	PGE_2, PGE_1, 15-HETE
?	PGE_2, PGE_1
LTB_4 - ?	PGE_2, PGE_1
PGE_2-$PGF_2\alpha$[b] (enhance the conversion of macrophages into tumor killing cells) 15-HPETE, LTC_4[c] (stimulate chemiluminescence, superoxide or H_2O_2 production)	PGE_2, PGI_2, PGE_1 (inhibit chemiluminescence, PAF productiom, tumoricidal activity)
?	?
Thromboxane A_2[d] $PGF_{2\alpha}$, LTC_4, LTD_4	PGI_2[d], PGE_1, PGE_2

[b]Mice cells only.
[c]Mice or guinea pig cells only.
[d]Production and effect varies with the site of origin. General trends only are shown. For further details see Chapter 14.

REFERENCES

1. B. L. Walker. *J. Nutr. 100*:355 (1970).
2. H. O. Bang, J. Dyerberg, and N. Hjorne. *Acta Med. Scand. 200*:69 (1976).
3. D. A. Peterson, J. M. Gerrard, G. H. R. Rao, T. P. Krick, and J. G. White. *Prostaglandins Med. 1*:304 (1978).
4. D. A. Peterson, J. M. Gerrard, and M. A. Benton. *Med. Hypotheses 7*: 1389 (1981).
5. D. A. Peterson, J. M. Gerrard, J. Peller, G. H. R. Rao, and J. G. White. *Prostaglandins Med. 6*:91 (1981).
6. M. Hamberg and B. Samuelsson. *J. Biol. Chem. 242*:5344 (1967).
7. D. H. Nugteren. *Biochim. Biophys. Acta 380*:299 (1975).
8. J. W. Edwards and W. L. Duax. *Prostaglandins 5*:275 (1974).
9. M. Hamberg, J. Svensson, T. Wakabayashi, and B. Samuelsson. *Proc. Natl. Acad. Sci. USA 71*:345 (1974).
10. B. Samuelsson. *Science 220*:568 (1983).
11. H. R. Morris, G. W. Taylor, P. J. Piper, and J. R. Tippins. *Nature (Lond.) 285*:104 (1980).
12. L. Orning, S. Hammarstrom, and B. Samuelsson. *Proc. Natl. Acad. Sci. USA 77*:2014 (1980).
13. R. C. Murphy, S. Hammarstrom, and B. Samuelsson. *Proc. Natl. Acad. Sci. USA 76*:4275 (1979).
14. R. N. Pinckard, L. M. McManus, and D. J. Hanahan. *Adv. Inflammation Res. 4*:147 (1982).
15. R. H. Michel. *Biochim. Biophys. Acta 415*:81 (1975).
16. G. Mauco, H. Chap, M. F. Simon, and L. Douste-Blazy. *Biochimie 60*: 653 (1978).
17. B. Maggio and J. A. Lucy. *Adv. Exp. Biol. Med. 83*:225 (1977).
18. A. Kishimoto, Y. Takai, T. Mori, U. Kikkawa, and Y. Nishizuka. *J. Biol. Chem. 255*:2273 (1980).
19. C. A. Tyson, H. V. Zande, and D. E. Green. *J. Biol. Chem. 251*:1326 (1976).
20. J. M. Gerrard, S. E. Kindom, D. A. Peterson, and J. G. White. *Am. J. Pathol. 97*:531 (1979).
21. H. T. Jonsson and R. E. Powers. *Progr. Lipid Res. 20*:787 (1982).
22. R. L. Jones. *Br. J. Pharmacol. 45*:144 (1972).
23. R. L. Jones. *J. Lipid Res. 13*:511 (1972).
24. R. L. Jones. *Nature (Lond.) 240*:1 (1972).
25. D. C. B. Mills and D. E. Macfarlane. *Thromb. Res. 5*:401 (1974).
26. R. Ueno, K. Honda, S. Inoue, and O. Hayaishi. *Proc. Natl. Acad. Sci. USA 80*:1735 (1983).

BIBLIOGRAPHY

J. Singer and G. Nicholson. *Science 175*:720 (1972).
E. J. Masoro. *Physiological Chemistry of Lipids in Mammals.* W. B. Saunders, Toronto (1968).
A. R. Johnson and J. B. Davenport (eds.). *Biochemistry and Methodology of Lipids.* Wiley-Interscience, Toronto (1971).
S. J. Wakil (ed.). *Lipid Metabolism.* Academic Press, New York (1970).

3
General Mechanisms

Understanding the complexity of prostaglandin-blood cell interaction is greatly facilitated by some knowledge of general processes and pathways which are common to all blood cell types. Processes which modulate cellular functions can be classified into activating and inhibiting ones. For example, with platelets which are relatively simple cells, activation—a change in cell shape, secretion of granule contents, and the development of a "sticky" external membrane—can be clearly and easily defined. Inhibitory processes interfere with events leading to cell activation and will tend to maintain the cell nearer to its resting quiescent form. In general, for other blood cells, activation (adherence, chemotaxis, phagocytosis, cytotoxicity, or mitogenesis) can similarly be defined in a relatively straightforward manner.

However, there are some situations where activation and inhibition may not be definable so clearly. For instance, random movement is sometimes measured to assess cell locomotion. If a cell is activated in the sense that its tendency to stick and adhere to the substratum or medium is increased, it will not move. But, if a cell is partially activated (or fully activated and partially inhibited) so that it has increased movement without much tendency to adhere, it may move farther than usual. For this reason, I have generally emphasized results using assays where activation is clearcut and avoided assays such as random motility where results may be more difficult to interpret. This does not mean that there may not be in vivo situations where cell movement without adherence is essential. Neutrophil migration to a site of infection may be an example.

A second area of blood cell biology where activation/inhibition processes may be more complex concerns cells which undergo a major transformation or differentiation involving a substantial synthesis of new protein following their initial activation. For example, B lymphocytes can be stimulated to become antibody-producing plasma cells. Similarly T cells and monocytes can change from relatively quiescent forms to metabolically much more active forms. Chemicals which are important for initial activation of the cell from a quiescent to an active state could be quite different from chemicals which regulate the function of the activated form. Also of considerable relevance to the present book, synthesis of prostaglandins and related chemicals could be quite different in the initial quiescent form and the transformed-activated form. One of the new proteins synthesized during activation, for example, could be a prostaglandin synthetic enzyme. As an example, some evidence suggests that quiescent monocytes synthesize primarily thromboxane A_2 and lipoxygenase products, while the activated monocyte synthesizes much more PGE_2. Sorting out the pattern of synthesis and effects of prostaglandins and related chemicals in cells which are chameleons can be difficult. I suspect that some of the current apparently contradictory data stem from this sort of problem. In presenting the chapter on lymphocytes and monocytes, these concerns are considered further. Notwithstanding these complexities, related general activation and inhibitory processes are present in most blood cells.

With most cell types, certain of the prostaglandins (or related compounds) act to promote cellular activation whereas others act to inhibit cellular activation. This group of chemicals taken together is thus like lawyers in a court, some promoting the prosecution, others promoting the defense. The overall effect of these chemicals in given situations therefore depends critically on the balance of production and effect.

Processes involved in cellular activation and inhibition are necessarily complex. It would be nice if activating prostaglandins worked through one general process while inhibitory prostaglandins worked through another. In this regard, it is now apparent, in most blood cells, that calcium fluxes to raise the cytoplasmic calcium level are central to cell activation. In contrast, raised cellular levels of cyclic adenosine monophosphate (cAMP) are a major mechanism of cellular inhibition. In general, activating prostaglandins and prostaglandin-like compounds appear to have as their principal effects modulation of cellular calcium levels or calcium-interactive events to promote activation, whereas inhibitory compounds have as a principal effect the stimulation of cellular adenylate cyclase to produce cell cAMP to raise the levels of this second messenger.

I. GENERAL CELLULAR ACTIVATION PROCESSES

Based on our present knowledge, there appear to be at least two and possibly as many as four or more major types of processes which lead to the activation of blood cells. The first of these processes is involved with the stimulation and the effects of elevated cytoplasmic calcium levels. The second group of processes is separate from, and yet interactive with, the elevated cytoplasmic calcium levels. In general, it would appear that processes directly leading to changes in intracellular calcium are closely connected to changes in cell shape and to cell movement. The second category of separate yet calcium-interactive processes appeares to contribute particularly to granule labilization and granule secretion, and may be important contributors to mitogenic events. There may be a third category of activation processes which have a role in promoting adhesion. A fourth category of cellular activation may concern processes which raise cellular cAMP levels and may be important for a certain stage of cell transformation.

It is also worth noting here that blood cells can be viewed as *responding to injury.* Noxious or damaging stimuli such as vessel wall injury, bacteria, viruses, foreign protein antigens, and tumor cells are examples. It is probable that along the course of evolution cellular responses have evolved from a nonspecific reaction to any injury to the present cell-specific response to a given stimulus. This view is mentioned further in the next chapter and the last one because I think it helps to understand how cells presently work and why prostaglandins and related chemicals have the role they do.

A. Calcium Flux-Mediated Events

1. Why Calcium?

A brief look at why calcium, rather than other ionic species, has a central role will facilitate understanding of this area (1, 2). First, for a particular ionic species to be of widespread importance to cellular activation, the cell must be able to regulate the intracellular level of the ion closely. In general, ionic species, because of their charged nature, pass poorly across the central lipid region of the bilayer membrane. However, the ease of passage varies inversely in proportion to the square of the valence, with the result that monovalent ions generally have too high a flux across biological membranes for close modulation, movement of trivalent ions is too restricted, but the movement of the divalent ions Ca^{2+} and Mg^{2+} can be regulated in a suitable fashion to suit cellular needs.

Second, the capacity for widespread interaction with biological molecules is critical. Cations are better in this regard than anions. Of the principal divalent cations, calcium is better than magnesium because its more irregular coordination geometry is better suited for interaction with proteins which frequently also have irregular geometries.

2. The Role of Calcium

An overview:studies with A23187, a calcium ionophore. The effect of raising the intracellular calcium concentration of various blood cells has been most clearly elucidated through the use of selective calcium ionophores such as A23187. Table 3-1 outlines some of the effects of A23187 on blood cells. It is now generally accepted that the resting cytoplasmic concentration of ionic calcium in blood cells is about 10^{-7} M. A23187 specifically raises the level of cytoplasmic calcium either by releasing calcium from an intracellular store or by transporting it across the outer plasma membrane into the cytoplasm. A23187 accomplishes this objective by binding the calcium internally so that the charge is buried and neutralized and the calcium-A23187 complex (with lipophilic groups now on the exterior surface) thus can pass readily across the lipid membrane. Because A23187 also has some affinity for magnesium, in the face of very high intracellular magnesium the calcium is unloaded in exchange for magnesium. The calcium can then interact with biological molecules inside the cell to promote cell activation.

An example of a specific process: platelet granule centralization. In many cases, calcium interacts with a small protein, calmodulin, to modify cellular responses. An example is the movement of platelet granules toward the center of this cell on stimulation. Several lines of evidence suggest that the major protein interaction involved in this process is the attachment of the contractile proteins actin and myosin to one another in such a fashion that each myosin filament can crawl along two actin filaments, beginning at the head end of each, so that structures tied to the tail ends of the two

Table 3-1 Some Effects of the Calcium Ionophore A23187 on Blood Cells

Blood cell type	Processes stimulated by A23187	References
Platelet	Shape change (pseudopod formation and granule centralization), aggregation, secretion, phospholipase activation to release membrane arachidonic acid	3-7
Erythrocyte	Spheroechinocyte formation, decreased deformability	8-11
Neutrophil	Aggregation, secretion, generation of oxygen radicals, enhancement of chemotaxis	12-14
Basophil/mast cell	Secretion, enhancement of leukotriene synthesis	15-18
Eosinophil	Enhancement of the formation of hydroxy derivatives of arachidonic acid	19
Lymphocyte	Mitogenesis	20, 21

actin molecules are pulled toward each other (22-24). The result of this actin-myosin interaction is the movement of the platelet granules to the platelet center (Fig. 3-1). Control over the ability of actin and myosin to interact with one another is exercised by calcium. When the cytoplasmic level of calcium is low (about 10^{-7} M) as it is in the resting cell, platelet myosin is not phosphorylated and remains separate from platelet actin. The latter exists largely in the gel form initially. When platelets are activated following stimulus by an agent such as thrombin, there is a resultant rise in the cytoplasmic calcium level to 10^{-5}–10^{-6} M. The cytoplasmic calcium now can interact with calmodulin to promote the activity of an enzyme, a protein kinase, which transfers a phosphate group from adenosine triphosphate (ATP) to myosin light chain (Fig. 3-2) (25,26). When myosin light chain becomes phosphorylated in this fashion, it will enable the whole myosin filament to interact with the newly forming actin filaments to produce contraction (27). The actin filaments have a tail end which sticks

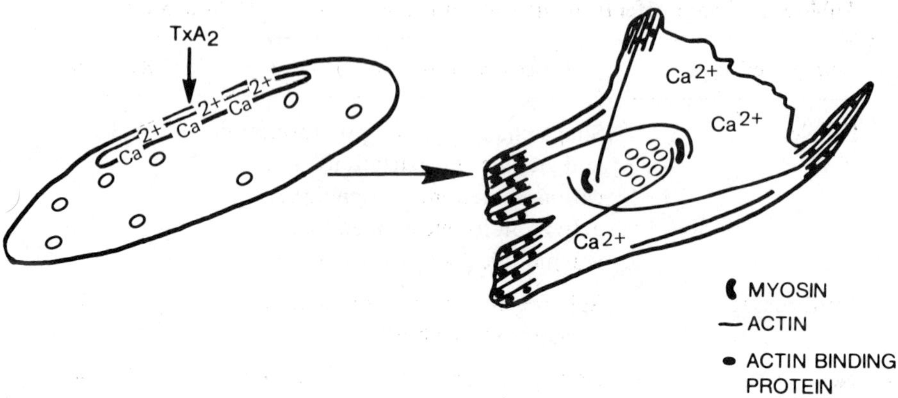

Fig. 3-1 A current concept of platelet activation resulting from a rise in cytoplasmic calcium induced by thromboxane A_2 (TxA_2). The rise in cytoplasmic calcium initiates actin-myosin contraction, currently believed to occur approximately as shown on the right. Each bipolar myosin interacts with two actin filaments. Increasing overlap of actin and myosin moves the granules to the platelet center. Actin-binding protein is shown as important in its interaction with actin for anchoring the tail ends of the actin filaments and for pseudopod formation.

to microtubules and granule membranes (this property of actin may require other proteins). Myosin is bipolar and pulls actin filaments together, bringing the granules and microtubules toward the cell center. Platelet actin-binding protein appears involved in platelet pseudopod formation and in anchoring the actin to the platelet membrane (27). A similar interaction of platelet actin and myosin appears essential for the platelet-mediated contraction of platelet-fibrin clots (28, 29).

The precise mechanism for calcium regulation of other processes is not yet so well established; however, calmodulin and protein kinase activation may be involved as well.

B. Activation of Protein Kinase C: A Process Separate from but Interactive with Calcium

Studies of the tumor promoter phorbol myristate acetate on blood cells showed that this agent specifically labilized granules in both platelets and

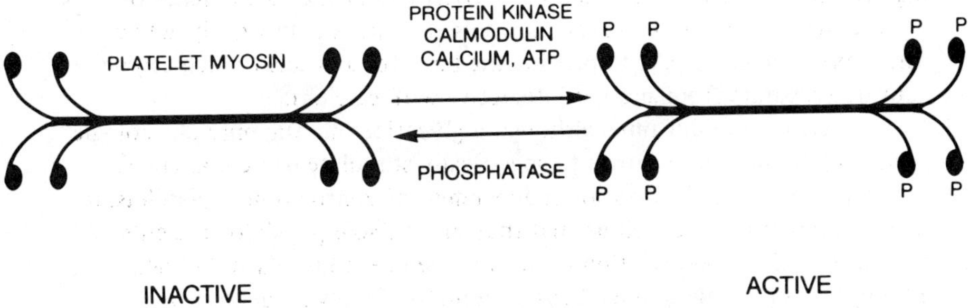

Fig. 3-2 In order for platelet actin to interact with platelet myosin to generate tension, myosin light-chain I must be phosphorylated as shown here by the addition of the phosphate (P) to myosin to make it active as shown on the right.

neutrophils (i.e., it appeared to facilitate fusion of the granule membranes with each other, with the plasma membranes, and in platelets with the surface-connected canalicular system) (30, 31a). In platelets, there was no significant centralization of granules produced, the primary effect of raising intracellular calcium levels. This effect was therefore very different from that produced by the calcium ionophore A23187. Furthermore, studies with PGG_2, which produces primarily granule centralization similar to A23187, showed that the combination of an agent which stimulated granule centralization and an agent which stimulated granule labilization resulted in a marked facilitation of granule secretion (31b). The only agents found to date with a morphologic effect on platelets similar to phorbol myristate acetate are diglycerides (24).

In the mid-1970s, studies of Haslam and Lynham suggested that platelet secretion was specifically associated with phosphorylation of a 47,000-dalton protein (32). More recent studies showed that phorbol myristate acetate is better at phosphorylating this protein than myosin light chain (27,33), that the protein kinase C which promotes phosphorylation of this protein copurifies with the phorbol myristate acetate receptor (34), and that the phorbol ester directly activates protein kinase C (35).

The results of extensive studies with protein kinase C show that in addition to phorbol myristate acetate, it is specifically stimulated by diglycerides and requires calcium for activity (36-38). In the absence of diglyceride, even with excess calcium, this enzyme is only weakly active. These experiments appear to provide the basis for a process which can be activated separate from and yet interactive with calcium.

At the present time, although diglycerides are the only physiologic agents which have been shown to specifically stimulate protein kinase C and to cause granule labilization independent of contraction in platelets, it may be premature to conclude that they are the sole physiologic agents responsible. The concentration of diglyceride needed is relatively high, although it is possible that a localized buildup of diglyceride may be sufficient to achieve this concentration. Nevertheless, the effect of oleoyl-acetyl-diglyceride, a synthetic diglyceride, to enhance secretion induced by A23187 and to activate platelets independent of a significant rise in cytoplasmic calcium levels suggest that the diglyceride-mediated activation of protein kinase C is an important component of physiologic platelet activation resulting from stimuli which promote breakdown of phosphoinositides to diglycerides (39-41).

The ability of phorbol myristate acetate to activate other blood cells besides platelets (Table 3-2) suggests a similar phorbol-myristate acetate-diglyceride activation of protein kinase C may be operative in other blood cells.

Table 3-2 The influence of Phorbol Myristate Acetate on Blood Cells

Blood cell	Processes stimulated by phorbol myristate acetate	References
Platelet	Selective granule labilization and aggregation	30
Neutrophils	Selective labilization of specific granules, stimulation of superoxide production and aggregation	31, 42, 43
Lymphocytes	A comitogen when added together with phytohemagglutinin (PHA), conconavalin A, or A23187	44-46

C. Cell-Cell Adhesion

Epinephrine can stimulate platelet-platelet adhesion (first-wave aggregation) in the absence of prostaglandin formation. Cell-cell adhesion is specifically stimulated without the changes seen internally in platelets with either the calcium ionophore A23187 or phorbol myristate acetate. Platelet-platelet adhesion involves fibrinogen binding, and this is true for epinephrine as well as for other agents. While it is possible that this effect of epinephrine results from a localized change in membrane calcium, there may be a more direct pathway for mediating this and perhaps other cellular adhesion events which does not necessarily require a change in intracellular calcium levels. This action of epinephrine on platelets is different from known effects of prostaglandin endoperoxides and thromboxane A_2 which stimulate shape change simultaneously with aggregation. However, it raises the possibility that these processes could be separable and that direct effects of arachidonate metabolites on cellular adhesion processes might occur.

D. cAMP and Cell Stimulation

With monocytes (see Ch. 11) there is some evidence that prostaglandin E_2, which stimulates monocyte cAMP, can convert monocytes/macrophages from a basal to a "transformed-active" state. Whether this is important in any other blood cells is not clear at present.

II. PROSTAGLANDINS AND RELATED CHEMICALS AND CELLULAR ACTIVATION

A. Calcium-Flux and Calcium-Interactive Processes

A considerable amount of evidence links the activating arachidonic acid metabolites produced in platelets, the prostaglandin endoperoxides, and thromboxane A_2 to an action to promote a flux of calcium. Addition of PGG_2, PGH_2, or thromboxane A_2 to platelets produces a pattern of response similar in many respects to that seen with exposure of the platelets to the calcium ionophore A23187 (31b). Production of PGH_2/thromboxane A_2 is in the dense tubular system, a membrane system which has a store of calcium for release into the cytoplasm on cell stimulation. Addition of PGG_2/PGH_2/thromboxane A_2 to a membrane fraction containing calcium-loaded dense tubular system vesicles causes a release of calcium from these vesicles (47-49). It can be concluded that one action of PGG_2/PGH_2/thromboxane A_2 is the initiation of the calcium flux needed for cellular activation. An action of PGG_2/PGH_2 and thromboxane A_2 to act as calcium ionophores has been considered (50). Their action is likely to be more complex, since structurally similar compounds can act as receptor antagonists (51, 52). It is time, also, to look for interactions of these compounds directly with proteins, or to influence the ionic requirements for protein action. For instance, PGG_2 has been shown to lower the calcium requirement for guanylate cyclase (53). Similar effects could be seen with many other proteins, and could explain in part the action of these active chemicals.

Hydroxy fatty acids and leukotrienes which activate neutrophils appear to act, as thromboxane A_2 does in platelets, at a step involving promotion of a flux of calcium or the effect of low calcium levels (54), with evidence that LTB_4 can act as a calcium ionophore (see Ch. 8). Since thromboxane A_2 does not activate neutrophils and leukotriene B_4 does not activate platelets, these chemicals are selective in the cell type affected. The basis for this selectivity is not yet clear, but certainly adds to the physiologic specificity of these active compounds.

B. Other Processes

1. Cyclic Guanosine Monophosphate (cGMP)

As mentioned previously, PGG_2 lowers the calcium requirement for the enzyme which produces cGMP. It has been considered that PGG_2/PGH_2/thromboxane A_2 might mediate their effects on platelets by raising cGMP levels (55). This is unlikely since the rise in cGMP occurs late during aggregation, and neither addition of cGMP analogues nor rises in cGMP produced by other agents such as ascorbic acid are associated with activation of platelets (56). The role of cGMP has yet to be determined, but in platelets, at least, cGMP is not an activation-producing messenger. It is possible that cGMP turnover may provide a localized energy source (57), but further studies in this direction are still needed.

2. Protein Phosphorylation Events

Addition of arachidonic acid or prostaglandin endoperoxide analogues to platelets is associated with increased phosphorylation of several platelet proteins, including actin-binding protein, a 47,000-dalton protein and myosin light chain (58). Aspirin, used to block endogenous synthesis of PGG_2/PGH_2/thromboxane A_2, will completely prevent phosphorylation of these proteins in response to arachidonic acid, while only partially inhibiting phosphorylation produced by the endoperoxide analogues or the calcium ionophore A23187. The effects of PGG_2/PGH_2/thromboxane A_2 may be secondary to an effect of these agents to promote calcium flux, but could involve a more direct interaction of PGG_2, PGH_2, or thromboxane A_2 with the enzymes involved in promoting phosphorylation. It is of interest that phosphorylation of the 47,000-dalton protein by A23187 seems particularly sensitive to aspirin inhibition, and is promoted particularly in arachidonic acid-treated platelets (58). This 47,000-dalton protein is the one phosphorylated by diglyceride stimulation of protein kinase C.

3. Inhibition of cAMP Phosphodiesterase

Miller and Gormon have demonstrated an effect of PGH_2 to inhibit the phosphodiesterase enzyme which degrades cAMP (59). The regulation of this enzyme by PGH_2 and thromboxane A_2 could occur secondary to a rise in cytoplasmic calcium levels, but there also appears to be a direct effect of these lipids on the enzyme.

4. Others

The role of PGG_2/PGH_2/thromboxane A_2 in promoting cell-cell attachment and cellular secretion is discussed in the chapter on platelets.

C. Inhibitory Effects of Prostaglandin-Related Chemicals

1. cAMP-Mediated Effects

The first demonstration of an inhibitory effect of a prostaglandin on the function of a blood cell was by Kloeze in 1967 (60). He showed that PGE_1 produced a rise in platelet cAMP levels. Using a membrane fraction, PGE_1 was next shown to act by stimulating the enzyme adenylate cyclase (61). Studies in other tissues then showed that the adenylate cyclase itself was the PGE_1 receptor.

More recently, adenylate cyclase has been characterized as having three components including a hormone receptor, a catalytic component, and a coupling component. The molecular mechanism by which prostaglandins stimulate adenylate cyclase is not known, although PGE_1 has been shown to act synergistically with (GTP) on the enzyme (62, 63). It has become clear that, at least in platelets, there are two receptors for prostaglandins. PGI_2 acts on one receptor. PGE_1 also acts on this receptor but is less potent. PGD_2 acts at a second receptor site.

Mechanism of the inhibitory effect of cAMP. cAMP appears to exert its principal effects through activation of protein kinases to stimulate phosphorylation of cellular proteins. In platelets, for example, phosphorylation of proteins of molecular weights 56,000, 48,000, 40,000, 24,000 and 22,000 (64-66) has been shown in response to agents which raise cellular cAMP. The connection between these phosphorylations and processes inhibited by cAMP is not clear, except for the action of cAMP on phospholamban and myosin light-chain kinase where some understanding is emerging.
Phospholamban. In 1977, Kaser-Glanzmann et al. showed that cAMP could act to promote the uptake of calcium by the platelet dense tubular system (a calcium-sequestering membrane analogous to the sarcotubule of skeletal muscle) (67). The enhancement of the calcium-sequestering pump could explain studies from several laboratories which showed that cAMP can antagonize the stimulatory effect of raised cytoplasmic calcium. Since then a protein, called phospholamban, has been suggested as critical to this process. cAMP stimulates phosphorylation of phospholamban in cardiac muscle. Phospholamban is then responsible according to this scheme for promoting calcium sequestration. Whether a similar process occurs in platelets and other blood cells is not yet certain.
Myosin light-chain kinase. Recent evidence from Adelstein and co-workers (68) suggests that cAMP can phosphorylate the kinase which stimulates phosphorylation of myosin light chain. When the kinase is phosphorylated, it can no longer phosphorylate myosin light chain. This action would prevent one of the important steps of platelet activation.

2. Other Inhibitory Effects of Prostaglandins

Sinha and Colman have proposed an alternative inhibitory effect of PGE_1 on platelets not mediated by cAMP but resulting from PGE_1-inhibiting factor Xa binding to platelets (69).

REFERENCES

1. D. W. Urry. *Ann. N.Y. Acad. Sci. 307*:3 (1978).
2. J. M. Gerrard, D. A. Peterson, and J. G. White. In *Platelets in Biology*

Pathology 2, J. L. Gordon (ed.). Elsevier/North Holland, Amsterdam (1981).
3. R. D. Feinman and T. C. Detwiler. *Nature 249*:172 (1974).
4. J. G. White, G. H. R. Rao, and J. M. Gerrard. *Am.J. Pathol. 77*:135 (1974).
5. J. M. Gerrard, J. G. White, and G. H. R. Rao. *Am. J. Pathol. 77*:151 (1974).
6. W. C. Pickett and P. Cohen. *J. Biol. Chem. 251*:2536 (1976).
7. S. Rittenhouse-Simmons and P. Deykin. *J. Clin. Invest. 60*:495 (1977).
8. J. G. White. *Am. J. Pathol. 77*:507 (1974).
9. J. G. White. *Semin. Hematol. 13*:121 (1976).
10. J. F. Kuettner, K. L. Dreher, G. H. R. Rao, J. W. Eaton, P. W. Blackshear, and J. G. White. *Am. J. Pathol. 88*:81 (1977).
11. K. L. Dreher, J. W. Eaton, K. P. Breslauve, P. Berger, P. L. Blackshear, and J. G. White. *Am. J. Pathol. 101*:543 (1980).
12. R. D. Estensen, M. E. Reusch, M. C. Epstein, and H. R. Hill. *Infect. Immun. 13*:146 (1976).
13. C. N. Serhan, H. M. Korchak, and G. Weissman. *J. Immunol. 125*: 2020 (1980).
14. C. N. Serhan, A. Radin, J. E. Smolen, H. Korchak, B. Samuelsson, and G. Weissman. *Biochem. Biophys. Res. Commun. 107*:1006 (1982).
15. L. M. Lichtenstein. *J. Immunol. 114*:1692 (1975).
16. J. C. Foreman, J. L. Mongar, and B. D. Gomperts. *Nature 245*:249 (1973).
17. R. C. Murphy, S. Hammarstrom, and B. Samuelsson. *Proc. Natl. Acad. Sci., USA 76*:4275 (1979).
18. H. R. Morris, G. W. Taylor, P. J. Piper, M. N. Samhoun, and J. R. Tippins. *Prostaglandins 19*:185 (1980).
19. D. M. Smith, L. Boies, E. Haus, M. Mikooi-Morehead, and J. G. White. *Fed. Proc. 42*:917 (1983).
20. J. R. Luckasen, J. G. White, and J. H. Kersey. *Proc. Natl. Acad. Sci. USA 71*:5088 (1974).
21. A. M. Mastro and M. C. Smith. *J. Cell. Physiol. 116*:51 (1983).
22. I. Cohen, J. M. Gerrard, R. N. Berman, and J. G. White. In *Protides of the Biological Fluids*, H. Peeters (ed.). Pergamon Press, Oxford (1979).
23. R. C. Carroll, R. G. Butler, P. A. Morris, and J. M. Gerrard. *Cell 30*: 385 (1982).
24. J. M. Gerrard, J. V. Schollmeyer, and J. G. White. In *Cytoskeletal Elements and Plasma Membrane Organization*, G. Poste and G. L. Nicholson (eds.). Elsevier/North Holland, Amsterdam (1981).
25. R. S. Adelstein and T. D. Pollard. *Prog. Hemostasis. Thromb. 4*:37 (1978).
26. D. R. Hathaway and R. S. Adelstein. *Proc. Natl. Acad. Sci. USA 76*: 1653 (1979).

27. E. A. Lebowitz and R. Cooke. *J. Biol. Chem. 253*:5443 (1978).
28. J. L. Daniel, I. R. Molish, H. Holmsen, and L. Salganicoff. *Cold Spring Harbor Conference on Cell Proliferation 8*:913 (1981).
29. I. Cohen, J. M. Gerrard, and J. G. White. *J. Cell. Biol. 93*:775 (1982).
30. R. D. Estensen and J. G. White. *Am. J. Pathol. 74*:441 (1974).
31a. J. G. White and R. D. Estensen. *Am. J. Pathol. 75*:45 (1974).
31b. J. M. Gerrard, D. Townsend, S. Stoddard, C. J. Witkop, and J. G. White. *Am. J. Pathol. 86*:99 (1977).
32. R. J. Haslam and J. A. Lynham. *Biochem. Biophys. Res. Commun. 77*: 714 (1977).
33. J. Yamanishi, Y. Takai, K. Kaibuchi, K. Sano, M. Castagna, and Y. Nishizuka. *Biochem. Biophys. Res. Commun. 112*:778 (1983).
34. J. E. Niedel, L. J. Kuhn, and G. R. Vandenbark. *Proc. Natl. Acad. Sci. USA 80*:36 (1983).
35. M. Castagna, Y. Takai, K. Kaibuchi, K. Sano, U. Kikkawa, and Y. Nishizuka. *J. Biol. Chem. 257*:7847 (1982).
36. Y. Takai, A. Kishimoto, Y. Iwasa, Y. Kawahara, T. Mori, and Y. Nishizuka. *J. Biol. Chem. 254*:3692 (1979).
37. A. Kishimoto, Y. Takai, T. Mori, U. Kikkawa, and Y. Nishizuka. *J. Biol. Chem. 255*:2273 (1980).
38. T. Mori, Y. Takai, B. Yu, J. Takahashi, Y. Nishizuka, and T. Figakwia. *J. Biochem. 91*:427 (1982).
39. K. Sano, Y. Takai, J. Yamanishi, and Y. Nishizuka. *J. Biol. Chem. 258*: 2010 (1983).
40. K. Kaibuchi, Y. Takai, M. Sawamura, M. Hoshijima, T. Fijukwia, and Y. Nishizuka. *J. Biol. Chem. 258*:6701 (1983).
41. T. J. Rink, W. Smith, and R. Y. Tsien. *FEBS Lett. 148*:21 (1982).
42. I. M. Goldstein, S. T. Hoffstein, and G. Weissman. *J. Cell. Biol. 65*:647 (1975).
43. C. N. Serhan, M. J. Broekman, H. M. Korchak, J. E. Smolen, A. J. Marcus, and G. Weissman. *Biochim. Biophys. Acta 762*:420 (1983).
44. A. M. Mastro and G. C. Mueller. *Exp. Cell Res. 88*:40 (1974).
45. C. H. Kwong and G. C. Mueller. *Cancer Res. 42*:2115 (1982).
46. A. M. Mastro and M. C. Smith. *J. Cell. Physiol. 116*:51 (1983).
47. J. M. Gerrard, A. M. Butler, G. Graff, S. F. Stoddard, and J. G. White. *Prost. Med. 1*:373 (1978).
48. L. D. Brace, D. L. Venton, and G. C. LeBreton. *Circulation 66* (Suppl. II):299 (1982).
49. J. R. Mayo, D. D. Miller, and D. R. Feller. *Biochem. Pharm. 32*:1952 (1983).
50. J. M. Gerrard, J. G. White, and D. A. Peterson. *Thromb. Hemostas. 40*: 224 (1978).

51. L. D. Brace, D.L. Venton, and G. C. LeBreton. *Circulation 66* (Suppl. II): 229 (1982).
52. S. C. Hung, D. L. Venton, and G. C. LeBreton. *Circulation 66* (Suppl. II):300 (1982).
53. G. Graff, J. H. Stephenson, D. B. Glass, M. K. Haddox, and N. G. Goldberg. *J. Biol. Chem. 253*:7662 (1978).
54. P. H. Naccache, T. F. P. Molski, E. L. Becker, P. Borgeat, S. Picard, P. Vallarand, and R. I. Sha'afi. *J. Biol. Chem. 257*:8608 (1982).
55. D. B. Glass, J. M. Gerrard, D. Townsend, D. W. Carr, J. G. White, and N. D. Goldberg. *J. Cyclic Nucl. Res. 3*:37 (1977).
56. N. D. Goldberg, G. Graff, M. K. Haddox, J. H. Stephenson, D. B. Glass, and M. E. Moser. *Adv. Enzyme Reg. 16*:165 (1977).
57. N. D. Goldberg, T. F. Walseth, S. J. Eide, and A. Ames III. *Fed. Proc. 42*:1847 (1983).
58. J. M. Gerrard and R. C. Carroll. *Prostaglandins 22*:81 (1981).
59. O. V. Miller and R. R. Gorman. *J. Cyclic Nucl. Res. 2*:79 (1976).
60. J. Koeze. In *Proc. 2nd Nobel Symposium, Interscience*, S. Bergstrom and B. Samuelsson (eds.). New York, (1967).
61. S. M. Wolfe and N. R. Shulman. *Biochem. Biophys. Res. Commun. 35*: 265 (1969).
62. G. Krishna, J. P. Harwood. *J. Biol. Chem. 247*:2253 (1972).
63. M. L. Steer and A. Wood. *J. Biol. Chem. 254*:10791 (1979).
64. R. J. Haslam, J. A. Lynham, and J. Fox. *Fed. Proc. 36*:566 (1977).
65. R. J. Haslam, M. M. L. Davidson, and J. V. Desjardins. *Biochem. J. 176*:83 (1978).
66. R. M. Lyons and J. O. Shaw. *J. Clin. Invest. 65*:252 (1980).
67. R. Kaser-Glanzman, M. Jakabova, J. N. George, and E. F. Luscher. *Biochom. Biophys. Acta 466*:429 (1977).
68. R. S. Adelstein, M. A. Conti, L. Rappaport, and C. R. Eaton. *Fed. Proc. 39*:2117 (1980).
69. A. K. Sinha and R. W. Colman. *Thromb. Res. 30*:553 (1983).

BIBLIOGRAPHY

H. Holmsen. In *Platelet Production, Function, Transfusion and Storage,* M. Baldwin and S. Ebbe (eds.). Grune and Stratton, New York (1974).

R. J. Haslam, M. C. Davidson, T. Davies, J. A. Lynham, and M. D. McClenaghan. *Adv. Cyclic. Nucl. Res. 9*:533 (1978).

J. M. Gerrard and J. G. White. *Prog. Thromb. Hemost. 4*:87 (1978).

A. J. Marcus. *J. Lipid Res. 19*:793 (1978).

R. R. Gorman. *Fed. Proc. 38*:83 (1979).
J. L. Gordon (ed.) *Platelets in Biology and Pathology 2.* Elsevier/North Holland, Amsterdam (1981).
A. K. Hall and H. R. Behrman. In *Prostaglandins,* J. B. Lee (ed.). Eslevier/North Holland, New York (1982).

4

Mechanisms Involved in the Release of the Fatty Acid Substrates for Prostaglandin Synthesis

Prostaglandins are not stored in cells; their synthesis is initiated by the release of substrate fatty acid from cellular lipids, usually phospholipids. Such hydrolysis of cellular lipids is normally the rate-limiting step in the formation of prostaglandins and related oxidized metabolites. This is because the intracellular level of precursor free fatty acids is very low (1). The release of arachidonic and related fatty acids from phospholipids involves the action of phospholipases. Activation of these phospholipases may occur nonspecifically with cell damage or injury, or may occur with specific receptor-coupled cell activation.

I. CELLULAR INJURY

Since fatty acids are integral components of the structure of phospholipids, any stimulus or insult which degrades cellular phospholipids will release fatty acids. In the most simplified fashion, cell or membrane damage should be associated with the release of fatty acids. That this is indeed the case is evident from studies of conditions associated with cell damage [i.e., burns, ischemia, and cell death, electroconvulsive shock, and mechanical trauma to the lungs

(2–5)]. As Piper and Vane conclude from their studies of lungs, "the common thread which runs through the different ways of causing release is the disturbance of the cell membrane. This may range from simple distortion to stretch to frank rupture" (5).

That the release of fatty acids and formation of prostaglandins with cell injury applies to blood cells as well as to other tissues is evident from studies of Salzman et al. (6). He found that platelets, even when subjected to mild stresses such as centrifugation, gel filtration, or stirring with siliconized glass beads, produced prostaglandins. Indeed, it is probable that the release of fatty acids and formation of oxidized products have evolved from a nonspecific result of cell injury to the very specific response seen with most cells which is tightly coupled to agonist receptor-mediated events.

Investigations of Hsueh and co-workers (7,8) suggest that the nonspecific lipase activities of heart and kidney (triggered by transient ischemia) are different from the specific lipase activity stimulated by the hormone bradykinin. The nonspecific lipase activity is more diffusely distributed, results in release of other fatty acids such as oleic acid as well as arachidonic acid, and is poorly coupled to the cyclooxygenase enzyme. These differences are all consistent with the concept that the prostaglandin system has evolved from a nonspecific cell response to injury to a specific (receptor-coupled) cell response to stimulation. While it is the latter that is of greatest interest, the former nonspecific process is still present and may be important for understanding some circumstances wherein prostaglandins or related chemicals have a role, as well as understanding the probable origin and evolution of this response.

II. SPECIFIC AGONIST-COUPLED RELEASE OF ARACHIDONIC ACID

Four types of phospholipases could potentially be involved in the release of fatty acids from cell phospholipids. Phospholipase A_1 cleaves the fatty acid from carbon 1 of phospholipids (see Ch. 2). Fatty acid species attached to carbon 1 are most frequently saturated fatty acids, and thus not the desired substrate fatty acids. While phospholipase A_1 is found in some blood cells, notably in platelet lysosomal granules, it is not involved in arachidonic acid release. Phospholipase A_2 cleaves the fatty acid from carbon 2 of cell phospholipids. Fatty acids on carbon 2 are usually unsaturated, with arachidonic acid being particularly prominent in certain phospholipids. Phospholipase A_2 species are usually not fatty acid specific (i.e., they cleave any fatty acid on carbon 2). Furthermore, while phosphatidylethanolamine is the preferred substrate for the isolated enzyme in intact blood cells, phophatidylcholine is the phospholipid which is usually hydrolyzed. Thus, it would appear that phosphatidylcholine containing primarily arachidonic acid and phospholipase A_2 must both be located at the same specific subcellular site. Evidence in support of this possibility is emerging for platelets and perhaps for neutrophils (see subsequent discussion).

Phospholipase C hydrolyzes phospholipids to produce diglyceride and phosphorylated base (i.e., inositol, choline, ethanolamine, or serine phosphate). Platelets and other blood cells have phospholipase C species which specifically attack the phosphatidylinositols (9). An immediate product of the activity of this phospholipase C is diglyceride (10). This diglyceride contains almost exclusively arachidonate and stearate as the two fatty acid species, and it is the substrate for a diglyceride lipase which hydrolyzes the ester bonds to release the fatty acids (11). This appears to be a second principal pathway for the release of arachidonic acid from cell phospholipids.

The diglyceride produced by hydrolysis of phosphatidylinositols is, however, mostly converted to phosphatidic acid. Billah et al. have provided evidence for a phosphatidic acid-specific phospholipase A_2 which can remove the arachidonic acid from phosphatidic acid (12). This could be a third pathway for the release of arachidonic acid for synthesis of prostaglandins.

Phospholipase D attacks phospholipids to remove the base (choline, inositol, ethanolamine, and serine) to leave phosphatidic acid. This enzyme is found in eosinophils. There is no evidence to date to implicate it in making arachidonic acid available for prostaglandin synthesis. A few further comments on each of the three potential pathways for release of arachidonic acid are in order.

A. Phospholipase C-Diglyceride Lipase

Phospholipase C is discussed first because there is evidence in platelets that this enzyme is activated first, and that enzyme activity is closely coupled to receptor occupancy by a stimulus. The evidence for this is: (a) the calcium ionophore A23187 which bypasses receptor activation by directly transporting calcium to raise the level of intracellular calcium in platelets causes little if any activation of phospholipase C (13–15); (b) ^{32}P and ^{3}H-arachidonic acid labeling of phosphatidic acid (an indirect product of the phospholipase C resulting from diglyceride) is closely coupled to receptor occupancy by thrombin (16).

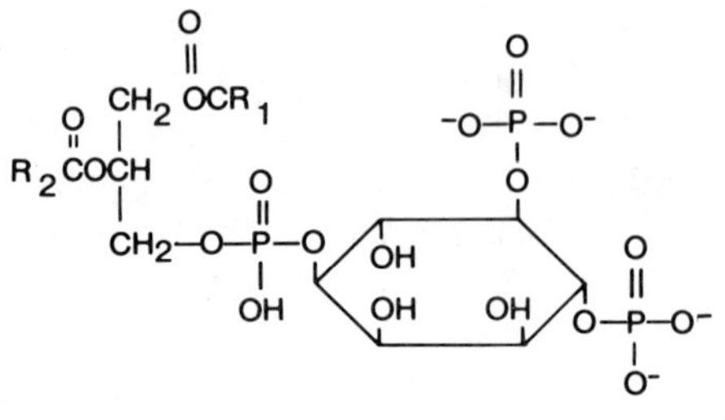

PHOSPHATIDYLINOSITOL - 4,5 BISPHOSPHATE (PIP_2)

Fig. 4-1 The structure of phosphatidylinositol-4,5-bisphosphate (PIP_2), formerly called triphosphatidylinositol, shows the polar inositol tris phosphate group attached to the glycerol backbone in the 3-position. R = the hydrocarbon chain of the fatty acids. Breakdown of this phospholipid now appears closely coupled to receptor-linked stimulation of platelets and perhaps other blood cells.

1. The First Reaction: Hydrolysis of Phosphatidylinositol or Phosphatidylinositol-4,5-Bisphosphate (PIP_2)

Until recently it was generally believed that phospholipase C initially acted on phosphatidylinositol. However, recent data clearly show that breakdown of phosphatidylinositol-4,5-bisphosphate (PIP_2)—formerly triphosphatidylinositol) Fig. 4-1 by phospholipase C occurs within seconds of the addition of thrombin to platelets (17-19). Furthermore, partially purified platelet phospholipase C has activity against PIP_2, phosphatidylinositol-4, phosphate (PIP, formerly diphosphatidylinositol), and phosphatidylinositol, with the measured Km and V_{max} values consistent with the PIP_2 and PIP being more actively hydrolyzed (20a). The preferencial hydrolysis of PIP_2 and PIP is also supported by studies of Vickers showing rapid initial production of inositol trisphosphate and inositol bisphosphate, but little inositol monophosphate in response to a low concentration of thrombin (20b). Thus, present indications are that the hydrolysis of PIP by phospholipase C (phosphodiesterase) is a very early receptor-coupled reaction.

The rapid fall in phosphatidylinositol content of stimulated platelets (21) could result from the rapid conversion of phosphatidylinositol to PIP_2 when the latter is cleaved by phospholipase C, as has been proposed

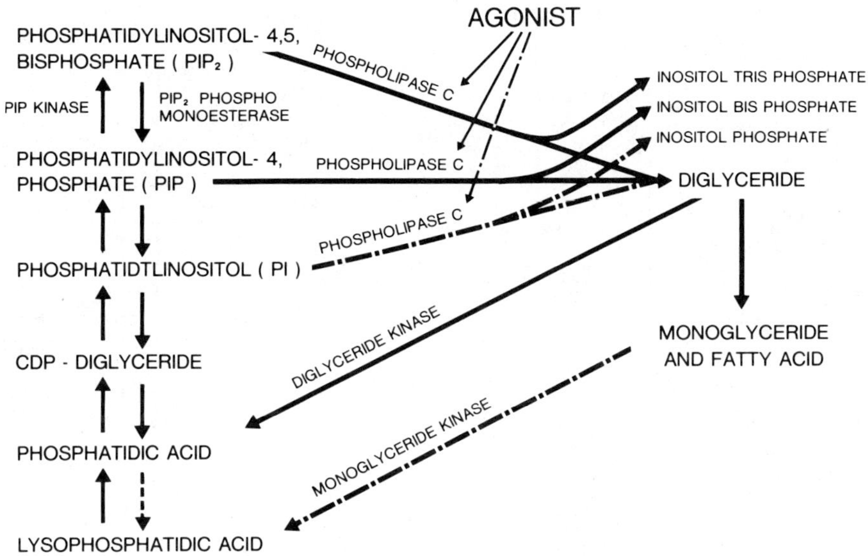

Fig. 4-2 Reactions involved in the breakdown and subsequent resynthesis of phosphatidylinositols. Current evidence suggests the activation of a phospholipase C which hydrolyzes phosphatidylinositol-4,5-biphosphate to produce diglyceride and inositol tris phosphate is the reaction most closely coupled to cellular stimulation by agonists.

with other cell systems (22,23). However, hydrolysis of phosphatidylinositol directly by phospholipase C (Fig. 4-2) may also occur simultaneously.

The inner surface of the plasma membrane of red blood cells has been said to be enriched in PIP_2 (24,25). A similar location of PIP_2 in the plasma membrane of other blood cells would be appropriate for a substance which responds rapidly to a receptor-linked activation process. The platelet dense tubular system may be enriched in phosphatidylinositol (see Ch. 6). Better definition of the subcellular localization of the polyphosphoinositides and the phospholipase C enzyme (a soluble enzyme in broken cells, but its localization in intact cells is not established) would clearly be useful. The role of a highly active phosphomonoesterase which degrades phosphatidylinositol-4,5-biphosphate to phosphatidylinositol-4-phosphate is also not clear.

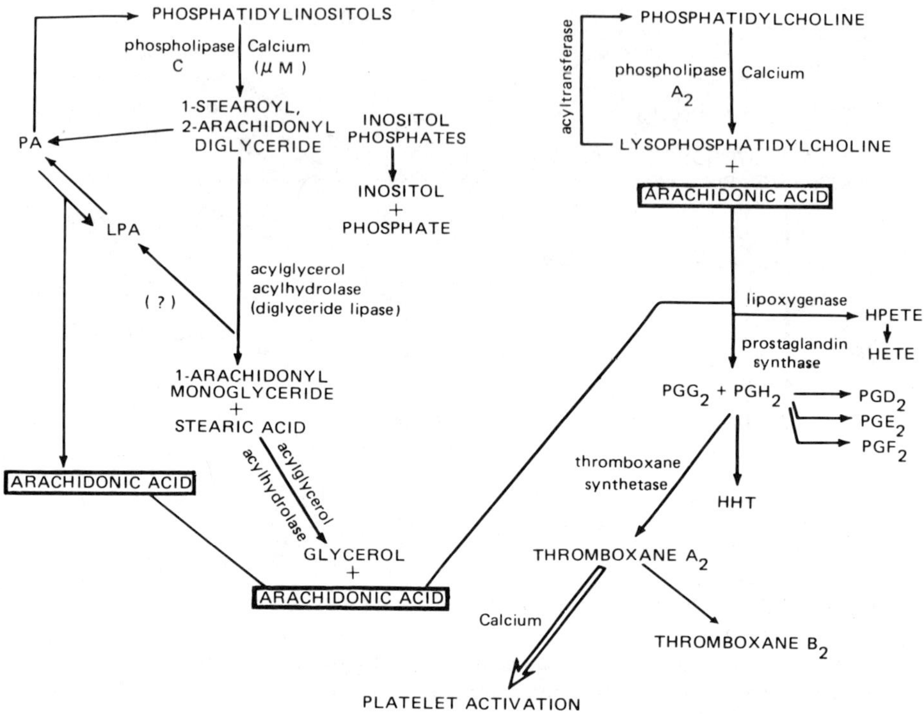

Fig. 4-3 An overview of the pathways leading to the release of arachidonic acid from platelet phospholipds and subsequent formation of metabolites. Current evidence suggests arachidonic acid is released both by the phospholipase A_2 on the right (major pathway) and phospholipase C-diglyceride lipase pathway (in the center) with a possible contribution from the phosphatidic acid specific phospholipase A_2 (on the left). Abbreviations: PA = phosphatidic acid; LPA = lysophosphatidic acid; PG = prostaglandin; HPETE = 12-hydroperoxy-eicosatetraenoic acid; HETE = 12-hydroxy-eicosatetraenoic acid; HHT = 12-hydroxy-heptadecatrienoic acid.

2. Metabolism of Diglyceride: The Second Step

Diglyceride (almost exclusively stearoyl-arachidonyl diglyceride) produced as a result of the phospholipase C activity is metabolized by one of two pathways (Fig. 4-3). A diglyceride kinase converts most of the diglyceride to phosphatidic acid (26). Some of the diglyceride is acted on by a diglyceride lipase enzyme which cleaves the stearic acid on carbon 1 (11). The same diglyceride lipase enzyme, or possibly a different enzyme, a monoglyceride lipase, then liberates arachidonic acid from its attachment at carbon 2 (27). Diglyceride lipase is located in the platelet endoplasmic reticulum (28), the same site as the prostaglandin endoperoxide synthase and thromboxane synthase (29,30), and thus its activity in releasing arachidonic acid could be closely coupled to the generation of prostaglandins and thromboxanes.

3. The Multifunctional Nature of the Phospholipase C-Activated Pathway

In addition to the release of arachidonic acid, this pathway probably facilitates cell activation in a number of ways.

1. The breakdown of membrane phosphoinositides may release proteins bound to the membrane via these phosphoinositides (31).
2. Diglyceride produced may be important for protein kinase C activation (32a).
3. Inositol trisphosphate may be an important messenger to cause additional mobilization of intracellular calcium (32b,32c).
4. Phosphatidic acid may be acted on by a specific phospholipase A_2 to form lysophosphatidic acid and additional free arachidonic acid (see below (12).
5. Phosphatidic acid or lysophosphatidic acid produced through this pathway may be an intracellular messenger promoting calcium flux and raising cytoplasm calcium levels (33,34).
6. Breakdown of the phosphoinositides may release calcium bound to these phosphoinositides in the membrane (17,33).
7. Phosphoinositides are inhibitory to the calcium-transporting activity of phosphatidic acid and lysophosphatidic acid (35) and perhaps to activities of certain intracellular enzymes. Breakdown of the membrane phosphoinositides may therefore release an inhibition by these compounds on cellular-activating processes.

The many potential important effects of this pathway may be a reason it is central to blood cell function and occurs rapidly after receptor-coupled stimulation in all blood cells which have been carefully studied.

B. The Phospholipase A_2 Pathway

Arachidonic acid, in addition to being derived from phosphatidylinositol, is also obtained from phosphatidylcholine (36) (Fig. 4-3) and possibly to a minor extent from phosphatidylethanolamine (37). A phospholipase A_2 has been implicated in the release of arachidonic acid from these two phospholipids (36,38).

Early studies of this enzyme suggested it was not active enough to account for the rapid release of arachidonic acid seen in thrombin-stimulated platelets (39). However, more recent studies of the purified enzyme show it has much more activity than previously found, and that there is an endogenous lipid inhibitor of the enzyme (40). The nature of the lipid inhibitor is unknown. This information and studies with diglyceride lipase inhibitors suggest that the phospholipase A_2 is the major mechanism for release of arachidonic acid for prostaglandin synthesis in platelets (40b,40c).

In platelets, phospholipase A_2 activity, like diglyceride lipase activity, has been localized to the endoplasmic reticulum (28). As discussed previously, this would be expected to provide close coupling of arachidonic acid release and formation of prostaglandins and thromboxanes.

In neutrophils, mast cells, and natural killer cells, Hirata, Axelrod, and co-workers have provided evidence for methylation of phosphatidylethanolamine to occur to give phosphatidylcholine as the initial reaction before release of arachidonic acid from phosphatidylcholine (41-43). However, labeled arachidonic acid is lost only from phosphatidylcholine, not phosphatidylethanolamine, in these cells. This would appear to make it unlikely that phosphatidylethanolamine containing arachidonic acid is first converted to phosphatidylcholine before the arachidonic acid is hydrolyzed. Hirata and Axelrod have further suggested that the phosphatidylcholine species which loses arachidonic acid is on the outer surface of the plasma membrane. This concept would explain how a large protein such as lipomodulin (40,000 daltons) added to the outside of neutrophils and natural killer cells can inhibit cellular release of arachidonic acid. Recent evidence of phospholipase A_2 in neutrophil granules which can be released on cell stimulation would also fit the concept that in neutrophils some of the phospholipase A_2 and the released arachidonic acid is external. Externally released arachidonic acid may be critically important for superoxide production (Ch. 8).

C. Phosphatidic Acid-Specific Phospholipase A_2

Billah et al. have described a pathway for the release of arachidonic acid from phosphatidylinositol in horse platelets. Phosphatidic acid formed from phosphatidylinositol (see previous discussion) is acted on by a phospholipase A_2 to give lysophosphatidic acid and arachidonic acid (12). Recently, by incubating human platelets at 23°C, Neufeld and Majerus have shown that arachidonic acid release largely occurs before formation of phosphatidic acid (44). This pathway is thus unlikely to be of major importance.

II. STUDIES WITH INHIBITORS

A. Raised cAMP Levels

Agents which raise intracellular cAMP levels (either by activating adenylate cyclase, or inhibiting a cAMP phosphodiesterase) produce an inhibition of the release of arachidonic acid from platelet phospholipids (45,46). Since phospholipase C requires calcium for activity (47), and since cAMP can promote sequestration of calcium in a storage organelle (48) believed to be the dense tubular system, cAMP could inhibit phospholipase C in part by restricting calcium availability. However, Billah et al. have provided evidence for an alternate direct or indirect inhibition of phospholipase C, probably mediated through an effect of cAMP on a protein kinase (49).

B. Steroids

Dexamethasone has been shown to inhibit the release of arachidonic acid from cellular phospholipids. The effect of this anti-inflammatory steroid is mediated through synthesis of proteins (macrocortin and lipomodulin) which inhibit the release of arachidonic acid (43,50).

C. Calmodulin Antagonists

Walenga et al. (51) have shown that trifluoroperazine, a calmodulin antagonist, inhibits phospholipase A_2 but not phospholipase C. The results suggest the former, but not the latter, requires calmodulin for activity. However, other evidence shows phenothiazines might act as direct inhibitors of the phospholipase.

D. Others

Phospholipase A_2 inhibitors can be inhibitors that bind to the enzyme, interact with the substrate, or antagonize calcium action; and they can be serine esterase inhibitors.

1. Inhibitors That Bind to the Enzyme

Bromophenacyl bromide. While this drug will inhibit phospholipase A_2 by binding to a histidyl residue at the active site of the enzyme it is nonspecific; it will also interact irreversibly with other enzymes and can irreversibly bind thiol groups.

Wallach and Brown Inhibitors. A series of potent phospholipase A_2 inhibitors with anti-inflammatory and platelet-inhibitory properties have been described (52).

Lipomodulin and macrocortin. These proteins, induced by glucocorticoids, are direct inhibitors of phospholipases A, C, and D.

2. Inhibitors That Interact with the Substrate

Mepacrine, chlorpromazine, propranalol, putrescine, and spermidine all appear to inhibit both phospholipase A_2 and C through interactions with the substrate lipids. It is possible that mepacrine may under some conditions be a selective inhibitor of phospholipase A_2, but this has been debated (53).

3. Inhibitors Which Antagonize Calcium Action

Ca^{2+} is necessary for both phospholipase A_2 and phospholipase C activity. Local anesthetics and related compounds and indomethacin (used at high concentrations, 100 μM) appear to act by preventing the binding of calcium to the enzyme (54,55).

4. Serine Esterase Inhibitors

These drugs have been shown to inhibit platelet phospholipase C (56).

REFERENCES

1. H. Kunze and W. Vogt. *Ann. N.Y. Acad. Sci. 180*:123 (1971).
2. M. I. Aveldano and N. G. Bazan, *Brain Res. 100*:99 (1975).
3. R. J. Cenedella, C. Galli, and R. Paoletti, *Lipids 10*:290 (1975).
4. N. G. Bazan and H. Rakowski. *Life Sci. 9*:501 (1970).
5. P. Piper and J. Vane. *Ann. N.Y. Acad. Sci. 180*:363 (1971).
6. E. W. Salzman, J. N. Lindon, and R. Rodvien, *J. Cyclic Nucl. Res. 2*:25 (1976)

7. W. Hsueh, P. C. Isakson, and P. Needleman. *Prostaglandins 13*:1073 (1977).
8. W. Hsueh and P. Needleman. *Prostaglandins 16*:661 (1978).
9. S. E. Rittenhouse. *Proc. Natl. Acad. Sci. USA 80*:5417 (1983).
10. S. Rittenhouse-Simmons. *J. Clin. Invest. 63*:580 (1979).
11. R. L. Bell, D. A. Kennerly, N. Stanford, and P. W. Majerus. *Proc. Natl. Acad. Sci. USA 76*:3238 (1979).
12. M. M. Billah, E. G. Lapetina, and P. Cuatrecasas. *J. Biol. Chem. 256*: 5399 (1981).
13. E. G.Lapetina, M. M. Billah, and P. Cuatrecasas. *J. Biol. Chem. 256*: 5037 (1981).
14. S. E. Rittenhause-Simmons. *J. Biol. Chem. 256*:4153 (1981).
15. M. M. Billah and E. G. Lapetina. *J. Biol. Chem. 257*:12705 (1982).
16. H. Holmsen, C. A. Dangelmaier, and H. K. Holmsen. *J. Biol. Chem. 256*:9393 (1981).
17. J. D. Vickers, R. L. Kinlough-Rathbone, and J. F. Mustard. *Blood 60*: 1247 (1982).
18. M. Billah and E. G. Lapetina. *J. Biol. Chem. 257*:12705 (1982).
19. B. W. Agranoff, P. Murphy, and E. B. Sequin. *J. Biol. Chem. 258*:2076 (1983).
20a. S. E. Rittenhouse. *Proc. Natl. Acad. Sci. USA 80*:5417 (1983).
20b. J. D. Vickers and J. F. Mustard. *Fed. Proc. 443*:979 (1978).
21. M. J. Broekman, J. W. Ward, and A. J. Marcus. *J. Clin. Invest. 63*:580 (1979).
22. M. J. Berridge, R. M. C. Dawson, P. Downes, J. P. Heslop, and R. E. Irvine. *Biochem. J. 212*:473 (1983).
23. M. J. Berridge. *Biochem. J. 212*:849 (1983).
24. R. H. Michell. *Biochem. Biophys. Acta 415*:81 (1975).
25. J. N. Hawthorne and D. A. White. *Vitam. Horm. 33*:529 (1975).
26. E. G. Lapetina and P. Cuatrecases. *Biochem. Biophys. Acta 573*:394 (1979).
27. S. M. Prescott and P. W. Majerus. *J. Biol. Chem. 258*:764 (1983).
28. M. Lagarde, S. Menashi, and N. Crawford. *FEBS Lett. 124*:23 (1981).
29. J. M. Gerrard, J. G. White, G. H. R. Rao, and D. Townsend. *Am. J. Pathol. 83*:283 (1976).
30. F. Carey, S. Menashi, and N. Crawford. *Biochem. J. 204*:847 (1982).
31. V. P. Torchilin, A. L. Klibanov, and V. N. Smirnov. *FEBS Lett. 138*:117 (1982).
32a. Y. Takai, A. Kishimoto, Y. Iwasa, Y. Kawahara, T. Mori, and Y. Nishizuka. *J. Biol. Chem. 254*:3692 (1979).
32b. S. K. Joseph, A. P. Thomas, R. J. Williams, R. F. Irvine, and J. R. Williamson. *J. Biol. Chem. 259*:3077 (1984).
32c. H. Streb, R. F. Irvine, N. J. Berridge, and I. Schultz. *Nature 306*:67 (1983).

33. J. M. Gerrard, D. A. Peterson, and J. G. White. In *Platelets in Biology and Pathology 2,* J. L. Gordon (ed.). Elsevier/North Holland, Amsterdam (1981).
34. C. Serhan, P. Anderson, E. Goodman, P. Dunham, and G. Weissman. *J. Biol. Chem. 256*:2736 (1981).
35. J. M. Gerrard, S. E. Kindom, D. A. Peterson, and J. G. White. *Am. J. Pathol. 97*:531 (1979).
36. T. K. Bills, J. B. Smith, and M. J. Silver. *Biochem. Biophys. Acta 424*: 303 (1976).
37. M. J. Broekman, J. W. Ward, and A. J. Marcus. *J. Clin. Invest. 66*:275 (1980).
38. M. L. McKean, J. B. Smith, and M. J. Silver. *J. Biol. Chem. 256*:1522 (1981).
39. R. L. Jesse and R. C. Franson. *Biochim. Biophys. Acta 575*:467 (1979).
40a. L. R. Ballou and W. Y. Cheung. *Proc. Natl. Acad. Sci. USA 80*: 5203 (1983).
40b. L. Y. Chau and H. H. Tai. *Biochem. Biophys. Res. Commun. 113*:241 (1983).
40c. J. M. Gerrard, G. Graff, P. C. Dedon, S. E. Kindom, and J. G. White. *Progr. Lipid Res. 20*:575 (1982).
41. F. Hirata and J. Axelrod. *Science 209*:1082 (1980).
42. F. Hirata. *J. Biol. Chem. 256*:7730 (1981).
43. F. Hirata, E. Schiffman, K. Venkatasubramanian, K. Salomon, and D. Axelrod. *Proc. Natl. Acad. Sci. USA 77*:2533 (1980).
44. E. J. Neufeld and P. W. Majerus. *J. Biol. Chem. 258*:2461 (1983).
45. M. Minkes, N. Stanford, M. M. Y. Chi, G. J. Roth, A. Raz, P. Needleman, and P. W. Majerus. *J. Clin. Invest. 59*:449 (1977).
46. J. M. Gerrard, J. D. Peller, T. P. Krick, and J. G. White. *Prostaglandins 14*:39 (1977).
47. G. Mauco, H. Chap, M. E. Simon, and L. Douste-Blazy. *Biochemistry 60*:653 (1978).
48. R. Kaser-Glanzmann, M. Jakabova, J. N. George, and E. F. Luscher. *Biochem. Biophys. Acta 466*:429 (1977).
49. M. M. Billah, E. G. Lapetina, and P. Cuatrecasas. *Biochem. Biophys. Res. Commun. 90*:92 (1979).
50. R. J. Flower and G. J. Blackwell. *Nature 278*:456 (1979).
51. R. W. Walenga, E. E. Opas, and M. B. Feinstein. *J. Biol. Chem. 256*: 12523 (1981).
52. D. P. Wallach and V. J. R. Brown. *Biochem. Pharm. 30*:1315 (1981)
53. S. L. Hofmann and P. W. Majerus. *J. Biol. Chem. 257*:14359 (1982).
54. S. Rittenhouse-Simmons and P. Deykin. *Biochem. Biophys. Acta 534*: 409 (1978).
55. R. C. Franson, D. Eisen, R. Jesse, and C. Lanni. *Biochem. J. 186*:633 (1980).

56. R. Wallenga, J. Y. Vanderhoek, and M. B. Feinstein. *J. Biol. Chem. 255*: 6024 (1980).

BIBLIOGRAPHY

G. J. Blackwell and R. J. Flower. *Br. Med. Bull. 39*:260 (1983).

5
Arachidonic Acid Metabolizing Enzymes and Inhibitors

Much of what has been learned about prostaglandins and their functions has come from the careful use of specific inhibitors. In this chapter, I shall review the actions of the most commonly used inhibitors, where possible discussing the inhibitors in terms of our current understanding of the enzymes. Many of the inhibitors mentioned are relatively specific. However, almost all probably have some additional actions. For example, even acetylsalicylate (aspirin), which is widely used as a specific and irreversible inhibitor of the prostaglandin endoperoxide synthase or cyclooxygenase enzyme, is known to acetylate additional platelet proteins. Whether such acetylation affects the function of these other proteins is not known but is certainly possible. With lipoxygenase inhibitors, specificity appears to be a major problem.

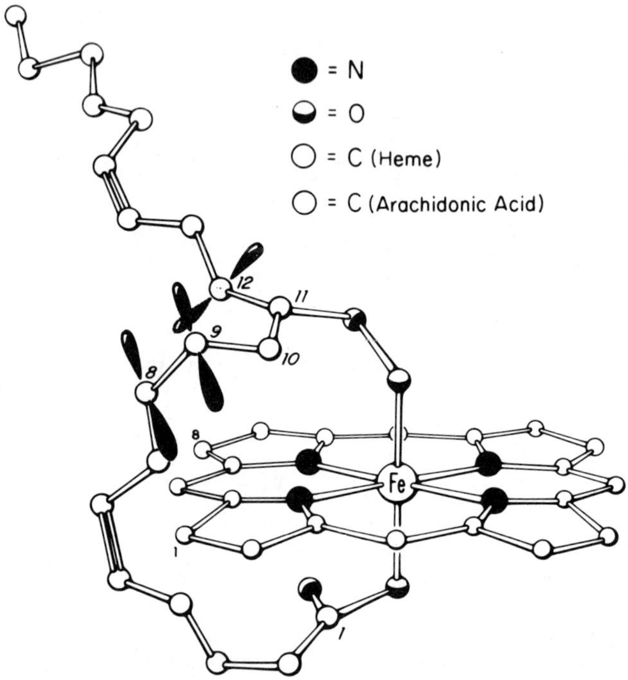

Fig. 5-1 A model of the interaction of iron (Fe) in heme (the protoporphyrin ring without the substituent groups is shown for clarity) with arachidonic acid. The oxygens attached to C_1 of arachidonic acid (the carboxylate group) are shown attaching to the Fe below the plane of the porphyrin ring. The arachidonic acid then winds around the porphyrin ring, and oxygen attached to the Fe above the porphyrin ring is attached to the arachidonic acid at carbon 11 of the fatty acid. The active site of the enzyme is therefore just above the Fe where the oxygen is bound and then transferred to the arachidonic acid. (Reprinted from Ref. 3.)

I. THE PROSTAGLANDIN ENDOPEROXIDE SYNTHASE (CYCLOOXYGENASE)

A. The Enzyme

Some knowledge of this enzyme and its active site is useful to understanding inhibitors and how they work. The prostaglandin synthase has a subunit molecular weight of about 70,000 daltons, with two identical subunits

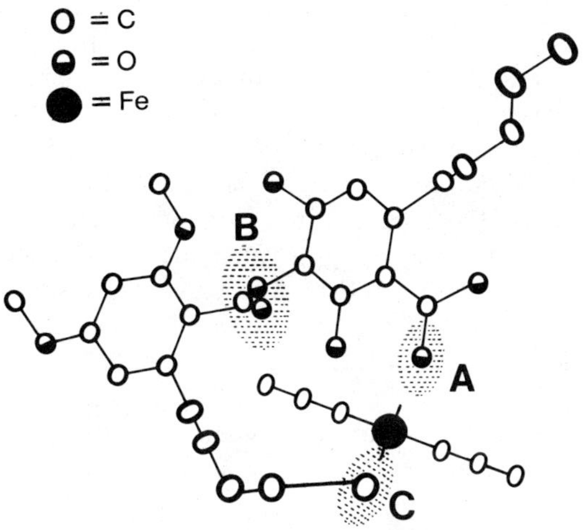

Fig. 5-2 The interaction of 4-O-methylcryptochlorophaeic acid with Fe^{2+}-heme, as proposed in Reference 6. In this view the Fe^{2+} within the porphyrin ring is shown from the side. Site A is the active site of the enzyme. Sites A and B are important for inhibitor action (see text), while site C is where the carboxylate group of arachidonic acid is proposed to attach.

associated together, and one heme group per subunit. There is known to be a serine group which can be acetylated by aspirin at the active site.

A number of models for the active site of the enzyme have been proposed (1-4). A model is shown in Fig. 5-1. Recent studies using the depside, 4-0-methylcryptochlorophaeic acid, a potent inhibitor of the cyclooxygenase enzyme which also has a rigid conformation, have extended knowledge of the probable interactions of substrates and inhibitors (Fig. 5-2) (5,6). Limitations in our present knowledge of the protein are such that we do not know if this model is an entirely accurate representation of the enzyme-heme-substrate interaction. However, it provides a useful framework for understanding inhibitors.

In this model, the carboxyl group of the arachidonic acid is seen as interacting with one of the available ligands on the Fe^{2+} of the heme on the enzyme (site C of Fig. 5-2). It is possible that the carboxyl group interacts with a cationic site elsewhere on the enzyme. However, interaction of the carboxyl of arachidonic acid with the Fe^{2+} in the heme would convey distinct advantages in terms of the control of substrate turnover, and the stereospecificity of the reaction, and is therefore probably correct (3).

The acyl chain of the arachidonic acid winds around the hydrophobic portion (Fig. 5-2, site B) of the heme, with the C-11 double bond positioned in close proximity to the second available ligand on the Fe^{2+} heme (Fig. 5-2, site A), so that O_2 transiently attached to the Fe^{2+} can be transferred to the carbon 11 of the arachidonic acid. Attachment of the O_2 at C-11 is followed by ring closure. With formation of the terminal endoperoxide structure, the O_2 attached across C9-11 swings around to bind at an oxygen binding site (Fig. 5-2, site B) on the enzyme, positioning the terminal acyl chain appropriately for the final O_2 addition at C-15. The active site A, site B, and the hydrophobic portion appear particularly important for inhibitor attachment. It should be mentioned here that there is not general agreement on the above mechanism; in particular it has been suggested, on the basis of a deuterium effect at C-13, where hydrogen is abstracted during the reaction, that addition of the oxygen at C-15 occurs before oxygen addition at C-11. However, the deuterium effect shows the hydrogen abstraction is rate limiting. It should not be used to indicate that O_2 addition at C-15 occurs first.

B. Modulation of Enzyme Activity by Peroxides

In an extensive series of studies, Lands and co-workers have characterized the activity of the cyclooxygenase enzyme and the influence of peroxides. The enzyme has unusual kinetics with an initial lag phase, a secondary accelerative phase leading to maximal activity, and finally a decelerating phase (self-catalyzed inactivation) until no further reaction occurs (7-9). Their studies have revealed that the low initial reaction rate seen was due to the absence (or extremely low levels) of peroxides. As the product peroxide PGG_2 was generated, it activated the enzyme to accelerate the rate of reaction. Peterson et al. have provided an explanation for this effect of peroxides (10). The active enzyme uses heme in the Fe^{2+} form, while the heme associated with the resting enzyme is in the Fe^{3+} form. Lipid peroxides can reduce heme from Fe^{3+}-heme to Fe^{2+}-heme. Thus, enzyme activation by peroxides may result from their ability to reduce heme to activate the enzyme according to the reaction $ROO^- + Fe^{3+} \rightarrow ROO^{\cdot} + Fe^{2+}$.

The mechanism of the self-deactivation of the enzyme has been investigated and appears related to the buildup of an active radical, with PGG_2 playing a critical role (11). Peterson et al. have suggested that as the reaction proceeds with a buildup of $ROO^{\cdot}$, the reverse reaction to he above $ROO^{\cdot} + Fe^{2+} \rightarrow ROO^- + Fe^{3+}$ occurs, leading to an inactive enzyme (10).

It is of interest that when eicosapentaenoic acid is used as the substrate, it appears to need more activating peroxide than when arachidonic acid is used (12).

From a physiologic point of view the self-destructive nature of the enzyme is probably important in that it assurs only a limited maximum amount of prostaglandin can be formed at one time, ensuring that there can not be a massive buildup of these active agents during an inflammatory response.

C. Inhibitors

Cyclooxygenase inhibitors are of three general types: (a) reversible competitive inhibitors, (b) irreversible inhibitors, and (c) inhibitors which have antioxidant or radical-traping properties. The latter are reversible noncompetitive inhibitors which act by decreasing the cellular level of peroxides.

1. Reversible Competitive Inhibitors

Fatty acids. Eicosapentaenoic acid, at peroxide levels less than 10^{-8} M, is primarily a reversible competitive inhibitor of arachidonic acid conversion to prostaglandin endoperoxides (12). Other fatty acids, including oleic (9,18:1), linoleic (9,2-18:2), and linolenic acids (9,12,15-18:3), can also competitively inhibit the cyclooxygenase, although higher concentrations are required (up to 5 mM) and a time-dependent irreversible component may be present. Positional isomers of dihomo-γ-linolenic acid (all cis 8,11,14-20:3), such as 8-cis, 12-trans, 14-cis-20:3, and of arachidonic acid (all cis-5,8,11, 14-20:4), such as 5-cis, 8-cis, 12-trans, 14-cis-20:4, are potent competitive inhibitors.

The acetylenic analogue of arachidonic acid, 5,8,11,14-eicosatetraynoic acid (with triple bonds instead of double bonds), is a competitive inhibitor of the cyclooxygenase (and the 12 and 15 lipoxygenases), but also has an irreversible effect.

Ibuprofen. Several compounds, including ibuprofen, mefenamic acid, and BL-2365 with a carboxylic acid group attached to a lipophilic constituent group containing one or more phenyl rings, are reversible competitive inhibitors. These drugs are probably effective because the carboxylate group attaches to the active-site Fe in the enzyme heme (site A, Fig. 5-2) while the lipophilic component locates in the hydrophobic region of the enzyme (13).

Salicylate. Salicylic acid effectively inhibits prostaglandin synthesis in vivo (14,15), whereas it is relatively ineffective in vitro. The reason for this is not understood. However, salicylate can clearly attach with similar affinity to aspirin to the active site, since it can prevent the irreversible effect of aspirin (see below) (16). The carboxylate of salicylate probably binds to the active-site Fe as with ibuprofen above (17).

Indomethacin. Indomethacin is a potent inhibitor of the cyclooxygenase. It is a competitive inhibitor. With sheep seminal vesicles there is a time-dependent irreversible action; however, the effect of indomethacin on the platelet cyclooxygenase is reversible in vivo (15). The carboxylate region of indomethacin has been suggested to interact with site A (Fig. 5-2), while the keto group interacts with site B.

2. Irreversible Inhibitors

Aspirin (acetylsalicylicate). Aspirin irreversibly inhibits the prostaglandin endoperoxide synthase enzyme by acetylating the OH on a serine located at the active site (18-20). Initial binding of aspirin to the enzyme, necessary before acetylation can occur, is competitively inhibited by salicylate, indomethacin, and ibuprofen.

Flurbiprofen, meclofenamic acid. Compounds with an aryl halogen (chlorine or fluorine), yet otherwise similar to reversible inhibitors, are irreversible cyclooxygenase inhibitors (21). These compounds probably interact with site A through their carboxylate group and with the chlorine or fluorine at site B (Fig. 5-2) (5,6).

3. Inhibitors Which Modify "Peroxide Tone"

Acetaminophen. Acetominophen is an inhibitor of prostaglandin synthesis in some tissues (i.e., brain and kidney) but not others (i.e., platelets, stomach) (22). Its effects on the prostaglandin synthase enzyme have been suggested to be due to an influence on peroxide tone (23).

Acetaminophen can inhibit the enzyme in tissues with low endogenous levels of peroxide (i.e., brain) by further lowering the available peroxide to a level below which the enzyme can function. In cells with a high endogenous level of peroxides, like platelets, acetaminophen is not inhibitory because the slight lowering of peroxide tone produced by acetaminophen is insufficient to affect cyclooxygenase activity.

II. THROMBOXANE SYNTHASE

The thromboxane synthase enzyme has been isolated, characterized, and a variety of inhibitors have been identified (24-26). In the platelet, the enzyme is found in the dense tubular system (smooth endoplasmic reticulum) (27). Compounds which are selective thromboxane synthetase inhibitors include imidazole, OKY-1581 (a substituted pyridine), and the imidazole derivatives dazoxiben and UK-38,485 (28-31). Other agents proposed as selective thromboxane synthetase inhibitors include nicotinic acid, hydralazine, diazoxide, and the H_2 receptor antagonist burimamide (32-34). Some agents which are thromboxane synthetase inhibitors are also cyclooxygenase inhibitors (i.e., L8027 and 1-nonyl-imidazole) or are also lipoxygenase inhibitors (i.e., sulfasalazine) (35,36).

III. PROSTACYCLIN SYNTHASE

This microsomal enzyme has been purified, and like the cyclooxygenase it contains heme iron (37). An important characteristic of this enzyme is its inhibition by alkyl hydroperoxides (38-41). The heme is at the active site of the enzyme, and the irreversible enzyme inactivation seen with alkyl hydroperoxides or with PGH_2 appears to result from a modification of the heme group (37).

Tranylcypromine has been used in vitro as a prostacyclin synthetase inhibitor (42,43). However, this drug has additional effects on intact cells and organisms which makes it difficult to use as a selective agent (44-47).

IV. LIPOXYGENASE ENZYMES

These enzymes are widely distributed in plants where they were first discovered. The finding of the 12-lipoxygenase in platelets; the 5-lipoxygenase in neutrophils, monocytes, and basophils; and the 15-lipoxygenase in eosinophils, immature erythrocytes, and lymphocytes (see Chs. 6-12) has led to much interest in these enzymes. The reaction kinetics for these enzymes has similarities to the cyclooxygenase with an initial product (peroxide) activation and later product inactivation (48). The basis for these characteristics may be similar to those of the cyclooxygenase (Sec. I) (49), but the iron may be in a nonheme state. The profile of substrate fatty acids and other characteristics of several of the blood cell enzymes have been reported (50, 51a).

A. Lipoxygenase Inhibitors

At the present time, caution must be urged in the use of lipoxygenase inhibitors. Many of these chemicals may have other effects on cells besides lipoxygenase inhibition as has been found for neutrophils (Ch. 8).

Acetylenic analogues of arachidonic acid (with triple bonds instead of double bonds) are competitive inhibitors of the lipoxygenase. With the triple bond present, hydrogen abstraction and peroxidation cannot occur. In addition to the two analogues discussed below (Sec. IV.A. 6 and 7), 5,6-11, 12-, and 14,15-dehydro arachidonic acid are selective inhibitors of the 5,11 or 15-lipoxygenases respectively (51b,c).

1. Retinoids

Retinoids (vitamin A derivatives), including retinol, retinal, trans-retinoic acid, and 13-cis retinoic acid, appear to be relatively selective inhibitors of the 5-lipoxygenase (I_{50}'s, 50, 10, 33, and 9 μM, respectively) (52).

2. Esculetin

Esculetin inhibits both the platelet 12-lipoxygenase and the basophil 5-lipoxygenase (53a,b). At high (mM) concentrations, the cyclooxygenase is also inhibited.

3. Phenidone

Phenidone inhibits the 5-lipoxygenase, the 12-lipoxygenase, and the cyclooxygenase (54a,b).

4. BW755C

BW755C, a pyrazoline analogue of phenidone, is a combined lipoxygenase and cyclooxygenase inhibitor (54a,c).

5. Nordihydroguiaretic Acid (NDGA)

NGDA has been used as an inhibitor of both 5- and 12-lipoxygenase, but also has inhibitory activity toward the cyclooxygenase (54a,d).

6. 5,8,11,14-Eicosatetraynoic Acid

This arachidonic acid analogue inhibits both lipoxygenase and cyclooxygenase enzymes.

7. 3,7,10,13-Eicosatetraynoic Acid

At low concentrations, this arachidonic acid analogue inhibits the lipoxygnease enzyme selectively, whereas at higher concentrations it inhibits both lipoxygenase and cyclooxygenase enzymes (55).

Both the above acetylenic analogues of arachidonic acid appear to have affects on cell function on neutrophils unrelated to their effects on lipoxygenase and cyclooxygenase enzymes.

8. Benoxaprofen

Benoxaprofen is a combined lipoxygenase and cyclooxygenase inhibitor (56).

V. ENZYMES INVOLVED IN LEUKOTRIENE C_4 AND D_4 FORMATION

Glutathione-S-transferase which converts LTA_4 to LTC_4 and γ-glutamyl transpeptidase appear to be membrane-bound enzymes in rat basophilic leukemia cells (57). However, in kidney, liver, and lung glutathione-S-transferase is a soluble enzyme (58), while γ-glutamyl transpeptidase is a particulate (cell membrane) enzyme (59).

Diethylcarbamazine inhibits LTC_4 and LTD_4 synthesis in murine mastocytoma cells, probably by blocking the conversion of (5-HPETE) to 5-hydroperoxyeicosatetraenoic acid LTA_4 (60).

VI. LIPASES

Phospholipases important for the release of arachidonic acid and their inhibitors are described in Ch. 4. The diglyceride lipase and its inhibitors will be briefly discussed here.

A. Diglyceride Lipase

Diglyceride lipase is found in the platelet dense tubular system (smooth endoplasmic reticulum) (61). The enzyme can be inhibited by high concentrations of indomethacin (62), by octyl-glyceryl ether (63), and by RHC 80267 (64).

VII. Receptor Antagonists

A. Thromboxane A_2 Receptor Antagonists

13-Azaprostanoic acid is a selective thromboxane receptor antagonist (65). Other compounds with thromboxane receptor antagonist action have been described, but some of these also have other effects (i.e., inhibition of thromboxane or prostacyclin synthase) (66-68).

B. LTD_4 Antagonists

FPL 55712 is a selective antagonist of LTD_4 (69).

REFERENCES

1. R. A. Scherrer. In *Antiinflammatory Agents: Chemistry and Pharmacology,* R. A. Scherrer and M. W. Whitehouse (eds.). Academic Press, New York (1974).
2. P. Gund and T. Y. Shen. *J. Med. Chem. 5*:683 (1976).
3. D. A. Peterson and J. M. Gerrard. *Med. Hypotheses 5*:683, (1979).
4. R. A. Appleton and K. Brown. *Prostaglandins 18*:29 (1979).
5. U. Sankawa, M. Shibuya, Y. Ebizuka, H. Noguchi, T. Kinoshita, and Y. Iitaka. *Prostaglandins 24*:21 (1982).
6. J. M. Gerrard and D. A. Peterson. *Prostaglandins Leukotrienes Med. 13*: 139 (1984).
7. W. L. Smith and W. E. M. Lands. *Biochemistry 11*:3276 (1972).
8. M. E. Hemler, G. Graff, and W. E. M. Lands. *Biochem. Biophys. Res. Commun. 85*:1325 (1978).
9. W. E. M. Lands. *J. Lipid Res. 20*:875 (1982).
10. D. A. Peterson, J. M. Gerrard, G. H. R. Rao, and J. G. White. *Prostaglandins Med. 4*:73 (1980).
11. R. W. Egan, J. Paxton, and F. A. Kuehl. *J. Biol. Chem. 251*:7329 (1976).
12. W. E. M. Lands and M. J. Byrnes. *Progr. Lipid Res. 20*:287 (1982).

13. D. A. Peterson, J. M. Gerrard, G. H. R. Rao, and J. G. White. *Prostaglandins Med. 2*:97 (1979).
14. G. A. Higgs, E. A. Harvey, S. H. Ferreira, and J. R. Vane. *Adv. Prostaglandin Thromboxane Res. 1*:105 (1970).
15. J. J. Kocsis, J. Hernandovitch, M. J. Silver, J. B. Smith, and C. Ingerman. *Prostaglandins 3*:141 (1973).
16. J. W. McDonald and M. Ali. *Clin. Res. 26*:A856 (1978).
17. D. A. Peterson, J. M. Gerrard, G. H. R. Rao, and J. G. White. *Prostaglandins Med. 6*:161 (1981).
18. J. B. Smith and A. L. Willis. *Nature (New Biol.) 231*:235 (1971).
19. G. J. Roth and P. W. Majerus. *J. Clin. Invest. 56*:624 (1975).
20. G. J. Roth and C. J. Siok. *J. Biol. Chem. 253*:3782 (1978).
21. L. H. Rome and W. E. M. Lands. *Proc. Natl. Acad. Sci. USA 72*:4863 (1975).
22. E. T. Tolman, B. A. Marinan, B. L. Fuller, and M. E. Rosenthale. *Fed. Proc. 42*:641 (1983).
23. W. E. M. Lands, H. W. Cook, and L. H. Rome. *Adv. Prostaglandin Thromboxane Res. 1*:7 (1976).
24. T. Yoshimoto, S. Yamamoto, M. Okuma, and O. Hayaishi. *J. Biol. Chem. 252*:5871 (1977).
25. S. Hammarstrom and P. Falardeau. *Proc. Natl. Acad. Sci. USA 74*:3691 (1977).
26. E. R. Hall and H. H. Tai. *Biochim. Biophys. Acta 665*:498 (1981).
27. F. Carey, S. Menashi, and N. Crawford. *Biochem. J. 204*:847 (1982).
28. S. Moncada, S. Bunting, K. Mullane, P. Thorogood, and J. R. Vane. *Prostaglandins 13*:611 (1977).
29. N. Feuerstein and P. W. Ramwell. *Eur. J. Pharmacol. 69*:533 (1981).
30. M. J. Randall, M. J. Parry, E. Hawkeswood, P. E. Cross, and R. P. Dickinson. *Thromb. Res. 23*:145 (1981).
31. S. Fischer, M. Struppler, B. Bohlig, C. Bernutz, W. Wober, and P. C. Weber. *Circulation 68*:821 (1983).
32. J. E. Vincent and F. J. Zulstra. *Prostaglandins 15*:629 (1978).
33. J. E. Greenwald, L. K. Wong, M. Rao, J. R. Blanchine, and R. V. Panganamala. *Biochem. Biophys. Res. Commun. 84*:1112 (1978).
34. G. Allan and K. E. Eakins. *Prostaglandins 15*:659 (1978).
35. A. V. Prancan, J. Lefort, M. Chignard, K. Gerozissis, F. Dray, and B. B. Vargaftig. *Eur. J. Pharmacol. 60*:287 (1979).
36. W. F. Stenson and E. Lobos. *Biochem. Pharmacol. 32*:2205 (1983).
37. D. L. DeWitt and W. L. Smith. *J. Biol. Chem. 258*:3285 (1983).
38. S. Bunting, R. Gryglewski, S. Moncada, and J. R. Vane. *Prostaglandins 12*:897 (1976).
39. J. A. Salmon, D. R. Smith, R. J. Flower, S. Moncada, and J. R. Vane. *Biochim. Biophys. Acta 523*:250 (1978).
40. R. J. Gryglewski, R. Korbut, and A. Ocetkiewicz. *Nature 273*:765 (1978).

41. E. A. Ham, R. W. Egan, D. D. Soderman, P. H. Gale, and F. A. Kuehl, Jr. *J. Biol. Chem. 254*:2191 (1979).
42. R. J. Gryglewski, S. Bunting, S. Moncada, R. J. Flower, and J. R. Vane. *Prostaglandins 12*:685 (1976).
43. R. I. Clyman, F. Mauray, M. A. Koerper, F. Wiemer, M. A. Heymann, and A. M. Rudolph. *Prostaglandins 16*:633 (1978).
44. S. L. Hong, T. Carty, and D. Deykin. *J. Biol. Chem. 255*:9538 (1980).
45. G. Rajtar and G. de Gaetano. *Thromb. Res. 14*:245 (1979).
46. G. H. R. Rao, S. Einzig, K. R. Reddy, and J. G. White. *Prostaglandins Med. 3*:201 (1979).
47. K. E. Clark and D. J. Harrington. *Prostaglandins 23*:227 (1982).
48. W. L. Smith and W. E. M. Lands. *J. Biol. Chem. 247*:1038 (1972).
49. D. A. Peterson and J. M. Gerrard. *Prostaglandins Med. 10*:107 (1975).
50. D. H. Nugteren. *Biochim. Biophys. Acta 380*:299 (1975).
51a. B. A. Jakschik, A. R. Sams, H. Sprecher, and P. Needleman. *Prostaglandins 20*:401 (1980).
51b. E. J. Corey and J. E. Munroe. *J. Am. Chem. Soc. 104*:1752 (1982).
51c. E. J. Corey and H. Park. *J. Am. Chem. Soc. 104*:1750 (1982).
52. C. Fielder-Nagy, J. G. Hamilton, C. Batula-Bernardo, and J. W. Coffey. *Fed. Proc. 42*:919 (1983).
53a. Y. Hamasaki and H. H. Tai. *Fed. Proc. 42*:641 (1983).
53b. K. Sekiya, H. Okuda, and S. Arichi. *Biochem. Biophys. Acta 713*:68 (1982).
54a. S. L. Levinson and C. C. Hedli. *Fed. Proc. 42*:443 (1983).
54b. G. J. Blackwell and R. J. Flower. *Prostaglandins 16*:417 (1978).
54c. G. A. Higgs, R. J. Flower, and J. R. Vane. *Biochem. Pharmacol. 28*: 1959 (1979).
54d. M. Hamberg. *Biochem. Biophys. Acta 431*:651 (1976).
55. R. J. Smith, F. F. Sun, S. S. Iden, B. J. Bowman, H. Sprecher, and J. C. McGuire. *Clin. Immunol. Immunopathol. 20*:157 (1981).
56. C. L. Armour, J. M. Hughes, J. P. Seale, and D. M. Temple. *Eur. J. Pharmacol. 72*:93 (1981).
57. B. A. Jakschik, T. Harper, and R. C. Murphy. *J. Biol. Chem. 257*:5346 (1982).
58. A. W. Wolkoff, R. A. Wiesiger, and W. B. Jakoby. *Progr. Liver Dis. 6*: 213 (1979).
59. S. S. Tate, G. A. Thompson, and A. Meister. In *Glutathione: Metabolism and Function,* T. M. Aries and W. B. Jakoby (eds.). Raven Press, New York (1976).
60. W. R. Mathews and R. C. Murphy. *Biochem. Pharmacol. 31*:2129 (1982).
61. M. Lagarde, S. Menashi, and N. Crawford. *Biochem. J. 204*:847 (1982).
62. S. Rittenhouse-Simmons. *J. Biol. Chem. 255*:2259 (1980).

63. J. M. Gerrard, G. Graff, P. C. Dedon, S. E. Kindom, and J. G. White. *Progr. Lipid Res. 20*:575 (1981).
64. C. A. Sutherland. *J. Biol. Chem. 257*:4006 (1982).
65. G. C. LeBreton, D. L. Venton, S. E. Enke, and P. V. Halushka. *Proc. Natl. Acad. Sci. USA 76*:4097 (1979).
66. F. A. Fitzpatrick, G. L. Bundy, R. R. Gorman, and T. Honohan. *Nature 275*:764 (1978).
67. D. N. Harris, M. B. Phillips, M. Michel, H. J. Goldenberg, J. E.Heikes, P. W. Sprague, and M. J. Antonaccio. *Prostaglandins 22*:295 (1981).
68. S-T Kam, P. S. Portoghese, E. W. Dunham, and J. M. Gerrard. *Prostaglandins Med. 3*:279 (1979).
69. J. Augstein, J. B. Farmer, T. B. Lee, P. Sheard, and M. L. Tattersall. *Nature (New Biol.) 245*:215 (1973).

BIBLIOGRAPHY

H. J. Robinson and J. R. Vane (eds.). *Prostaglandin Synthetase Inhibitors.* Raven Press, New York (1974).

H. J. M. Barnett, J. Hirsch, and J. F. Mustard. *Acetylsalicylic Acid: New Uses for an Old Drug.* Raven Press, New York (1982).

II

SPECIFIC BLOOD CELL TYPES

6
Blood Platelets

Platelets are small blood cells, discoid in shape, which have no nucleus and are involved principally in the response of the blood to vessel wall injury. When platelets are exposed to a damaged vessel wall, they become sticky and promote the formation of a hemostatic platelet-fibrin plug. Prostaglandin endoperoxides and thromboxane A_2 produced when platelets are stimulated promote cell activation and involvement in hemostatic plug formation.

I. PLATELET ANATOMY

A. Morphology

Internal platelet structure is shown in Fig. 6-1. Platelets are surrounded by a plasma membrane with numerous invaginations penetrating into the cell interior—the surface-connected canalicular system (SCCS). Microtubules are found as a circumferential band beneath the plasma membrane around the circumference of the disk. Randomly dispersed inside the platelet are mitochondria and several types of granules. Alpha granules containing fibrinogen, thrombospondin, platelet factor 4, beta-thromboglobulin, factor VIII,

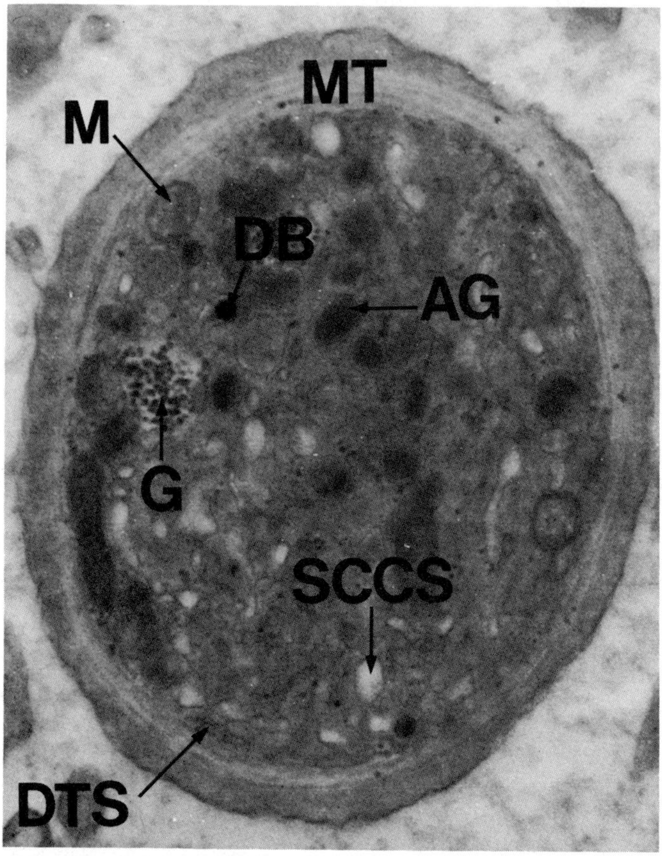

Fig. 6-1 A transmission electron microscopic view of the platelet interior. Around the periphery of this platelet, cut in the equatorial plane, is a band of microtubules (MT) positioned just beneath the plasma membrane. In the cell interior there is a dense body (DB), numerous alpha granules (AG), several mitochondria (M), and clusters of glycogen (G) particles. Channels of the surface-connected canalicular system (SCCS) and the dense tubular system (DTS) are also visible. (×20,700.)

fibronectin, and platelet-derived growth factor predominate. Dense granules contain ADP, ATP, serotonin, calcium, and pyrophosphate. Lysosomes containing hydrolytic enzymes and peroxisomes containing catalase are also found. In the cytoplasm, platelets have a large quantity of contractile proproteins including actin, myosin, actin-binding protein, and alpha-actinin. Membranes of smooth endoplasmic reticulum called the dense tubular system are found throughout the platelet, and particularly in association with SCCS membranes and with microtubules. The dense tubular system membranes are an important site for storage of calcium (1a). Indeed the SCCS and the dense tubular system may be analogous to skeletal muscle t-tubules and sarcotubules, respectively, in the regulation of cytoplasmic calcium (Fig. 6-2).

B. Lipids

Platelet lipid composition is summarized in Table 6-1 (1b-5). Phosphatidylcholine is the most abundant phospholipid. The distribution of phospholipids in platelet membranes is uneven. Most of the sphingomyelin of the platelet is located on the outer bilayer of the plasma membrane (6,7). This bilayer also has a large amount of phosphatidylcholine, but only minor amounts of phosphatidylethanolamine and phosphatidylserine (6-9). Curiously, this half of the plasma membrane has very little arachidonic acid (7).

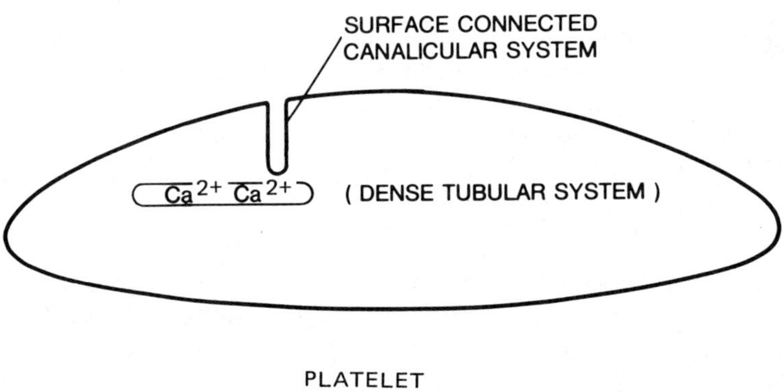

Fig. 6-2 A schematic diagram emphasizing the close association of the surface-connected canalicular system, an invagination of the platelet plasma membrane, and the dense tubular system, an internal membrane system where calcium is stored.

Table 6-1 Platelet Phospholipid Composition and Arachidonic Acid Content

Phospholipid	Lipid phosphorus %[a]	Nanomoles phospholipid Per 10^9 Platelets[b]	Nanomoles arachidonic acid Per 10^9 Platelets[c]
Phosphatidylcholine	39.2 ± 1.2	168	40
Phosphatidylethanolamine	27.9 ± 2.6	119	76
Sphingomyelin	17.3 ± 1.2	74	0
Phosphatidylserine	9.7 ± 1.0	42	19
Phosphatidylinositol	4.1 ± 0.8	17.5	14.6
Lysophosphatidylcholine	1.2 ± 0.5	5.1	0
Diphosphatidylglycerol	0.9	3.9	
Phosphatidylinositol-4-phosphate	0.187	0.8	
Phosphatidylinositol-4-5, bisphosphate	0.072	0.31	
Total		428	150

[a]The mean ± SD of data given in Refs. 1, 2, 4, 5, 7 except for DPI and TPI which is from Ref. 3.

[b]Total platelet phospholipid is estimated using data from Ref. 1 and using 1.5 mg platelet protein/10^9 platelets (123). Values for individual phospholipids are calculated using the percentages shown in the first column. Direct measurement of PI in one study (124), gave a value for PI of 17.5 nmol/10^9 platelets, identical to the number calculated in this table. Values given are generally higher than those reported by Broekman et al. (125), who did not use an internal standard to correct for recovery.

[c]Values are calculated using figures in the second column and the fatty acid composition of individual phospholipids as given in Ref. 1.

The inner half of the plasma membrane contains phosphatidylethanolamine and phosphatidylcholine as the predominant phospholipids. Smaller but significant amounts of phosphatidylserine and phosphatidylinositol also appear to be present in this half of the bilayer.

Intracellular smooth endoplasmic reticulum or dense tubular system membranes have been compared with plasma membranes (10). They contain very little sphingomyelin, less cholesterol, and less protein than the plasma membrane. Of importance for platelet arachidonic acid metabolism, the dense tubular system is relatively enriched in phosphatidylcholine and phosphatidylinositol and contains relatively more of the arachidonic acid in these two phospholipids than the plasma membrane. The distribution of phosphatidylcholine, phosphatidylethanolamine, and phosphatidylinositol within the dense tubular system is unknown at present, although a comparison with other endoplasmic reticulum has been used to suggest the inside bilayer might be enriched in phosphatidylcholine and phosphatidylinositol (11).

Phosphatidylserine appears to be relatively decreased in plasma and dense tubular system membranes (10) and may be an important phospholipid in granule membranes. Diphosphatidylglycerol, a minor phospholipid, appears enriched in mitochondria (4).

Ethanolamine phospholipids contain approximately equal amounts of diacyl and alkenylacyl (plasmalogen) species. In contrast, choline phospholipids contain very little alkenylacyl (1.4%) or alkylacyl (4.5%) species (5). The latter is of potential importance as the precursor of platelet-activating factor.

II. PLATELET FUNCTION

A. Adhesion to an Injured Vessel Wall

In response to vessel wall injury platelets rapidly attach to the site of exposed subendothelium, become activated, and spread along the injured surface. Platelets appear to attach primarily to injury-exposed collagen present in the subendothelial layer. Such attachment involves platelet membrane glycoprotein Ib, von Willebrand factor, and calcium and is affected by the local flow conditions (i.e., von Willebrand factor is more important with high shear stress).

B. Aggregation

When platelets are activated by collagen or other stimuli (i.e., epinephrine, ADP, thrombin, bacteria), their surface becomes sticky and they aggregate together. Aggregation involves membrane glycoprotein IIb and IIIa interaction with fibrinogen and thrombospondin. Current evidence suggests the latter two proteins act as bridging ligands forming the cross-bridges between adjacent platelets necessary for platelet-platelet attachment.

C. Shape Change and Granule Centralization (Internal Contraction)

An early event in the response of platelets to most stimuli is a change in platelet shape. The cell becomes rounded, pseudopods are extended, and granules are redistributed toward the platelet center. Closely surrounding the centrally packed granules is a constricted band of microtubules and a contracting web of platelet actin and myosin filaments. Present evidence suggests that the interaction of actin with a 260,000-dalton actin-binding protein is important for pseudopod formation, whereas actin-myosin interaction is important for the centralization of platelet granules and constriction of the microtubule ring (see Fig. 3-1) (12). Actin interaction with actin-binding proteins appears to be regulated, in part, by the phosphorylation state of actin-binding protein (12,13). Actin-myosin interaction has been well studied and is regulated by the level of cytoplasmic calcium. When the level of cytoplasmic calcium is raised, calcium interacts with calmodulin to activate a protein kinase which phosphorylates myosin light chain (14). When myosin light chain is phosphorylated, actin-myosin interaction and tension development occur (15).

D. Secretion

Activated platelets secrete the contents of dense granules, alpha granules, and lysosomes. Secretion depends on the extent of the stimulus; in general, a stronger stimulus is required for secretion than for aggregation. Secreted products, particularly ADP, may augment the extent of aggregation. Secretion requires labilization of the granules and the interaction of platelet contractile proteins. Considerable evidence supports the presence of a specific mechanism involved in granule labilization (fusion of granule membranes with membranes of the SCCS or the plasma membrane) so that granule contents can be extruded. Phorbol myristate acetate, an agent which can specifically labilize platelet granules (16), has been found to activate platelet protein kinase C, giving a specific phosphorylation of a 47,000-dalton protein (47P) (12,17). Diglycerides, which also specifically stimulate phosphorylation of this protein (18), produce similar morphological changes when added to platelets (19,20). These findings suggest that the 47,000-dalton protein, when phosphorylated, may be responsible for labilizing platelet granules. This concept fits with other evidence that phosphorylation of this protein is closely associated with secretion of platelet granules (21,22). However, agents that promote calcium flux and myosin light-chain phosphorylation potentiate secretion. It would appear that while granule labilization (due to 47P action) may be essential for secretion, the process is ordinarily facilitated or driven by an internal platelet contraction which squeezes the granule contents out through the channels of the surface-connected canalicular system.

E. Promotion of Fibrin Formation

The platelet surface acts to promote two reactions important for blood coagulation, the conversion of factor X into Xa by factor IXa with factor VIIIa as cofactor, and the cleavage of prothrombin to give thrombin by factor Xa with factor Va as cofactor. In the latter reaction, platelets bind factors Va and Xa to facilitate the cleavage of prothrombin to form thrombin. The thrombin then cleaves fibrinogen to form fibrin. Fibrin monomers polymerize to give fibrin strands which can interact with platelets and stabilize platelet aggregates at sites of injury.

F. Clot Retraction

Platelets contract the platelet-fibrin clot. In this process, platelet contractile proteins play an important role.

III. METABOLISM OF ARACHIDONIC ACID AND RELATED FATTY ACIDS IN PLATELETS

A. Arachidonic Acid (20:4)

Under the usual circumstances the major metabolites of arachidonic acid in platelets are thromboxane A_2 and 12-hydroxy-heptadecatrienoic acid (HHT) produced by the combined action of the prostaglandin synthase and thromboxane synthase and 12-hydroperoxy eicosatetraenoic acid (12-HPETE) and 12-hydroxy eicosatetraenoic acid (12-HETE) produced by the platelet lipoxygenase enzyme (Fig. 2-10) (23,24). PGD_2, PGE_2, and $PGF_{2\alpha}$ are minor products. Prostaglandin endoperoxide synthase and thromboxane synthase enzymes are located in the dense tubular system membranes (25,26). The 12-lipoxygenase enzyme appears to be cytosolic (25), but might be loosely membrane bound.

When small amounts of labeled arachidonic acid are added to platelets in the presence of plasma or medium containing similar high levels of albumin, the arachidonic acid is largely taken up into platelet phospholipids (27). However, when small amounts of arachidonic acid are added to platelets in the absence of albumin, the arachidonic acid is largely converted directly to products of the platelet cyclooxygenase and lipoxygenase enzymes (28).

B. Dihomo-γ-Linolenic Acid (20:3)

Dihomo-γ-linolenic acid (20:3), a fatty acid, is incorporated into platelet phospholipids in a similar fashion to arachidonic acid, but in response to thrombin, 20:3 is released from platelet phosphatidylinositol but not from phosphatidylcholine (29). The difference is unlikely to be due to the acyl chain specificity of platelet phospholipase A_2, but might result from the incorporation of 20:3 and 20:4 into phosphatidylcholine localized at different sites within the platelet. The major product of dihomo-γ-linolenic acid metabolism in platelets is the 12-lipoxygenase product; 12h-17:2 is also a significant product (31). Smaller amounts of 20:3 are converted to the cyclooxygenase metabolites, PGD_1, PGE_1, and thromboxane B_1, and to dihydroxy and trihydroxy fatty acids derived from the lipoxygenase pathway. The latter compounds were identified as 8,15-dihydroxy-9,11,13-eicosatrienoic acid, 14,15-dihydroxy-8,10,12-eicosatrienoic acid, 8,9,12-trihydroxy-10,14-eicosadienoic acid, and 8,11,12-trihydroxy-9,14-eicosadienoic acid.

C. Eicosapentaenoic Acid (20:5)

Eicosapentaenoic acid is incorporated into human platelet phospholipids, and released by thrombin in a similar fashion to arachidonic acid (32). Human platelets can convert eicosapentaenoic acid to the lipoxygenase product 12-HEPE (12h-20:5) and the cyclooxygenase products HHTE (12h-17:4) and thromboxane A_3 (32,33). The conversion of eicosapentaenoic acid to these products is much less efficient than the conversion of arachidonic acid, and production of the lipoxygenase product 12-HEPE in proportion to cyclooxygenase products is higher than with arachidonic acid metabolites (33). The arachidonic acid metabolite 12-HPETE promotes the conversion of eicosapentaenoic acid (34). Though eicosapentaenoic acid is converted to cyclooxygenase products less efficiently than arachidonic acid, it can compete effectively with arachidonic acid for the enzyme to inhibit production of PGH_2 and thromboxane A_2 (32). Species variability exists; rat and rabbit platelets do not convert eicosapentaenoic acid to lipoxygenase or cyclooxygenase products (33,35).

IV. THE INFLUENCE OF PROSTAGLANDIN PRECURSORS ON PLATELET FUNCTION

A. Arachidonic Acid

Arachidonic acid stimulates a change in platelet shape, centralization of platelet granules, aggregation of platelets, and secretion of granule contents (28, 36-38). The concentration of arachidonic acid needed is proportional to the amount of albumin in the suspending media, varying from approximately 1 μM with no albumin to about 1 mM with platelets in plasma. All effects of arachidonic acid on platelets can be prevented by the prostaglandin synthetase inhibitors, aspirin and indomethacin, with two notable exceptions: (a) When the amount of arachidonic acid used is disproportional to the concentration of albumin in the media suspending the platelets (i.e., high arachidonic acid, low albumin), arachidonic acid can cause lysis of platelets and this effect is not inhibited by aspirin (39). (b) When arachidonic acid is used together with epinephrine, the combination can stimulate platelet aggregation that cannot be inhibited by aspirin (40).

Curiously, under some conditions, high concentrations of arachidonic acid added to washed platelets will inhibit platelet aggregation to collagen, thrombin, and ADP (41). The mechanism of this effect is not well understood.

B. Dihomo-γ-Linolenic Acid (20:3)

Addition of dihomo-γ-linolenic acid to washed human platelets can, under some circumstances, stimulate a change in platelet shape that is inhibitable by aspirin (42). This effect is probably due to production of PGH_1 which has weak proaggregatory properties (see below). On the other hand, addition of dihimo-γ-linolenic acid to platelets will inhibit aggregation stimulated by ADP, collagen, epinephrine, and arachidonic acid (43,44). This inhibitory effect may be due to a combination of: (a) inhibition of platelet cyclooxygenase (see Ch. 5); (b) production of PGE_1 (see below); (c) possibly the diversion of arachidonic acid metabolism from thromboxane A_2 toward PGE_2 and PGD_2 (45); and (d) perhaps as well a nonspecific perturbation of the platelet membrane.

C. Eicosapentaenoic Acid (20:5)

Incubation of eicosapentaenoic acid with platelets results in inhibition of platelet aggregation (46-50). Similarly, a diet enriched in eicosapentaenoic acid will produce platelets with phospholipids enriched in this fatty acid which are less aggregable (51,52). Inhibition of platelet function by eicosapentaenoic acid appears to result from a combination of: (a) replacement of arachidonic acid by 20:5 in platelet phospholipids (Sec. III.C); (b) inhibition by 20:5 of arachidonic acid conversion to PGH_2 (Ch. 5); (c) decreased conversion of 20:5 to PGH_3 and thromboxane A_3 (Sec. III.C); (d) the weak proaggregatory effect of PGH_3; and (e) the production of PGD_3 which is a potent inhibitor of platelet aggregation (see below) (53).

V. THE INFLUENCE OF METABOLITES ON PLATELETS

A. Platelet-Derived Metabolites of Arachidonic Acid

1. Prostaglandin G_2/H_2/Thromboxane A_2

The action of the prostaglandin endoperoxides and thromboxane A_2 will be dealt with together since both are active on platelets. Thromboxane A_2 may be slightly more active than the endoperoxides, but selective inhibitors of thromboxane synthetase (without any effects on receptors or other platelet processes) have minimal inhibitory effect on platelet function (54-57), except for arachidonic acid aggregation (see Sec. VI.B). Whether there might be minor or even significant differences in the mechanism of action of the endoperoxides and thromboxane A_2 has not been established. Slight and variable inhibition of human platelet aggregation in response to epinephrine and collagen using thromboxane synthetase inhibitors could be due to enhanced conversion of PGH_2 to PGD_2, in some instances in the presence of these compounds, or could be due to slight, as yet undefined, differences in the mechanisms of their effects on platelets.

Addition of prostaglandin endoperoxides or thromboxane A_2 to platelets produces a change in platelet shape, platelet aggregation, and secretion of platelet granules (23,24,58). Each of these processes will be considered separately.

Platelet aggregation. Prostaglandin endoperoxides and thromboxane A_2 can stimulate platelet aggregation. The effect of these agents is associated with the binding of fibrinogen to the platelet surface (59). Controversy has existed with regard to a role for secreted ADP. The accumulated evidence is now compelling. Secreted ADP is not required for prostaglandin endoperoxide and thromboxane A_2-induced platelet aggregation (60-65). It is remotely possible that a tiny amount of ADP (~10 nM) already present in plasma might be required for such aggregation (66), but even this is unlikely. However, ADP can act synergistically with prostaglandin endoperoxides and thromboxane A_2 to promote aggregation (67).

The mechanism by which prostaglandin endoperoxides and thromboxane A_2 promote platelet fibrinogen binding is unknown. It is possible that it is related to an effect on intracellular calcium flux (see below), but it could also result from other actions of these agents.

Granule centralization. Prostaglandin endoperoxides and thromboxane A_2 added to platelets stimulate a redistribution of platelet granules toward the platelet center and the formation of pseudopods (68,69). The granule centralization (internal contraction) is associated with, and almost certainly results from (Sec. II.C), the phosphorylation of myosin light chain (70), which causes actin-myosin interaction to produce the contraction. As well as causing phosphorylation of myosin light chain, prostaglandin endoperoxides and thromboxane A_2 stimulate a rise in cytoplasmic calcium (71). This flux of calcium almost certainly mediates the phosphorylation of myosin light chain (Ch. 3). Investigations of the mechanism of the prostaglandin enoperoxide and thromboxane A_2-mediated calcium flux have shown that these agents can stimulate the release of calcium from the platelet dense tubular system (72-74). Indeed, the fact that synthesis of the endoperoxides and thromboxane A_2 occurs in this same dense tubular system led to the initial suggestion that such calcium release was a central and principal mechanism of their action (25). The mechanism of the thromboxane-induced calcium efflux could be the result of its action as a calcium ionophore (75), or a result of a more indirect receptor-mediated event such as stimulation of phosphoinositide metabolism (76).

Granule secretion. Production of prostaglandin endoperoxides and thromboxane A_2 by platelets is closely associated with the secretion of serotonin. Granule secretion by platelets needs granules labilized so that the granule membranes fuse with the membranes of the surface-connected canalicular system or the plasma membranes. Recent evidence links activation of protein kinase C and phosphorylation of a 47,000-dalton protein to granule labilization and secretion (Sec. II.D). Activation of this protein kinase needs diglyceride as well as calcium. Prostaglandin endoperoxide-induced platelet aggregation is associated with some breakdown of phosphatidylinositol and production of diglyceride and phosphatidic acid, but is much weaker, in this regard, than thrombin (76,78). It is possible that the small amount of diglyceride produced is enough to activate protein kinase C. Alternatively, it is possible that prostaglandin endoperoxides/thromboxane A_2 can perform the same function as the diglyceride in activating protein kinase C. In support of this possibility, addition of arachidonic acid or prostaglandin endoperoxides to platelets produces a rapid phosphorylation of the 47,000-dalton protein.

As shown from studies using inhibitors, production of $PGG_2/H_2/$ thromboxane A_2 by platelets is an important pathway for platelet activation. However, alternate pathway(s) exist(s); the relative importance of this and the alternate pathway(s) to various functions can be dissected using specific inhibitors (see subsequent discussion).

Clot retraction. When a platelet-rich plasma clot is formed using reptilase (which does not activate platelets), retraction of the clot occurs on addition of prostaglandin endoperoxides (79).

2. Prostaglandin D_2

PGD_2 acts on platelets to stimulate adenylate cyclase (80). The resulting increase in platelet cAMP acts to inhibit most platelet functions (81). PGD_2 is a minor product in platelets; it is therefore of little importance, except perhaps under some circumstances where it might serve a minor role as a negative feedback mechanism.

3. Prostaglandin E_2

Early studies suggested PGE_2 might under some circumstances potentiate platelet aggregation. The small amounts of PGE_2 produced by platelets relative to thromboxane A_2 and the weak activity of PGE_2 suggest it is unimportant in a global consideration of platelet function.

B. Platelet-Metabolites of Dihomo-γ-Linolenic Acid

1. Prostaglandin E_1

PGE_1 produced from dihomo-γ-linolenic acid (DHGLA) by platelets inhibits platelet function. DHGLA is a minor constituent of platelet phospholipids, and production of PGE_1 is likely of little importance. However, some investigators suggest that unactivated platelets may produce enough PGE_1 under basal conditions for the PGE_1 to have a role in maintaining the resting inactive state of platelets.

2. Prostaglandin H_1

PGH_1 is a much weaker platelet agonist than PGH_2.

C. Platelet Metabolites of Eicosapentaenoic Acid

1. Prostaglandin H_3

PGH_3 added to platelets inhibits aggregation. This effect is due to conversion to PGD_3 (below). If the platelets are pretreated with dideoxyadenosine to block the effect of the PGD_3 produced, then PGH_3 itself has a weak pro-aggregatory effect (53).

2. Prostaglandin D_3

PGD_3 is a potent inhibitor of platelet aggregation (IC_{50} = 7 ng/ml), being slightly more potent than PGD_2 (IC_{50} = 20 ng/ml) (53).

3. Thromboxane A_3

Thromboxane A_3 is weak or inactive as an inducer of platelet aggregation (82,83a).

D. Arachidonate Metabolites Derived From Other Cells

1. Prostaglandin I_2 (Prostacyclin)

PGI_2, synthesized primarily by endothelial cells, is a potent inhibitor of platelet adhesion to an injured vessel wall, platelet aggregation, platelet phospholipase activity, and platelet granule secretion. Prostacyclin acts by stimulating platelet adenylate cyclase to raise cellular cAMP levels. Elevated cellular cAMP levels inhibit platelet processes through activation of specific protein kinases to phosphorylate proteins which then act to sequester calcium to lower the cytoplasmic calcium level or to inhibit cellular contractile protein interactions (83b,c).

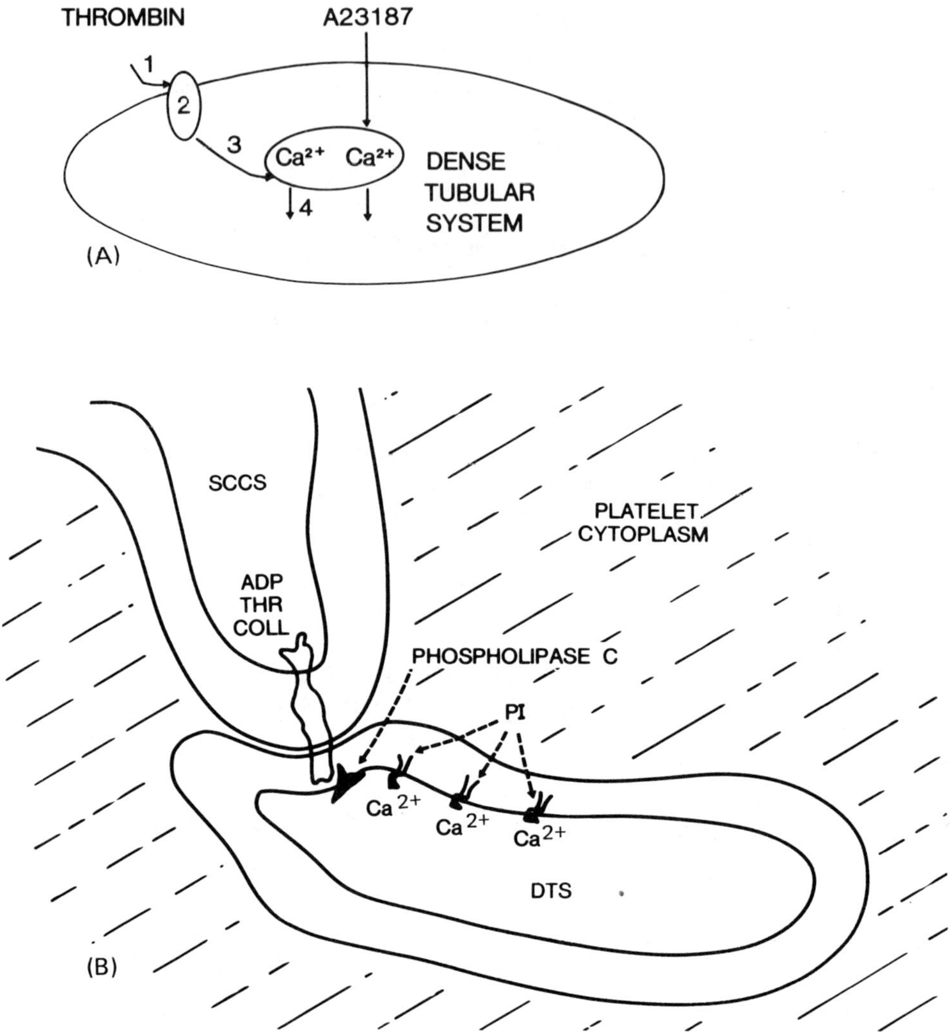

Fig. 6-3 Two mechanisms for linking receptor coupled cell stimulation to an efflux of calcium from the dense tubular system have been suggested. In A, thrombin binds on the inner surface of the plasma membrane (2), giving rise to a messenger (3) which causes release of calcium from the dense tubular system (4). The calcium ionophore, A23187, can bypass the receptor-coupled steps and directly release calcium. An alternate possibility, shown in B, is that thrombin (THR) collagen (COLL) and ADP interact with a protein inside the surface connected canalicular system which is directly coupled to activation of proteins such as a phospholipase C inside the dense tubular system which hydrolyses phosphoinositides (PI) and releases calcium (121).

VI. STIMULATION OF THE RELEASE OF ARACHIDONIC ACID FROM PLATELET MEMBRANE PHOSPHOLIPIDS

A. Phospholipase C-Diglyceride Lipase Pathway

Platelet phospholipase C can act on phosphatidylinositol, phosphatidylinositol-4-phosphate, and phosphatidylinositol-4,5-bisphosphate (85). The principal substrate in the intact platelet is unknown; however, at least phosphatidylinositol-4,5-bisphosphate is cleaved (86). In disrupted platelets, phospholipase C is a soluble enzyme, and is generally presumed to be cytoplasmic; but it may be loosely bound to the plasma-membrane (Fig. 6-3A) and could possibly be within the dense tubular system (Fig. 6-3B). It requires micromolar calcium for activity.

Diglyceride, the initial product, is predominantly converted to phosphatidic acid, but some is acted on by diglyceride lipase located in the dense tubular system which first cleaves the one-position fatty acid (almost exclusively stearic acid) and then the enzyme, or an associated monoglyceride lipase cleaves the two-position fatty acid (almost exclusively arachidonic acid) (87,88). Inhibition of the diglyceride lipase enzyme prevents thrombin-stimulated formation of monoglyceride, but appears not to significantly inhibit the amount of arachidonic acid released, presumably because most arachidonic acid is released by the phospholipase A_2 pathway (89,90a), although evidence for an opposite view has been presented (90b,c).

B. The Phospholipase A_2 Pathway

Platelets contain a phospholipase A_2 which can hydrolyze phosphatidylethanolamine, phosphatidylcholine, and phosphatidylinositol to liberate the fatty acid in the two-position. Initial concern that there is insufficient phospholipase A_2 activity in platelets has recently been mitigated by the findings of a lipid inhibitor which gave erroneously low values in earlier studies (91). In intact platelets, loss of arachidonic acid through the phospholipase A_2 pathway occurs primarily from phosphatidylcholine (92,93). Furthermore, while the isolated enzyme cleaves all two-position fatty acids, only arachidonic acid is lost from phosphatidylcholine in intact cells. Thus, the phospholipid specificity in intact cells most likely results from the intracellular location of phosphatidylcholine containing arachidonic acid being adjacent to the enzyme within the dense tubular system. A phospholipase A_2 specific for phosphatidic acid has been described in horse platelets, but its presence and role in human platelets is still uncertain (see Ch. 4).

VII. STUDIES WITH INHIBITORS

A. Prostaglandin Synthase Inhibitors

1. General Effects on Aggregation and Secretion

Aspirin and other cyclooxygenase inhibitors have been used to define the role of prostaglandin endoperoxides and thromboxane A_2 in the actions of various agonists on platelets (94-99). Whereas these inhibitors will block most of the effects of arachidonic acid on platelets (Sec. IV.A), other agonists are less affected. With epinephrine as agonist, the second wave of aggregation and associated granule centralization and secretion are blocked by cyclooxygenase inhibitors. With collagen as agonist, at low doses of collagen, aspirin and indomethacin produce a considerable inhibition of aggregation, granule centralization, and secretion. With high doses of collagen, the inhibitory effects of aspirin can be overcome. With ADP as agonist, aspirin inhibits the second wave of platelet aggregation and associated secretion, but has little effect on ADP-stimulated granule centralization. With low-dose thrombin, aspirin can inhibit the second wave of aggregation and the associated secretion. At higher concentrations of thrombin, aspirin has no effect on aggregation or secretion. Aspirin has little effect on thrombin-stimulated granule centralization. With the calcium ionophore A23187 as agonist, aspirin usually has little inhibitory effect (101); however, under some conditions where A23187 produces a second wave of aggregation, aspirin will inhibit this (102). In general, the inhibitory effect of aspirin is greater when platelets are suspended in a medium with low external calcium, and less when platelets are in a medium with physiologic calcium externally. With platelet-activating factor, the role of extracellular calcium is particularly pronounced. With low external calcium, aspirin inhibits secretion and produces significant inhibition of aggregation. With high extracellular calcium, aspirin has little influence on the effect of platelet-activating factor (103,104).

Studies using aspirin and indomethacin to evaluate ADP-induced platelet aggregation under conditions of varying shear stress, suggest that prostaglandin endoperoxides/thromboxane A_2 may be particularly important in vivo for promoting the formation and stability of platelet aggregates under conditions of high shear stress (104a,b).

2. Effects on Calcium Flux, Phosphorylation of Myosin Light Chain, and Granule Centralization

Aspirin inhibits the effects of arachidonic acid, collagen (low concentrations), and epinephrine to cause platelet granule centralization, myosin light-chain phosphorylation, and an increase in cytoplasmic calcium (21,70,100,105, 106). Aspirin does not inhibit the effects of ADP, thrombin, and A23187 to produce granule centralization, myosin light-chain phosphorylation, or a rise in cytoplasmic calcium (70,100,105).

3. Effects on Secretion, 47P Phosphorylation, and Diglyceride Production

Aspirin inhibits the effect of arachidonic acid, ADP, collagen, and epinephrine on secretion and 47P phosphorylation, but does not inhibit the effect of phorbol myristate acetate on 47P phosphorylation or on secretion (21,105).

B. Thromboxane Synthetase Inhibitors

Thomboxane synthetase inhibitors are discussed in Sec. IV.A.1. It is worthwhile noting here that while thromboxane synthetase inhibitors usually have little effect on collagen and epinephrine aggregation, in a proportion of individuals arachidonic acid aggregation will be fully inhibited—"responders" (107). In other individuals, arachidonic acid aggregation is not affected—"nonresponders." The difference between the two appears to result from production of PGD_2 which stimulates platelet adenylate cyclase to raise cell cAMP since responders can be converted to nonresponders with inhibition of adenylate cyclase.

C. Lipoxygenase Pathway Inhibitors

To date, perhaps because of the nonselective nature of most lipoxygenase inhibitors, good evidence using inhibitors for a role of platelet lipoxygenase in platelet function is not available. Studies of Okuma on patients deficient in lipoxygenase activity showed enhanced rather than inhibited aggregation (108). However, Schaffer, also studying patients with similar myeloproliferative disorders and a lipoxygenase deficiency, found deficient patients had prolonged bleeding times (109a). Perhaps the lipoxygenase products are important for platelet adhesion to an injured vessel wall rather than for platelet aggregation.

In one particular situation, individuals on high saturated fatty acid diets, with platelets enriched in the fatty acid-20:3w9, this fatty acid has been shown to be converted to the lipoxygenase product 12-OH-5,8,10-20:3 which can potentiate platelet aggregation. Under conditions where platelets are first incubated with 20:3w9, a lipoxygenase inhibitor will block the associated enhanced platelet response to thrombin (109b).

VIII. OTHER LIPIDS

A. Diglycerides

Oleoyl-acetyl-diglyceride has been shown to cause platelet aggregation (18, 110). Such aggregation, similar to that induced by phorbol myristate acetate, is associated with labilization of platelet granules (20) and with a relatively selective activation of protein kinase C and stimulation of a 47,000-dalton protein phosphorylation. However, the concentration of diglyceride needed for stimulation of platelets is high. It is possible that this reflects poor penetration of the diglyceride into the platelet. Alternately, the local production of diglyceride inside the membrane may be high enough to activate protein kinase C within the cell. A third possibility is that other factors (prostaglandin endoperoxides for example) can activate protein kinase C in addition to the diglyceride.

B. Phosphatidic Acid/Lysophosphatidic Acid

Lysophosphatidic acid added to platelets can cause platelet aggregation in relatively low doses (0.1-1.0 μM) (111). Such activation appears to proceed primarily through stimulation of calcium flux and activation of phosphorylation of platelet proteins (112,113). Breakdown of phosphatidylinositol is largely bypassed (20). It is not clear at present whether sufficient lyosphosphatidic acid is produced early in response to agonists such as thrombin, or whether the lysophosphatidic acid is just acting to mimic the action of phosphatidic acid within platelets.

C. Platelet-Activating Factor (PAF)

PAF aggregates platelets, appearing to work by stimulating breakdown of phosphatidylinositol (102,103). PAF production by human platelets is very small and may not be sufficient to have a significant effect (113). At present,

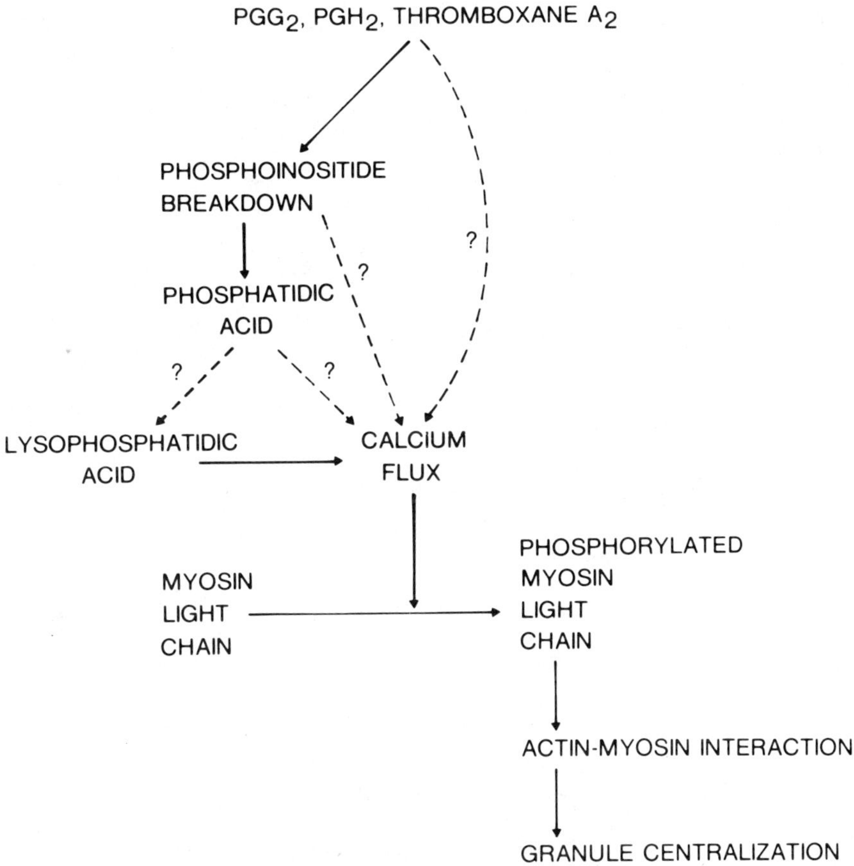

Fig. 6-4 The sequence of events involved in the centralization of platelet granules. The precise mechanism whereby PGG_2, PGH_2, and thromboxane A_2 promote a rise in cytoplasmic calcium levels is not yet clear.

though there has been much speculation that PAF production might be a mechanism through which thrombin acts, this is unlikely in human platelets.

IX. OVERVIEW

Prostaglandin endoperoxides and thromboxane A_2 have an important and fundamental role in platelet function which can be summarized as follows.

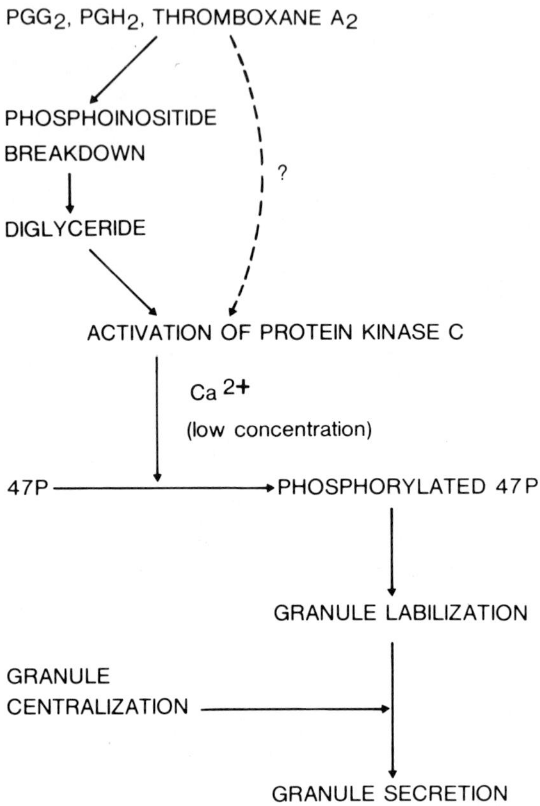

Fig. 6-5 The influence of PGG_2, PGH_2, and thromboxane A_2 on granule labilization appears to occur through activation of protein kinase C and 47P phosphorylation.

1. Prostaglandin endoperoxides and thromboxane A_2 stimulate platelet granule centralization. The sequence of events appears to need calcium flux initiating phosphorylation of myosin light chain (Fig. 6-4). The mechanism of thromboxane A_2-induced stimulation of calcium flux whether direct or indirect (via phosphoinositide breakdown) is uncertain.

2. Prostaglandin endoperoxides and thromboxane A_2 stimulate granule labilization, one of the essential steps in granule secretion (Fig. 6-5). The biochemical sequence appears to require phosphorylation of 47P. The mechanism of thromboxane A_2-induced phosphorylation of 47P whether

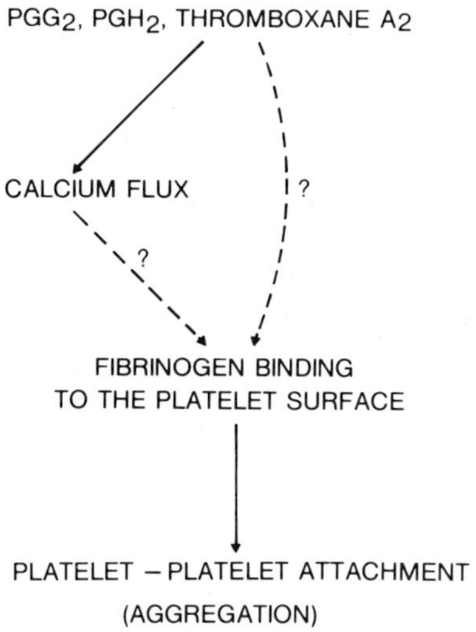

Fig. 6-6 Although, PGG_2, PGH_2, and thromboxane A_2 will stimulate fibrinogen binding to the platelet surface followed by aggregation, the mechanism for this is uncertain.

direct activation of protein kinase C or indirect (via phosphoinositide breakdown and diglyceride production) is currently uncertain.

3. Prostaglandin endoperoxides and thromboxane A_2 stimulate platelet aggregation. The sequence of events appears to require fibrinogen binding, and could be secondary to a rise in cytoplasmic calcium (Fig. 6-6).

4. All the above three effects can be produced independent of secreted ADP.

5. The role of endogenous thromboxane production in platelet function varies with the agonist used. Two examples are shown in Figs. 6-7 and 6-8. For epinephrine, thromboxane production is necessary for both granule centralization and granule labilization, with a lesser contribution to aggregation (second wave only). For ADP which can directly stimulate significant aggregation and granule centralization, thromboxane A_2 is required primarily for 47P phosphorylation, granule labilization, and secretion, and makes only a small contribution to aggregation (second wave only) and granule centralization.

For agonists such as collagen, thrombin, and platelet-activating factor which can stimulate significant phosphoinositide breakdown directly,

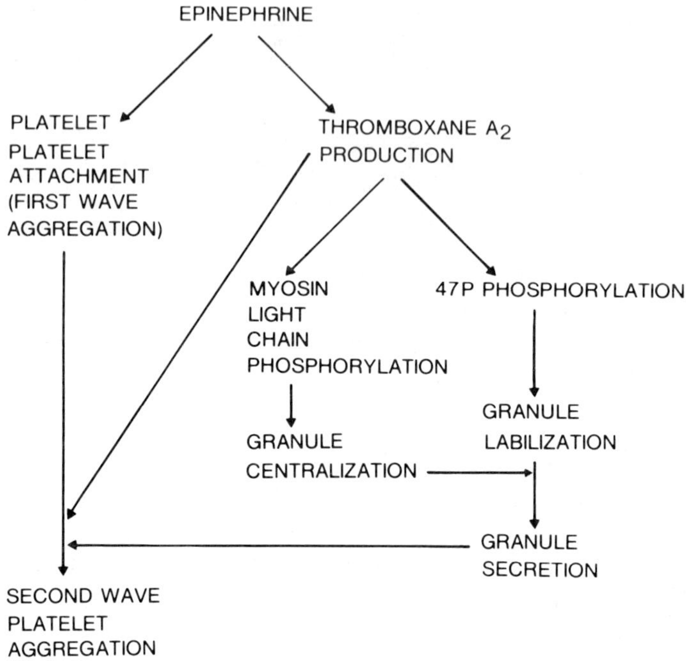

Fig. 6-7 The role of thromboxane A_2 in the effect of epinephrine on platelets.

the role of thromboxane A_2 appears to be an amplifying one. At low agonist concentrations this effect may be very important, while at high agonist concentrations the production of thromboxane A_2 has little impact on the overall effect. In addition, the effect of low concentrations of collagen differs from that of low concentrations of thrombin in that there is not a first wave-second wave pattern to the aggregation response. The primary wave of thrombin could be due to a direct effect of thrombin on calcium flux independent of phospholipase C-induced phosphoinositide breakdown. Alternatively, collagen might induce more phospholipase A_2 activation relative to phospholipase C activity so that thromboxane production is more important for the single-wave collagen response.

6. Platelets have activation pathways independent of thromboxane production. The precise nature of these pathways and the role of nonthromboxane components are not yet established with certainty. Phosphoinositide breakdown as discussed in Ch. 4 appears to be a multifunctional mechanism.

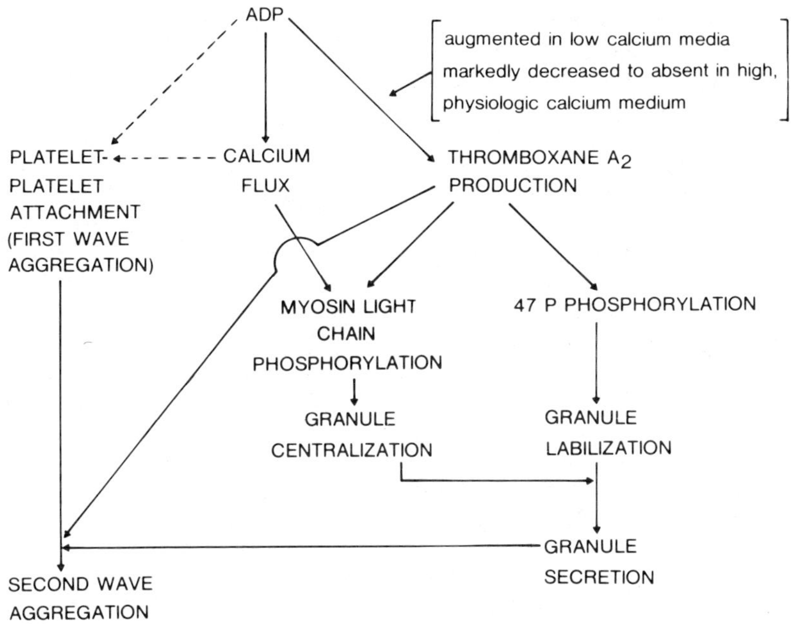

Fig. 6-8 The role of thromboxane A_2 in the effect of ADP on platelets. It should be noted that there is still some controversy with regard to the effect of ADP to stimulate myosin light chain phosphorylation in the absence of thromboxane A_2, even though an ADP initiated calcium flux and granule centralization has been adequately confirmed. It is possible that under some conditions ADP can aggregate platelets without stimulating significant Ca^{2+} flux, myosin phosphorylation and granule centralization.

Release of membrane-bound calcium and proteins when phosphoinositides are broken down and production of diglycerides, inositol tris phosphate, phosphatidic acid, and lysophosphatidic acid may all contribute to the thromboxane-independent component of platelet activation.

APPENDIX 6-1 IMPORTANT SPECIES DIFFERENCES

Phospholipase A_2: Dog platelets have little or no phospholipase A_2, whereas rat platelets have a significant amount (114). These differences could relate to the presence of an inhibitor in dog platelets similar to that recently described in human platelets (115).

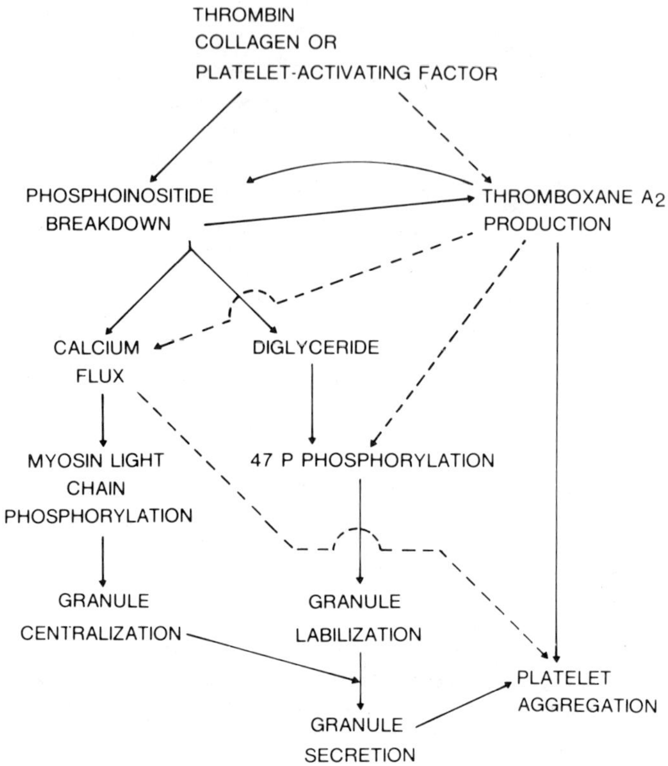

Fig. 6-9 The role of thromboxane A_2 in collagen, thrombin, and platelet-activating factor-induced aggregation.

Arachidonic Acid Aggregation: Platelets from many dogs (about 70%) will not aggregate irreversibly with arachidonic acid in spite of adequate conversion to thromboxane A_2 (116-118). The defect in these nonresponder dogs is not explained, although micromolar concentrations of epinephrine will convert this to an arachidonic acid-responsive state (118).

Platelets from rats, like nonresponder dogs, will not aggregate on addition of prostaglandin endoperoxides in spite of adequate conversion to thromboxane A_2 (119a).

Eicosapentaenoic acid: Rat and rabbit platelets do not convert eicosapentaenoic acid to lipoxygenase or cyclooxygenase products, while human platelets do (33,35).

Prostaglandin D_2: PGD_2 is a potent inhibitor of human, monkey, horse, and sheep platelets, but is only weakly inhibitory toward rabbit, dog, and pig platelets, and is inactive on rat platelets and chicken thrombocytes (81,119b, 119c).

Lysophosphatidic Acid: Platelets from dogs and rabbits will not aggregate with lysophosphatidic acid, unless they have been previously exposed to ADP (112,120). Rat and pig platelets similarly are unresponsive to lysophosphatidic acid, while cat and human platelets respond well to this agent (120).

PAF (AGEPC): Rabbit platelets are extremely responsive to PAF (10^{-10} M). Human platelets are less responsive (10^{-7} M). Rat platelets are unresponsive (78). Recent studies suggest carefully prepared washed human platelets may respond to somewhat lower concentrations of PAF (79).

REFERENCES

1a. S. Menashi, C. Davis, and N. Crawford. *FEBS. Lett. 140*:298 (1982).
1b. A. J. Marcus, H. L. Ulman, and L. B. Safier. *J. Lipid Res. 10*:108 (1969).
2. P. Cohen and A. Derksen. *Br. J. Haematol. 17*:359 (1969).
3. P. Cohen, M. J. Broekman, A. Verkley, J. W. W. Lisman, and A. Derksen. *J. Clin. Invest. 50*:762 (1971).
4. M. J. Broekman, R. I. Handin, A. Derksen, and P. Cohen. *Blood 47*: 963 (1976).
5. V. Natarajan, M. Zuzarte-Augustin, H. H. O. Schmid, and G. Graff. *Thromb. Res. 30*:119 (1983).
6. H. J. Chap, R. F. A. Zwall, and L. L. M. Van Deenen. *Biochim. Biophys. Acta 467*:146 (1977).
7. B. Perret, H. J. Chap, and L. Douste-Blazy. *Biochim. Biophys. Acta 556*:434 (1979).
8. P. K. Schick, K. B. Kurica, and G. K. Chacko. *J. Clin. Invest. 57*:1221 (1976).
9. S. Rittenhouse-Simmons, F. A. Russell, and D. A. Deykin. *Biochem. Biophys. Res. Commun. 70*:295 (1976).
10. M. Lagarde, M. Guichardant, S. Menashi, and N. Crawford. *J. Biol. Chem. 257*:3100 (1982).
11. J. M. Gerrard, J. G. White, and D. A. Peterson. *Thromb. Hemostas. 42*: 224 (1978).
12. R. C. Carroll, R. G. Butler, P. A. Morris, and J. M. Gerrard. *Cell 30*: 385 (1982).
13. R. C. Carroll and J. M. Gerrard. *Blood 59*:466 (1982).

14. D. R. Hathaway and R. S. Adelstein. *Proc. Natl. Acad. Sci. USA 76*: 1653 (1979).
15. E. A. Lebowitz and R. Cooke. *J. Biol. Chem. 253*:5443 (1974).
16. R. D. Estensen and J. G. White. *Am. J. Pathol. 74*:441 (1974).
17. M. Castagna, Y. Takai, and K. Kaibuchi. *J. Biol. Chem. 257*:7847 (1982).
18. K. Kaibuchi, Y. Takai, M. Sawamura, M. Hoshijima, T. Fujikura, and Y. Nishizuka. *J. Biol. Chem. 258*:6701 (1983).
19. J. M. Gerrard, J. V. Schollmeyer, and J. G. White. *Cell Surface Rev. 7*: 217 (1981).
20. J. M. Gerrard. Unpublished observations.
21. R. J. Haslam and J. A. Lynham. *Biochem. Biophys. Res. Commun. 77*: 714 (1977).
22. R. J. Haslam and J. A. Lynham. *Thromb. Res. 12*:619 (1978).
23. M. Hamberg and B. Samuelsson. *Proc. Natl. Acad. Sci. USA 71*:3400 (1974).
24. M. Hamberg, J. Svensson, and B. Samuelsson. *Biochem. J. 204*:847 (1982).
25. J. M. Gerrard, J. G. White, G. H. R. Rao, and D. W. Townsend. *Am. J. Pathol. 83*:283 (1976).
26. F. Carey, S. Menashi, and N. Crawford. *Biochem. J. 204*:847 (1982).
27. T. K. Bills, J. B. Smith, and M. J. Silver. *Biochim. Biophys. Acta 424*: 303 (1976).
28. J. M. Gerrard, J. D. Peller, T. P. Krick, and J. G. White. *Prostaglandins 14*:39 (1977).
29. T. K. Bills, J. B. Smith, and M. J. Silver. *J. Clin. Invest. 60*:1 (1977).
30. P. Falardeau, M. Hamberg, and B. Samuelsson. *Biochim. Biophys. Acta 441*:193 (1976).
31. U. Diczfalusy, P. Falardeau, and S. Hammarstrom. *FEBS Lett. 84*: 271 (1977).
32. P. Needleman, A. Raz, M. S. Minkes, J. A. Ferrendelli, and H. Sprecher. *Proc. Natl. Acad. Sci. USA 76*:944 (1979).
33. G. Hornstra, E. Haddeman, G. A. A. Kivits, and J. A. Don. *Thromb. Haemostas. 50*:275 (1983).
34. I. Morita, R. Takahashi, Y. Saito, and S. Murota. *J. Biol. Chem. 258*: 10197 (1983).
35. I. Morita, Y. Saito, W. C. Chang, and S. Murota. *Lipids 18*:42 (1983).
36. M. J. Silver, J. B. Smith, C. Ingerman, and J. J. Kocsis. *Prostaglandins 4*:863 (1973).
37. A. W. Sedar, M. J. Silver, J. B. Smith, C. M. Ingerman, and J. J. Kocsis. *Blood 44*:177 (1974).
38. B. B. Vargaftig and P. Zirinis. *Nature* [*New Biol.*] *244*:114 (1973).
39. C. Tsao and C. M. Holly. *Prostaglandins 17*:775 (1979).

40. G. H. R. Rao, J. M. Gerrard, C. J. Witkop, and J. G. White. *Prostaglandins Med.* *6*:459 (1981).
41. M. Cattaneo, R. L. Kinlough-Rathbone, D. W. Perry, A. Chahil, J. D. Vickers, S. C-T Lam, M. A. Packham, and J. F. Mustard. *Blood 60*: 1179 (1982).
42. W. Siess and E. G. Lapetina. *Thromb. Haemostas. 50*:275 (1983).
43. A. L. Willis, K. Comai, D. C. Kuhn, and J. R. Paulsrud. *Prostaglandins 8*:509 (1974).
44. K. C. Srivastava. *Z. Ernaehrungswiss 17*:248 (1978).
45a. P. B. A. Kernoff, A. L. Willis, K. J. Stone, J. A. Davies, and G. P. McNicol. *Br. Med. J. 2*:1441 (1977).
44b. D. E. MacIntyre, R. L. Hoover, M. J. Karnovsky, and E. W. Salzman. *Thromb. Haemostas. 46*:277 (1981).
46. J. Dyerberg and H. O. Bang. *Lancet 1*:152 (1978).
47. J. Dyerberg, H. O. Bang, E. Stoffersen, S. Moncada, and J. R. Vane. *Lancet 2*:117 (1978).
48. R. J. Gryglewski, J. A. Salmon, F. B. Ubatuba, B. C. Weatherly, S. Moncada, and J. R. Vane. *Prostaglandins 18*:453 (1979).
49. J. A. Jakubowski and N. G. Ardle. *Thromb. Res. 16*:205 (1979).
50. J. Dyerberg, K. A. Jorgensen, and T. Arnfred. *Prostaglandins 22*:857 (1981)
51. J. Dyerberg and H. O. Bang. *Lancet 2*:433 (1979).
52. W. Seiss, P. Roth, B. Scherer, I. Kurzmann, B. Bohlig, and P. C. Weber. *Lancet 1*:441 (1980).
53. M. O. Whitaker, A. Wyche, F. Fitzpatrick, H. Sprecher, P. Needleman. *Proc. Natl. Acad. Sci. USA 76*:5919 (1979).
54. P. Needleman, A. Raz, A. Ferrendelli, and M. Minkes. *Proc. Natl. Acad. Sci. USA 74*:1716 (1977).
55. E. J. Hornby and I. F. Skidmore. *Biochem. Pharm. 31*:1158 (1982).
56. V. Berrtele, C. Cerletti, A. Schiepatti, G. diMinno, and G. deGaetano. *Lancet 1*:1057 (1981).
57. J. B. Smith and W. Jubiz. *Prostaglandins 22*:353 (1981).
58. L. J. Grimm, D. R. Knapp, D. Senator, and P. V. Halushka. *Thromb. Res. 24*:307 (1981).
59. J. S. Bennett, G. Vilaire, and J. W. Burch. *J. Clin. Invest. 68*:981 (1981).
60. I. F. Charo, R. D. Feinman, T. C. Detwiler, J. B. Smith, C. M. Ingerman, and M. J. Silver. *Nature 269*:66 (1977).
61. J. M. Gerrard, D. Townsend, S. Stoddard, C. J. Witkop, and J. G. White. *Am. J. Pathol. 86*:99 (1977).
62. M. S. Minkes, H. J. Joist, and P. Needleman. *Thromb. Res. 15*:169 (1979).
63. J. M. Gerrard and J. G. White. *Progr. Hemostas. Thromb. 4*:87 (1978).

64. G. DiMinno, P. Thiagarajan, B. Perussia, J. Martinez, S. Shapiro, G. Trinchieri, and S. Murphy. *Blood 61*:140 (1983).
65. J. W. Burch and R. J. Lamb. *Thromb. Res. 31*:747 (1983).
66. E. M. Huang and T. C. Detwiler. *J. Lab. Clin. Med. 95*:59 (1980).
67. R. L. Kinlough-Rathbone, M. A. Packham, and J. F. Mustard. *Thromb. Res. 11*:567 (1977).
68. J. M. Gerrard and J. G. White. *Am. J. Pathol. 80*:189 (1975).
69. J. M. Gerrard, D. Townsend, S. Stoddard, C. J. Witkop, and J. G. White. *Am. J. Pathol. 86*:99 (1977).
70. J. M. Gerrard and R. C. Carroll. *Prostaglandins 22*:81 (1981).
71. N. E. Owen and G. C. LeBreton. *Fed. Proc. 39*:425 (1980).
72. J. M. Gerrard, A. M. Butler, G. Graff, S. F. Stoddard, and J. G. White. *Prostaglandins Med. 1*:373 (1978).
73. J. R. Mayo, D. D. Miller and D. R. Feller. *Biochem. Pharm. 32*:1952 (1983).
74. J. P. Rybicki, D. L. Venton, and G. C. LeBreton. *Biochim. Biophys. Acta. 751*:66 (1980).
75. J. M. Gerrard, D. A. Peterson, and J. G. White. *Thromb. Haemostas. 40*:224 (1978).
76. W. Siess, F. L. Siegel, and E. G. Lapetina. *J. Biol. Chem. 258*:11236 (1983).
77. J. B. Smith, C. Ingerman, J. J. Kocsis, and M. J. Silver. *J. Clin. Invest. 53*:1468 (1974).
78. J. M. Gerrard and P. Robinson. *Biochim. Biophys. Acta.* (in press).
79. V. Bertele, G. DiMinno, and G. DeGaetano. *Thromb. Res. 18*:543 (1980).
80. D. C. B. Mills and D. E. MacFarlane. *Thromb. Res. 5*:401 (1974).
81. J. B. Smith, M. J. Silver, C. M. Ingerman, and J. J. Kocsis. *Thromb. Res. 5*:291 (1974).
82. A. Raz, M. S. Minkes and P. Needleman. *Biochim. Biophys. Acta. 488*:305 (1977).
83a. R. J. Gryglewski, J. A. Salmon, F. B. Ubatuba, B. C. Weatherly, S. Moncada, and J. R. Vane. *Prostaglandins 18*:453 (1979).
83b. R. Kaser-Glanzmann, E. Gerber, and E. F. Luscher. *Biochim. Biophys. Acta 558*:344 (1979).
83c. M. B. Feinstein, J. J. Egan, R. I. Sha'afi, and J. White. *Biochem. Biophys. Res. Commun. 113*:598 (1983).
84. P. Needleman, P. S. Kulkarni, and A. Raz. *Science 195*:409 (1977).
85. S. E. Rittenhouse. *Proc. Natl. Acad. Sci. 80*:5417 (1983).
86. B. W. Agranoff, P. Murphy, and E. B. Sequino. *J. Biol. Chem. 258*: 2076 (1983).
87. L. Y. Chau and H. H. Tai. *Biochem. Biophys. Res. Commun. 100*: 1688 (1981).
88. S. M. Prescott and P. W. Majerus. *J. Biol. Chem. 258*:764 (1983).

89. L. Y. Chau and H. H. Tai. *Biochem. Biophys. Res. Commun. 113*: 241 (1983).
90a. J. M. Gerrard, G. Graff, P. C. Dedon, S. E. Kindom, and J. G. White. *Prog. Lipid Res. 20*:575 (1981).
90b. M. Lagarde, E. Verichel, M. Guichardant, and M. Dechevanne. *Biochem. Biophys. Res. Commun. 99*:1398 (1981).
90c. T. M. Bross, S. M. Prescott, and P. W. Majerus. *Biochem. Biophys. Res. Commun. 116*:68 (1983).
91. L. L. Ballou and W. Y. Cheung. *Proc. Natl. Acad. Sci. USA 80*:5203 (1983).
92. M. L. McKean, J. B. Smith, and M. J. Silver. *J. Biol. Chem. 256*:1522, (1981).
93. E. Neufeld and P. W. Majerus. *J. Biol. Chem. 258*:2461 (1983).
94. H. J. Weiss and L. M. Aledort. *Lancet 2*:495 (1967).
95. J. R. O'Brien. *Lancet 1*:204 (1968).
96. J. R. O'Brien. *Lancet 1*:779 (1968).
97. G. Evans, M. A. Packham, E. A. Nishizawa, J. F. Mustard, and E. A. Murphy. *J. Exp. Med. 128*:877 (1968).
98. M. B. Zucker and J. Peterson. *Proc. Soc. Exp. Biol. Med. 127*:547 (1968).
99. J. M. Gerrard and J. G. White. *Am. J. Pathol. 82*:513 (1976).
100. J. G. White, G. H. R. Rao, and J. M. Gerrard. *Am. J. Pathol. 77*:135 (1974).
101. O. Oelz, H. R. Knapp, L. J. Roberts, R. Oelz, B. J. Sweetman, J. A. Oates, and P. W. Reed. *Adv. Prostaglandin Thromboxane Res. 3*:147 (1978).
102. E. G. Lapetina. *J. Biol. Chem. 257*:7314 (1982).
103. S. D. Shukla and D. J. Hanahan. *Biochem. Biophys. Res. Commun. 106*:697 (1982).
104a. T. J. Hallam, T. J. Rink, and A. Sanchez. *J. Physiol. 343*:97P (1983).
104b. W. Yung and M. M. Frojmovic. *Thromb. Res. 28*:379 (1982).
105. R. C. Carroll and J. M. Gerrard. Unpublished results.
106. T. J. Rink, A. Sanchez, and T. J. Hallam. *Nature 305*:317 (1983).
107. J. R. A. Mitchell. *Br. Med. Bull. 39*:289 (1983).
108. M. Okuma and H. Uchino. *Blood 54*:1258 (1979).
109a. A. I. Schaffer. *N. Engl. J. Med 306*:381 (1982).
109b. M. Lagarde, M. Burtin, H. Sprecher, M. Dechevanne, and S. Renaud. *Lipids 18*:219 (1983).
110. A. M. Benton, J. M. Gerrard, T. Michiel, and S. E. Kindom. *Blood 60*: 642 (1983).
111. J. M. Gerrard, S. E. Kindom, D. A. Peterson, J. Peller, K. E. Krantz, and J. G. White. *Am. J. Pathol. 96*:423 (1979).
112. J. M. Gerrard, S. E. Kindom, D. A. Peterson, and J. G. White. *Am. J. Pathol. 97*:531 (1979).
113. I. Alam, J. B. Smith, and M. J. Silver. *Thromb. Res. 30*:71 (1983).

114. C. A. Sutherland and D. Amin. *J. Biol. Chem. 257*:14007 (1982).
115. L. R. Ballou and W. Y. Cheung. *Proc. Natl. Acad. Sci. USA 80*:5203 (1983).
116. M. Chignard and B. B. Vargaftig. *Eur. J. Pharmacol. 38*:7 (1961).
117. M. Chignard and B. B. Vargaftig. *Prostaglandins 14*:222 (1977).
118. G. J. Johnson, L. A. Leis, G. H. R. Rao, and J. G. White. *Thromb. Res. 14*:147 (1979).
119a. C. E. Dutilh, E. Haddeman, G. H. Jouvenaz, F. Ten Hoor, and D. H. Nugeren. *Lipids 14*:241 (1979).
119b. B. J. R. Whittle, S. Moncada and J. R. Vane. *Prostaglandins 16*:363 (1978).
119c. T. Watanabe, T. Shimizu, S. Narumiya and O. Hayaishi. *Arch. Biochem. Biophys. 216*:372 (1982).
120. K. U. Benner, K. A. Schumacher, and H. G. Classen. *Thromb. Diath. Haemorrh. 31*:354 (1974).
121. J. M. Gerrard, D. A. Peterson, and J. G. White. In *Platelets in Biology and Pathology, 2,* J. L. Gordon (ed.). (1981).
122. R. Castillo, L. M. McManus, and R. N. Pinckard. *Fed. Proc. 42*:693 (1983).
123. R. L. Nachman. *Sem. Hematol. 5*:18 (1968).
124. R. L. Bell and P. W. Majerus. *J. Biol. Chem. 255*:1790 (1980).
125. M. J. Broekman, J. W. Ward, and A. J. Marcus. *J. Clin. Invest. 66*:275 (1980).

BIBLIOGRAPHY

J. L. Gordon (ed.). *Platelets In Biology and Pathology. 2*. Elsevier/North Holland, Amsterdam (1981).

J. G. White and J. M. Gerrard. In *The Biology of Inflammation,* G. Weissman (ed.). p. 83 (1980).

7

The Red Blood Cell

The red blood cell, or erythrocyte, is present in the bloodstream as a biconcave disk about 7 μ in diameter (Fig. 7-1). Its primary function is to pick up oxygen in the lung and deliver it to the tissues.

I. ANATOMY OF THE ERYTHROCYTE

Inside the membrane of the erythrocyte the major cellular constituent is hemoglobin, the protein responsible for oxygen transport. In addition, the red cell interior contains structural proteins such as spectrin and actin which are critical for maintaining the cell shape, as well as glycolytic enzymes needed to use glucose to maintain cellular ATP, and enzymes and other factors required to keep the hemoglobin in a reduced (Fe^{2+}) form.

II. THE LIPIDS OF THE ERYTHROCYTE

Phosphatidylcholine is the predominant phospholipid found in human red blood cells (30-36%), with phosphatidylethanolamine (25-29%), sphingomye-

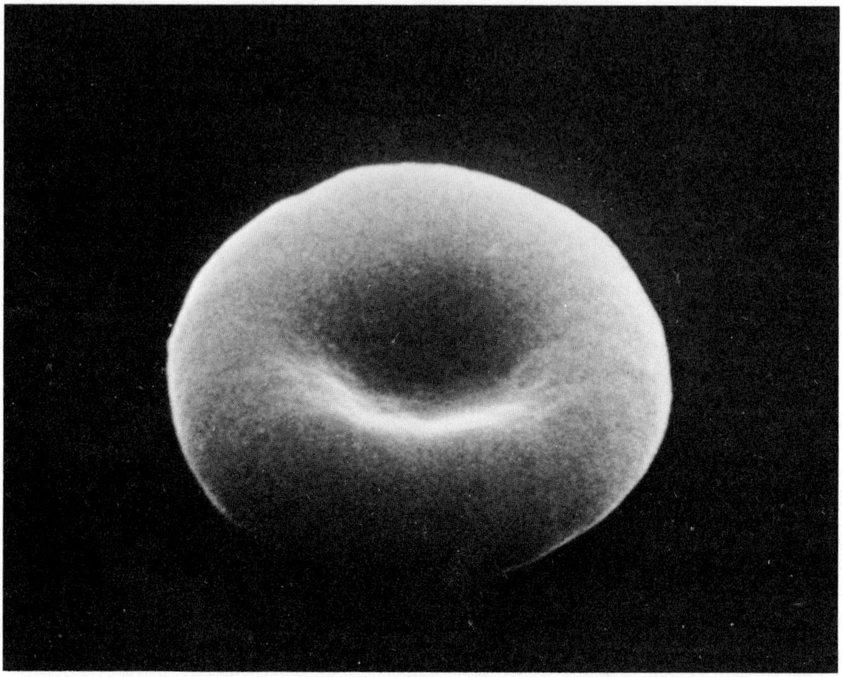

Fig. 7-1 A Scanning electron micrograph of a normal human erythrocyte showing its bioconcave shape. (Photo courtesy of Dr. J. G. White.) (X9,000.)

lin (21-23%), and phosphatidylserine (10-15%) less prominent (1-4). Phosphatidylinositol is only a very small percent (1%). Plasmalogen phospholipids make up about 45% of phosphatidylethanolamine and 3% of phosphatidylcholine. Relative to platelets, arachidonic acid is much lower in erythrocytes, constituting only 5-6% of the fatty acids in phosphatidylcholine (platelets have about 15%), and only 22-25% of the fatty acids in phosphatidylethanolamine (platelets have 32-37%) (1,3,5). The absence of intracellular membranes in red cells has greatly facilitated the study of its plasma membrane. The outer leaflet of the membrane is rich in phosphatidylcholine and sphingomyelin. The inner leaflet is rich in phosphatidylethanolamine and phosphatidylserine, with some phosphatidylchole also present (6,7).

III. FUNCTION OF THE ERYTHROCYTE

The primary function of red cells is oxygen transport. Since prostaglandins do not appear to have significant effects on hemoglobin oxygen uptake and release, the reader is referred elsewhere for a consideration of this aspect of erythrocyte function. In order to transport oxygen to tissues, erythrocytes require a second function, deformability, to allow them to pass through small capillaries.

A. Deformability

Deformability appears to depend on the fluidity of the lipids in the membrane and on the interactions of the structural proteins with the lipid membrane. A role of cellular calcium in deformability change has been implicated.

When eythrocytes exist in conditions of flowing blood, they undergo deformation which depends on the nature of the flow and the size of the blood vessels. In tiny capillaries, deformation may result in the erythrocytes changing from their usual biconcave disk into a sausage shape, with a cylindrical diameter approximately that of the capillary. Such deformation is essential to the normal flow of blood. When red cell deformability is decreased, blood viscosity is significantly increased, and this may be associated with a tendency to thrombosis as well as a shortened cell life span.

IV. SYNTHESIS OF PROSTAGLANDINS AND RELATED CHEMICALS BY RED BLOOD CELLS

Mature red blood cells do not synthesize any prostaglandins. This is consistent with the absence of endoplasmic reticulum, the usual subcellular site of prostaglandin synthesis, in mature red blood cells.

The rabbit reticulocyte, the immediate precursor of the mature erythrocyte, has recently been found to synthesize the hydroperoxy derivative of arachidonic acid, 15-HPETE, and the hydroxy derivative of arachidonic acid, 15-HETE, through the action of a 15-lipoxygenase enzyme. This enzyme was not present in mature rabbit red blood cells (8).

V. ERYTHROCYTE METABOLISM OF PROSTAGLANDINS AND RELATED CHEMICALS

A. PGI_2

Erythrocytes bind and inactivate PGI_2 (9). When red blood cells are present together with platelets, PGI_2 has less of an inhibitory effect on platelet function (10).

B. PGA

When PGA or PGA_2 are incubated with red blood cells, there is a fairly rapid metabolism (half-life about 5 min) of these prostaglandins (11,12). The metabolites formed using PGA_1 have been identified as glutathione conjugates of PGA_1 (13). Other prostaglandins, including PGB_1, PGB_2, PGE_1, and $PGF_{2\alpha}$ are not metabolized to any significant extent by red blood cells. The importance of this reaction is unclear. PGAs are potent vasodepressor chemicals, whereas their metabolites are inactive. However, PGA_2 is not known to be formed in vivo, although this possibility exists.

C. Hydroperoxy Fatty Acids

Hydroperoxy fatty acids are rapidly degraded to a variety of end products in the presence of hemoglobin (14,15).

VI. EFFECTS OF PROSTAGLANDINS AND RELATED CHEMICALS ON RED BLOOD CELLS

A. Prostaglandin Precursors

To date, no effects of physiologic concentrations of arachidonic acid, dihomo-γ-linolenic acid, and eicosapentaenoic acid on red blood cells have been described. High concentrations of fatty acid salts used in medium with a low albumin level will act in a "detergent" fashion to cause lysis of red cells.

B. Prostaglandins

1. Deformability

PGE_2 has been found to decrease erythrocyte deformability when measured at 10^{-9} M (16). The effect of PGE_2 was associated with a redistribution of ATP, a decrease in the cytosol ATP (17), a decrease in cytosol calcium (17), and an increase in the cell water (and cell volume) (18).

Johnston et al. (19) also found that low levels of PGE_2 (10^{-11} M in their studies) decreased erythrocyte deformability in most donors; 10^{-5} and 10^{-7} M PGA_2, 10^{-5}, and 10^{-9} M $PGF_{2\alpha}$, and 10^{-5} and 10^{-7} M $PGF_{1\alpha}$ also decreased deformability in most donors, whereas PGA_1 and PGE_1 at 10^{-5}, 10^{-7}, 10^{-9}, and 10^{-11} M had no effects on red cell deformability in the majority of donors studied. In all their studies, considerable variation was seen in the response of erythrocytes from different individuals or from the same individuals studied at different times.

PGI_2 has been tested at a single dose (1.6×10^{-6} M) and had no effect on erythrocyte filterability (20). The dose used, however, was high, and no firm conclusion can be drawn regarding the effect of PGI_2. The mechanism of these effects of prostaglandins on red blood cells is unknown. Studies using a micropipette method failed to demonstrate any effect of PGE_2 on red cell deformability (21). Studies using a fatty acid spin-label, however, showed results consistent with an effect of 10^{-10} - 10^{-11} M PGE_2 to decrease the order parameter (i.e., make the cell membranes less flexible), and render the cell less deformable (12). Low concentrations of PGE_1 had the opposite effect. External calcium was required for both these actions.

Opposing effects of PGE_2 and PGE_1 have since been found by others. Johnson and Ramwell (quoted in Ref. 12) found that PGE_2 diminished and PGE_1 enhanced the prostaglandin antagonist-(7-oxa-13-prostynoic acid) induced swelling of erythrocytes. Baar found that thermally injured red cells showed decreased deformability and calcium extrusion in response to PGE_2 and the opposite with PGE_1 (23).

Meyers and Swislocki (24), using circular dichroism, provided evidence for effects of PGE_1 and $PGF_{2\alpha}$ on erythrocyte membrane protein conformation, specifically to decrease by 13 and 20%, respectively, the membrane protein helicity. Since these authors found no effect of PGE_2 and since the effective concentration range was much broader in this study than in the studies of deformability, the relation between these findings and the deformability changes are unclear.

The mechanism by which prostaglandins influence erythrocyte deformability is not known. PGE_2 can activate red blood cell adenylate cyclase to raise cellular cAMP (18,25). The fact that human, rat, and mouse red cells show decreased deformability in response to PGE_2, whereas only the rat and mouse cells show an elevation of cAMP, has been put forward to show that these two phenomena are unrelated (18). However, no data were presented, and this point can therefore not be critically evaluated.

The effects of prostaglandins on membrane fluidity and cell deformability might relate to changes in phospholipid methylation (26,27), or to metabolism of the phosphoinositides; however, to date there is no published data to support an action of prostaglandins on either process in erythrocytes.

The significance in vivo of the changes in erythrocyte deformability is not yet certain but could be a consideration in thrombotic disorders. For example, PGE_1 and PGI_2 infused in vivo to subjects with Raynaud's phenomenon and systemic sclerosis were both found to increase red cell deformability as well as provide clinical improvement (28). Effects of prostaglandins on deformability could also potentially relate to the differential effect of PGE_1 and PGE_2 on myocardial infarct size after coronary occlusion (29), but other effects of these prostaglandins are likely more important.

2. Red Blood Cell cAMP

A number of studies have evaluated the influence of PGE_1 on frog erythrocytes. When PGE_1 is added together with isobutylmethylxanthine, an inhibitor of the phosphodiesterase which breaks down cAMP, a significant increase in cellular cAMP is seen, associated with increased phosphorylation of a protein with an apparent molecular weight of 240,000, and an increase in sodium and potassium influx into the cells (30). Time-course studies suggest these latter three processes may be linked with the phosphorylated protein being responsible for the cation influx. PGE_1 has no effect on turkey erythrocyte cAMP or cation flux (30).

Studies of the PGE_1 receptor on frog erythrocytes show that it is closely coupled to adenylate cyclase and that it exists in a high-affinity, slowly dissociable form suggested to represent a "desensitized" conformation, and a lower-affinity, rapidly dissociable "biologically active" form (31). Guanine nucleotides can shift the equilibrium toward the latter active form.

3. Red Cell Storage

Effects of PGE_1 added to red cells which were then stored for 1 week were evaluated. No effects were seen on cell concentrations of 2,3-diphosphoglycerate, adenosine triphosphate, sodium ion, or potassium ion, or on the red cell pH, osmotic fragility, filterability, or the oxyhemoglobin dissociation curve (32).

C. Effects of Inhibitors of Prostaglandin Synthesis on Red Blood Cells

Prostaglandin synthetase inhibitors have not been extensively evaluated for their effects on red blood cells, largely presumably because these cells lack the capacity to synthesize prostaglandins. Abnormalities of erythrocyte electrolyte transport in Bartter's syndrome are not affected by treatment of the patient with cyclooxygenase inhibitors, showing that this abnormality is not secondary to excess prostaglandin production in this disorder (33). Studies using prostaglandin synthesis inhibitors in vivo in an animal model might help to evaluate claims that low concentrations of prostaglandins produced in vivo under some conditions (i.e., burns) (23) have an important effect on red cell deformability, and thus potentially on the predisposition to thrombosis.

VII. EFFECTS OF OTHER ACTIVE LIPIDS ON RED BLOOD CELLS

A. Polyphosphoinositides, Diglyceride, Lysophosphatidic Acid

When erythrocytes from most species are exposed to A23187 in the presence of calcium, the cells change from discocytes to echinocytes and become stiff (34,35). Associated with these changes, a polyphosphoinositide phosphodiesterase (a phospholipase C) cleaves phosphatidylinositol-4,5 bisphosphate to give an increase in membrane diglyceride (36,37). The increased membrane diglyceride was proposed as mediating the echinocyte formation resulting from an increased intracellular calcium (38). More recent studies of Burris et al. have largely disproved this concept (39). Burris added the diglyceride dipalmitin to red blood cells and found no changes in cell shape or stiffness. However, he did not consider the possibility that both diglyceride and raised intracellular calcium might be required (see Ch. 3), and he did not try the unsaturated diglycerides which have been found more effective in other cell types. Nevertheless, Burris studied lamb erythrocytes which did not accumulate diglyceride and yet changed shape when exposed to A23187 and calcium. The latter experiment, at least, rules out diglyceride, even with calcium as the effective lipid in lamb red cells. Either diglyceride has no role in this process, or another lipid can substitute for it.

More recent studies have addressed the possibility that phosphatidylinositol-4-phosphate (40) or lysophosphatidic acid (41) might be involved in these processes. The studies implicate decreased membrane phosphatidylinositol-4-phosphate or increased lysophosphatidic acid as possibly contributing to echinocyte formation. At the present time, these points are not resolved. They are mentioned here because erythrocytes do have very active synthesis of phosphatidylinositol-4,5-bisphosphate and phosphatidylinositol-4-phosphate, and because the breakdown of polyphosphoinositides has in other cell types been linked to cellular activation.

VIII. AN OVERVIEW

At the present time, the importance of prostaglandins to erythrocyte function would appear to be minor. Red blood cells do not synthesize prostaglandins, and they appear to respond relatively weakly and somewhat variably to PGE_2 with an increase in cellular deformability. In spite of considerable investigation in this area in the early 1970s, the role of this effect of PGE_2 in vivo is uncertain.

On the other hand, erythrocytes do have a very active synthesis of polyphosphoinositides. Such synthesis uses considerable cellular ATP and is likely to be important. Breakdown of polyphosphoinositides has been linked to the echinocyte transformation and increased cellular rigidity seen with cells treated with A23187 and calcium; however, to date no hypothesis for the linkage of these events is supported by sufficient experimental data to be convincing, although continued investigation in this area might be rewarding.

Erythrocytes clearly have a role to metabolize and inactivate PGI_2. It is possible that to some extent this serves as a mechanism to limit the potential adverse consequences of release of significant quantities of PGI_2 into the bloodstream.

The newly discovered production of lipoxygenase products by reticulocytes suggests that the role of this product in the bone marrow production of erythrocytes and other blood cells should be investigated.

APPENDIX 7-1 IMPORTANT SPECIES DIFFERENCES

Considerable differences in the phospholipid composition of erythrocytes exist from one species to another. Sheep, cow, ox, and goat erythrocytes have little or no phosphatidylcholine and a very high level of sphingomyelin (42, 43).

PGE_1 and/or PGE_2 stimulate erythrocyte adenylate cyclase in rat, mouse, and frog red blood cells, but not in those from humans or turkeys (18,25,30).

REFERENCES

1. P. Cohen and A. Derksen. *Br. J. Haematol. 17*:359 (1969).
2. C. F. Reed, S. N. Swisher, G. V. Marinetti, and E. G. Eden. *J. Lab. Clin. Med. 45*:281 (1960).
3. J. W. Farquhar. *Biochim. Biophys. Acta 60*:80 (1962).
4. J. T. Dodge and C. B. Phillips. *J. Lipid Res. 8*:667 (1967).
5. A. J. Marcus, H. L. Ullman, and L. B. Safier. *J. Lipid Res. 10*:108 (1969).
6. R. F. A. Zwaal, B. Roelofson, and C. M. Colley. *Biochim. Biophys. Acta 300*:159 (1973).
7. A. J. Verkleij, R. F. A. Zwaal, B. Roelofsen, P. Comfurius, D. Kastelijn, and L. L. M. Van Deenen. *Biochim. Biophys. Acta 323*:178 (1973).
8. R. W. Bryant, J. M. Bailey, T. Schewe, and S. M. Rapoport. *J. Biol. Chem. 257*:6050 (1982).
9. C. Willems, H. V. Stel, W. Van Aken, and. J. A. Van Mourik. *Br. J. Haematol. 54*:43 (1983).
10. J. A. Jakubowski, C. B. Thompson, and D. Deykin. *Br. J. Haematol. 54*: 659 (1983).
11. M. S. Golub, P. K. Zia, and R. Horton. *Prostaglandins 8*:13 (1974).
12. J. B. Smith, M. J. Silver, C. M. Ingerman, and J. J. Kocsis. *Prostaglandins 9*:135 (1975).
13. L. M. Cagen, H. M. Fales, and J. J. Pisano. *J. Biol. Chem. 251*:6550, (1976).
14. M. Hamberg. *Lipids 10*:87 (1975).
15. R. W. Bryant and J. M. Bailey. *Progr. Lipid. Res. 20*:279 (1981).
16. J. E. Allen and H. Rasmussen. *Science 174*:512 (1971).
17. J. E. Allen and H. Rasmussen. In *Prostaglandins in Cellular Biology*, P. W. Ramwell and B. B. Pharriss (eds.). Plenum Press, New York (1972).

18. J. E. Allen and R. Valeri. *Arch. Intern. Med. 133*:86 (1974).
19. C. C. Johnston, S. L. Dowers, and R. J. Urbanski. *Prostaglandins 13*: 281 (1977).
20. J. H. Slott, K. Hall, D. A. Clark, and M. J. Stuart. *Prost. Leuk. Med. 8*: 21 (1982).
21. A. W. L. Jay, S. Rowlands, and L. Skibo. *Prostaglandins 3*:871 (1973).
22. P. G. Kury, P. G. Ramwell, and H. M. McConnell. *Biochem. Biophys. Res. Commun. 56*:478 (1974).
23. S. Baar. *Br. J. Exp. Pathol. 63*:644 (1982).
24. M. B. Meyers and N. I. Swislocki. *Arch. Biochem. Biophys. 164*:544 (1974).
25. H. Sheppard and C. R. Burghardt. *Mol. Pharmacol. 6*:425 (1970).
26. B. V. R. Sastry, C. N. Statham, R. G. Meeks, and J. Axelrod. *J. Pharmacol. 23*:211 (1981).
27. J. Hirata and J. Axelrod. *Science 209*:1082 (1980).
28. P. M. Dowd, I. B. Kovacs, C. J. H. Bland, and J. D. T. Kirby. *Br. Med. J. 283*:350 (1981).
29. B. I. Jugdutt, G. M. Hutchins, B. H. Bulkley, and L. C. Becker. *Circ. Res. 49*:685 (1981).
30. S. A. Rudolph and P. Greengard. *J. Biol. Chem. 255*:8534 (1980).
31. R. J. Lefkowitz, D. Mullikin, C. L. Wood, T. B. Gore, and C. Mukherjee. *J. Biol. Chem. 252*:5295 (1977).
32. C. R. Valeri, C. G. Zaroulis, J. C. Rogers, R. I. Handin, and L. D. Marchionni. *Science 175*:539 (1972).
33. C. H. Cole and S. O'Regan. *Pediatr. Res. 15*:926 (1981).
34. J. G. White. *Am. J. Pathol. 77*:507 (1974).
35. J. F. Kuettner, K. L. Dreher, G. H. R. Rao, J. W. Eaton, P. W. Blackshear, and J. G. White. *Am. J. Pathol. 88*:81 (1977).
36. U. B. Seiffert and B. W. Agranoff. *Biochim. Biophys. Acta 98*:574 (1965).
37. D. Allan and R. H. Michell. *Biochim. Biophys. Acta 508*:277 (1978).
38. D. Allan and R. H. Michell. *Nature 258*:348 (1975).
39. S. M. Burris, J. W. Eaton, and J. G. White. *J. Lab. Clin. Med. 96*:749 (1980).
40. E. E. Quist and K. L. Reece. *Biochem. Biophys. Res. Commun. 95*: 1023 (1980).
41. S. M. Burris, J. M. Gerrard, J. G. White, and C. C. Clawson. *Fed. Proc. 39*:740 (1980).
42. J. DeGier and L. L. M. Van Deenan. *Biochim. Biophys. Acta 49*:286 (1961).
43. G. L. Nelson. *Biochim. Biophys. Acta 144*:221 (1967).

8
Neutrophils

The neutrophil circulates in the bloodstream as a spherical smooth-surfaced blood cell (Fig. 8-1). The primary function of the neutrophil is to seek out sites of infection and to phagocytose and kill bacteria.

I. ANATOMY OF THE RESTING NEUTROPHIL

In the approximate geometric center of the neutrophil is the centrosome (two centrioles with microtubules radiating outward, and the golgi complex). The lobes of the nucleus (most commonly three, but varying from one to five or more) are arrayed in a circle around the centrosome. The centrosome is the most rigid part of the cell, suggesting an important cytoskeletal or organizing function. Scattered in the periphery of the neutrophil cytoplasm are azurophilic (primary) granules (specialized lysosomes containing lysozyme, myeloperoxidase, sulfated glycoconjugates, and phospholipids, in addition to a variety of hydrolytic enzymes including acid phosphatase and elastase) and specific (secondary) granules. Lactoferrin, for some time believed to be in specific granules, has now been localized to a subpopulation of primary granules (1a). Neutrophils rely primarily on glycolysis and have much glyco-

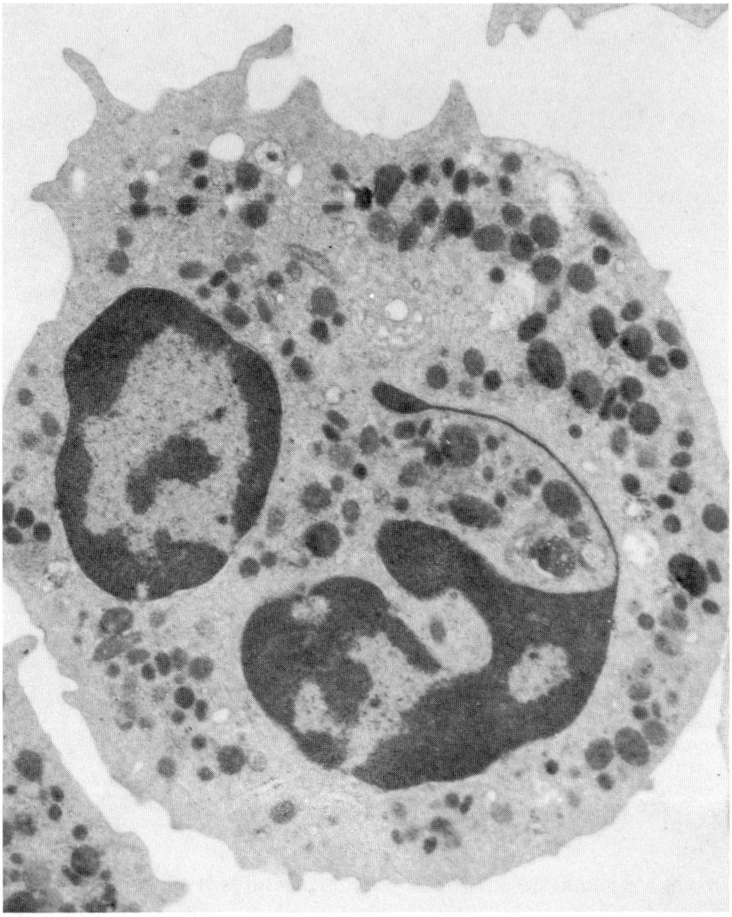

Fig. 8-1 A neutrophil showing two nuclear lobes, central golgi region, and many periphally located granules. (×11,300.)

gen and few mitochondria. A small and limited amount of smooth and rough endoplasmic reticulum is present.

II. THE LIPIDS OF THE RESTING NEUTROPHIL

The reported proportion of phospholipid as phosphatidylcholine has varied from 32-40%, that of phosphatidylethanolamine 32-34%, sphingomyelin

9-13%, phosphatidylserine 10-11%, and phosphatidylinositol 6-8% (1b-3). Compared with other blood cells, phosphatidylethanolamine is slightly higher. Neutrophils contain a relatively lower proportion (12-14%) of the total lipid fatty acid species as arachidonic acid compared with other blood cells (2,4,5). The membranes of phagocytic vesicles have less arachidonic acid than the rest of the cell and are enriched in saturated fatty acids (4,5). Membranes with an increased saturated fatty acid content are more rigid and less permeable to water-soluble substances. The increased saturated fatty acid content of phagocytic vesicles is thus likely a mechanism to protect the cell from exposure to noxious chemicals dumped from lysosomes into the phagocytic vesicles. In addition, there is considerable potential for lipid peroxidation during phagocytosis. Having membranes with a high saturated fatty acid content will decrease the potential for cell damage due to peroxidation. An alternative view of the reason for the low arachidonic acid in these membranes is that this fatty acid is selectively utilized during phagocytosis.

III. FUNCTIONS OF THE NEUTROPHIL

Neutrophils show directed movement toward certain stimuli (chemotaxis), they ingest bacteria and other particles (phagocytosis), and they fuse their lysosomes with phagocytic vesicles to expose any ingested bacteria to injurious enzymes and chemicals (killing).

A. Chemotaxis

Neutrophils sense the presence of a gradient of certain chemicals and move toward the highest concentration of the chemical. Receptors for the chemotactic chemicals C5a, CCF (an 8,400-dalton neutrophil granule glycoprotein), and N-formylated chemotactic peptides (i.e., Formyl-methionine-leucine-phenylalanine or FMLP) have been described. Following exposure of the neutrophil to a chemoattractant, and interaction of the chemicals with the cellular receptors, the neutrophil flows along a surface in the direction of the highest chemical concentration. Membrane-receptor interaction, stimulus-transmission coupling, and lipid protein and calcium changes at the leading edge, the protopod (Fig. 8-2), appear critical in the cellular chemotactic response. Arachidonic acid metabolites appear to play an important role in this process.

Similarities in the stimuli which cause aggregation of neutrophils and those which initiate chemotaxis suggest the biochemical responses involved in these two processes are similar.

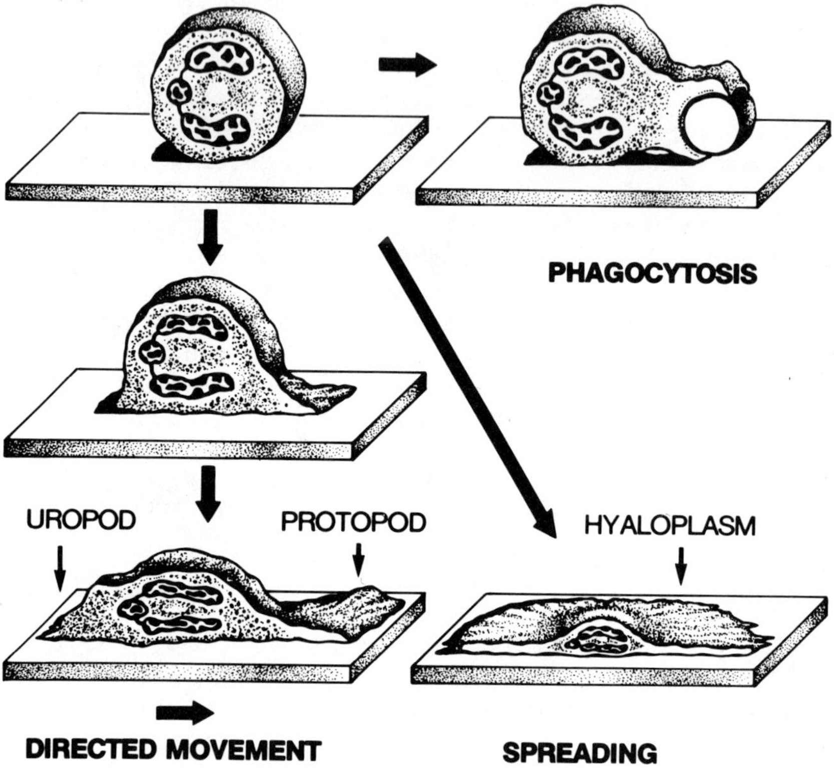

Fig. 8-2 Directed movement, spreading, and phagocytosis are important functions of neutrophils.

B. Phagocytosis

Phagocytosis involves the attachment of the neutrophil surface membrane to the particle, followed by a flowing of the cell membrane around the particle or bacterium to engulf it (Fig. 8-2). Spreading of a neutrophil on a glass slide may be somewhat analagous in that it may represent the attempt of a neutrophil to phagocytose an object bigger than itself. Opsonic activity (IgG antibodies, or C3b fixed to the bacteria or particle to be phagocytosed) is important for the initial adherence of the neutrophil to the particle. Membrane fluidity and intracellular contractile proteins are also important for phagocytosis.

C. Degranulation and Killing

After ingestion of a bacterium and formation of a phagocytic vesicle, intracellular granules fuse with the membrane of the phagosome and dump their contents into it. Specific granules fuse first (starting about 30 sec after ingestion), followed by azurophilic granules (starting at about 3 min after ingestion) (6). Lipid alterations in the membrane are probably critical to such membrane fusion. Killing of bacteria results from the actions of enzymes within the neutrophil granules and the generation of toxic oxygen-derived radicals. There are a multiplicity of potential "killing" mechanisms, perhaps, in part, the variety of such mechanisms is needed to attack the many different organisms which neutrophils may encounter.

IV. SYNTHESIS OF PROSTAGLANDINS AND RELATED CHEMICALS IN NEUTROPHILS

A. Arachidonic Acid Metabolism

The major pathway of arachidonic acid metabolism in neutrophils is via a lipoxygenase enzyme. When labeled arachidonic acid is added to human peripheral blood neutrophils, the major product is 5-HETE (7). 15-HETE is also found, but it may be produced primarily by contaminating eosinophils. When A23187 is added together with arachidonic acid, conversion of the arachidonic acid is enhanced (8), and significant amounts of leukotrienes, particularly leukotriene B_4, are produced (Table 8-1). Small amounts of a variety of other lipoxygenase products have also been detected. (Fig. 8-3) (9).

Table 8-1 Conversion of Arachidonic Acid by Human Peripheral Blood Neutrophils in the Presence of A23187

	Percent of added arachidonic acid in each product				
Reference	5-HETE	15-HETE	LTB_4	PGE_2	TxB_2
7	10	2.4	1.4	*	*
8	7	*	*	4.0	0.6

*Not assayed or not identified with certainty. The proportion of TxB_2 produced by contaminating platelets was subtracted to give the 0.6% TxB_2 shown.

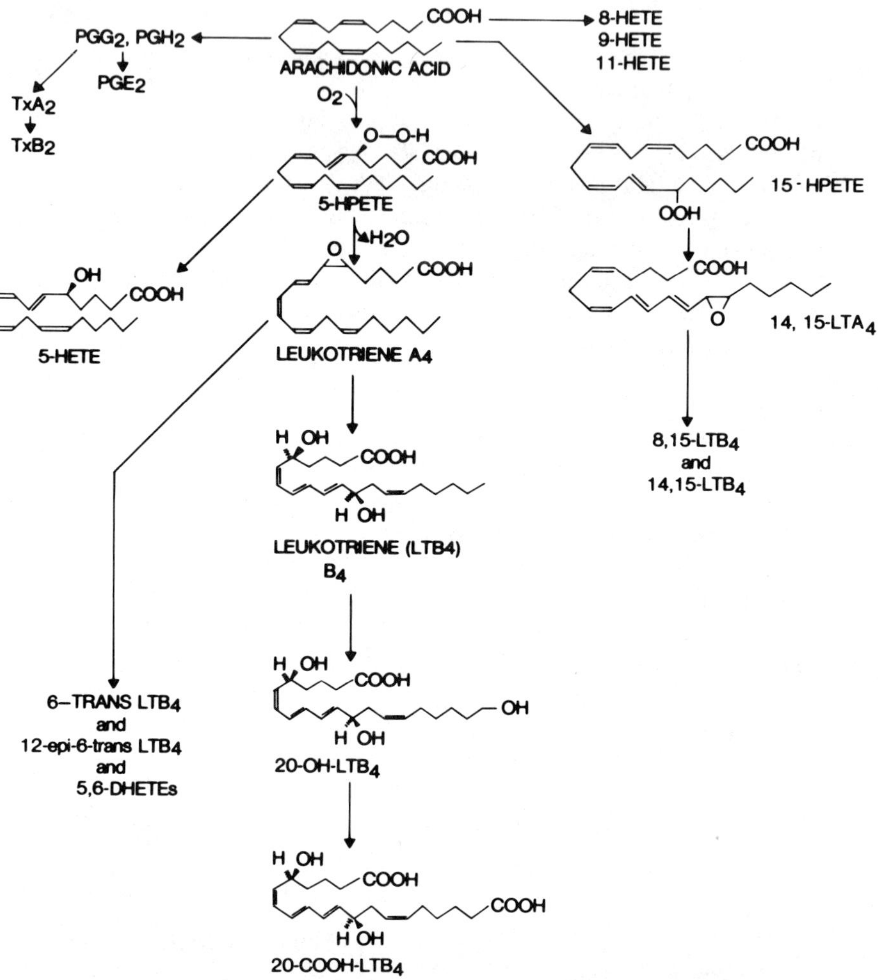

Fig. 8-3 The principal metabolites of arachidonic acid in human neutrophils. The compound of most importance is leukotreine B_4 (LTB_4). The 15-lipoxygenase occurs predominantly in eosinophils, and it is possible that eosinophil contamination of the neutrophil preparations is responsible for reports of its synthesis in neutrophils.

Conversion of arachidonic acid by the prostaglandin endoperoxide synthase enzyme does occur but is less prominent. PGE_2 is the major end product of this pathway, with some thromboxane A_2 also being formed (8).

In the absence of exogenous arachidonic acid, human neutrophils will respond to stimuli such as serum-treated zymosan by the release of arachidonic acid from phospholipids (10) and the formation of both lipoxygenase and cyclooxygenase products (11-13a). The calcium ionophore A23187 can also serve as a significant stimulus, with 5-HETE and leukotriene B_4 (LTB_4) being the major products resulting (7).

In the presence of thrombin or collagen-stimulated platelets, neutrophils will convert platelet-derived 12-HETE to 12,20-DiHETE (12S,20-dihydroxyeicosatetraenoic acid) (13b).

B. Dihomo-γ-Linolenic Acid

Dihomo-γ-linolenic acid is converted by neutrophils primarily to 8-D-hydroxy-9,11,14-eicosatrienoic acid (14). Lesser amounts of the lipoxygenase products 8,15-leukotriene B_3, 14,15-leukotriene B_3 and the cycloxygenase products PGE_1, $PGF_{1\alpha}$, and thromboxane B_1 are produced (14b).

V. THE INFLUENCE OF PROSTAGLANDINS AND RELATED CHEMICALS ON NEUTROPHIL FUNCTION

A. The Influence of Prostaglandin Precursors on Neutrophil Function

1. Arachidonic Acid

Arachidonic acid stimulates neutrophil chemotaxis (15), degranulation (16, 17), and calcium flux (rabbit peritoneal neutrophils) (14,15), as well as metabolic activity and chemiluminescence (canine neutrophils) (16). These effects of arachidonic acid (excluding chemiluminescence which is blocked by cyclooxygenase inhibitors can be blocked by inhibitors of the lipoxygenase, consistent with a neutrophil lipoxygenase metabolite being a mediator of these effects (15-19). While these data are impressive, it is the experience of the author that considerable caution should be exercised when using arachidonic acid on neutrophils in buffers with low albumin levels because cell damage can be produced by the arachidonic acid as well as physiologic effects. In the above studies, appropriate caution with regard to cell injury has not always been taken.

2. Eicosapentaenoic Acid and Dihomo-γ-Linolenic Acid

Eicosapentaenoic acid and oxidized products were found to be chemotactic similar to arachidonic acid (15). A diet enriched in eicosapentaenoic acid does not lead to impaired neutrophil function, consistent with eicosapentaenoic acid metabolites being as effective as those of arachidonic acid (20). A full analysis of eicosapentaenoic acid and dihomo-γ-linolenic acid and their effects on neutrophils is not currently available.

B. Endogenous Arachidonic Acid Metabolites

1. Leukotriene B_4 (LTB_4)

LTB_4 is the most potent of the neutrophil-derived arachidonic acid metabolites, producing chemotaxis at picomolar concentrations, with a maximal effect at 0.02-0.1 μM (21,22). LTB_4 is also potent in stimulating aggregation, degranulation, and superoxide generation in neutrophils which have been preincubated with cytochalasin B (23-25). In the absence of cytochalasin B, effects of LTB_4 on aggregation and degranulation are limited. These effects are very similar to those of the calcium ionophore A23187 (26). Evidence that LTB_4 can act as a calcium ionophore in transporting calcium across liposome bilayers (27) and can stimulate a flux of calcium to raise the neutrophil cytoplasmic calcium level (28) is consistent with a role of LTB_4 as a calcium ionophore. Other evidence suggests LTB_4 acts in a more complex, perhaps calcium-related, receptor-mediated mechanism (29-32).

2. Mono-HETEs

Hydroxy derivatives of arachidonic acid with one hydroxy group (mono-HETEs) stimulate the chemotaxis of human neutrophils. The rank order of potency is 5-HETE > 8-HETE = 9-HETE > 11-HETE = 12-HETE > 15-HETE (33,34). The activity of these compounds is much less than that of LTB_4, and thus the contribution of the endogenous production of mono-HETEs is probably less than that of LTB_4. However, 5-HETE does potentiate the granule secretion stimulated by platelet-activating factor, LTB_4, and phorbol myristate acetate (though not that produced by C5a or A23187) (33,34). Thus, 5-HETE could be one of several products contributing to the full neutrophil response.

3. Prostaglandin E_2

PGE_2 has been shown to suppress aggregation, granule secretion, and LTB_4 production by neutrophils in response to FMLP (37a,b), probably by elevating cellular cAMP. The relative effect of other prostaglandins $PGE_2 \simeq PGE_1 > PGA_1 \simeq PGA_2 > PGF_{2\alpha} > PGD_2$ suggests neutrophils have a PGE_2 receptor (37). Reports of the effects of PGE_2 on neutrophil chemotaxis range from promotion in the presence of albumin (38) to inhibition (39).

4. Thromboxane A_2

Thromboxane A_2 increases neutrophil adhesiveness (40). Thromboxane B_2, the stable metabolite of thromboxane A_2, is chemotactic for neutrophils (41). 13-Azaprostanoic acid, a thromboxane A_2 receptor antagonist, partially inhibits neutrophil secretion of lysosomal enzymes in response to zymosan (42).

C. Exogenously Derived Arachidonic Acid Metabolites

1. Prostaglandin E_1

PGE_1 raises neutrophil cAMP levels and inhibits superoxide and LTB_4 production, aggregation, and lysosomal enzyme release from stimulated human neutrophils (37a,b,41,43,44).

2. Prostaglandin I_2

PGI_2 has been shown to inhibit neutrophil adhesiveness to endothelial cells and nylon fibers (45,46), and to inhibit chemotaxis, aggregation, secretion (43,47) and neutrophil synthesis of LTB_4 in response to serum-treated zymosan (48). A PGI_2 analogue has also been shown to inhibit FMLP stimulation of neutrophil LTB_4 production (37). These inhibitory effects of PGI_2, like those of PGE_1 and PGE_2, are probably mediated through an elevation of neutrophil cAMP. A recent study has questioned data showing PGI_2 inhibition of neutrophil adherence to endothelial cells, and suggests that PGI_2-

mediated inhibition is an indirect effect, perhaps the result of PGI_2 inhibiting platelet thromboxane A_2 production (48b).

3. Leukotriene C_4 and D_4

LTC_4 and LTD_4 both enhance the adherence of human neutrophils to Sephadex G-25 (48c). Concomitantly, neutrophil thromboxane B_2 production is increased. The effects of LTC_4 and LTD_4 on neutrophil adherence are inhibited by indomethacin, consistent with a role for thromboxane A_2 (see above) mediating this response.

4. 12-Hydroperoxyeicosatetraenoic Acid (12-HPETE)

12-HPETE, synthesized by platelets, can stimulate neutrophil production of 5-HETE, LTB_4, and 5,12-diHETE (48d).

VI. THE ROLE OF ARACHIDONIC ACID METABOLITES AS MEDIATORS OF THE RESPONSE OF NEUTROPHILS TO AGONISTS OTHER THAN ARACHIDONIC ACID

A. The Release of Arachidonic Acid and Synthesis of Metabolites in Response to Neutrophil Agonists

Neutrophils stimulated by A23187 and serum-treated zymosan clearly release arachidonic acid from their phospholipids and synthesize 5-HETE and LTB_4 (49-51). Results using neutrophils stimulated by FMLP have been variable, with some investigators reporting production of 5-HETE and LTB_4 (37,52-54) and others not (51,55). It is possible that the source of neutrophils and the conditions used for the study may have some impact on the results. Palmer and Salmon, measuring LTB_4 using a radioimmunoassay, suggest that FMLP may not cause synthesis of LTB_4 without externally added arachidonic acid being present (51).

B. The Influence of Inhibitors of Prostaglandin and Leukotriene Synthesis on Neutrophil Function

As outlined earlier (Sec. V), inhibitors of the lipoxygenase enzyme block neutrophil synthesis of leukotrienes and most of the effects of arachidonic acid on neutrophils. However, results with lipoxygenase enzyme inhibitors on the effects of A23187, FMLP, and serum-treated zymosan have been more variable.

From careful studies with a variety of inhibitors, it seems clear that neither 5-HETE nor LTB_4 has a major role in neutrophil granule secretion induced by FMLP, serum-treated zymosan, or A23187 (50,51). Similarly, LTB_4 appears to have little if any role in neutrophil aggregation induced by platelet-activating factor (56), A23187, and phorbol myristate acetate (57). A selective role for LTB_4 in the neutrophil aggregation induced by FMLP and C5a has been suggested and is perhaps possible (57). Studies of calcium flux in neutrophils suggest that the lipoxygenase inhibitors inhibit FMLP-stimulated calcium uptake but not the initial release of calcium from an intracellular pool stimulated by FMLP (58). One result of the studies with lipoxygenase inhibitors in neutrophils has been the realization that many of the compounds used probably have effects other than just lipoxygenase inhibition (50,51,59).

VII. THE MECHANISM OF THE RELEASE OF ARACHIDONIC ACID FROM NEUTROPHIL PHOSPHOLIPIDS

Stimulation of endogenous LTB_4 production results from an initial release of arachidonic acid from neutrophil phospholipids and an activation of the LTB_4 synthetic pathway (51). The precise mechanism involved in the release of arachidonic acid from neutrophil phospholipids is not yet known. Attention has been focused on two pathways, one involving the breakdown of phosphatidylinositols by phospholipase C and the second involving a phospholipase A_2 activity. The two pathways may be closely related and could be activated sequentially.

A. Phosphatidylinositol Metabolism: The Phospholipase C Pathway

Occupancy by FMLP of its receptors on the neutrophil surface is associated with a rapid breakdown of phosphatidylinositol (PI) and formation of diglyceride and phosphatidic acid (60-63). External calcium facilitates but is not essential for PI breakdown (60,63). Calcium-depleted neutrophils show neither PI breakdown nor secretion in response to FMLP (60). Studies using labeled arachidonic acid in horse neutrophils suggest that the arachidonyl moiety of phosphatidic acid can turn over rapidly and selectively, suggesting a mechanism (phospholipase A_2?) exists for selective release of arachidonic acid (64). The presence of diglyceride lipase has not yet been established in neutrophils. This pathway is outlined in Fig. 8-4.

B. The Phospholipase A_2 Pathway

A receptor-coupled plasma membrane phospholipase A_2 which is activated by FMLP, C5a and LTB_4 has been described (64b).

Hirata et al. suggest the following mechanism for phospholipase A_2 activation (65). When neutrophils are stimulated by chemoattractants, one of the early events is the activation of protein carboxy-O-methyltransferase and the methylation of phosphatidylethanolamine to form phosphatidylcholine (65). Phosphatidylcholine can be degraded to release arachidonic acid (presumably by the action of phospholipase A_2), and the fraction of phosphatidylcholine which is formed by the methylation pathway appears to be selectively utilized for this purpose (66a). This evidence suggests carboxy-O-methyl transferase activation precedes phospholipase A_2, but does not completely rule out a more direct phospholipase A_2 activation step. Data of Serhan et al. showing a rapid decrease in phosphatidylethanolamine and an increase in phosphatidylcholine within the first few seconds after addition of FMLP provide support for the concept that carboxy-O-methyl transferase is activated on neutrophil stimulation (62a).

The precursor of platelet activating factor, 1-0 alkyl-2-acyl-sn-glycerol-3-phosphorylcholine, is enriched in arachidonic acid suggesting the release of arachidonic acid and the formation of platelet activating factor may be closely connected (66b).

The secretion of some phospholipase A_2 when neutrophils are stimulated by FMLP (62b) raises the question as to the function of extracellularly secreted phospholipase A_2. Polyunsaturated fatty acids released on the outside of the cell or in a phagocytic vacuole could be important for the production of superoxide and other oxygen radicals (62c,d).

C. Lipomodulin

Lipomodulin is a 40,000 molecular weight protein which inhibits various phospholipases, including phospholipase A_2, C, and D (67). Synthesis of

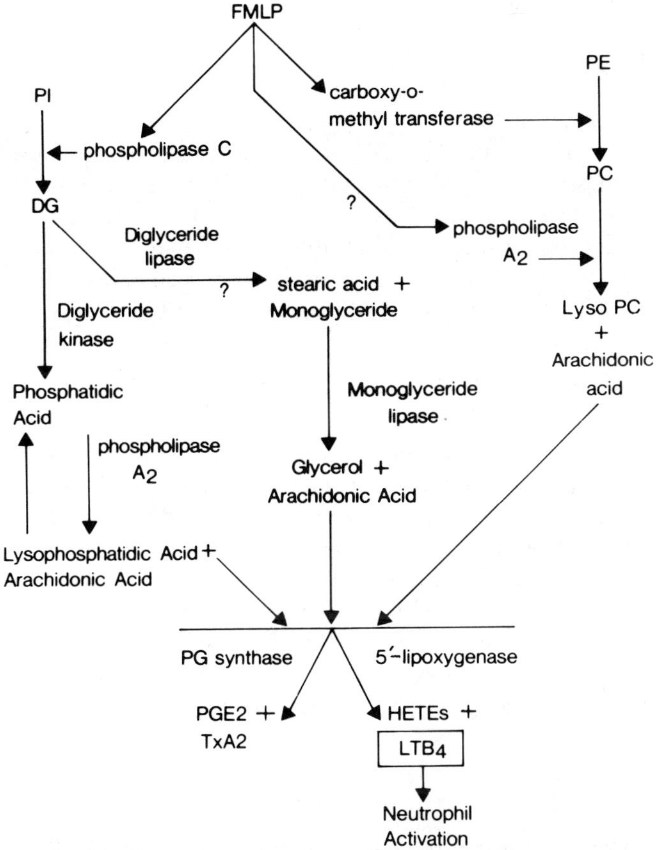

Fig. 8-4 Potential pathways by which agonists such as formyl-methionine-leucine-phenylalanine (FMLP) may degrade neutrophil phospholipids and give rise to active lipid species. PI = phosphatidylinositol; PE = phosphatidylethanolamine; PC = phosphatidylcholine; DG = diglyceride.

lipomodulin is induced by glucocorticoids, and this appears to account for the inhibitory effect of these steroids on arachidonic acid release and subsequent prostaglandin synthesis (68). The inhibitory effect of lipomodulin can be prevented by phosphorylation of this protein (67).

VIII. OTHER LIPID MEDIATORS

A. Platelet-Activating Factor

Platelet-activating factor is produced by neutrophils (69,70). Alone, it will stimulate neutrophil chemotaxis and aggregation. When added in the presence of cytochalasin B, it induces superoxide production and granule secretion (70-73a). FMLP-stimulated PAF production is enhanced by the presence of albumin in the medium (73b). The role of this lipid in endogenous neutrophil activation is not clear. It may have a role in the neutropenia seen in IgE anaphylaxis, immune-complex disorders, and acute serum sickness (70,74,75).

B. Phosphatidic Acid and Lysophosphatidic Acid

Phosphatidic acid is produced in significant quantities in neutrophils stimulated by FMLP (61-63,76). Evidence that the arachidonic acid group of phosphatidic acid can turn over rapidly suggests lysophosphatidic acid may also be produced in significant quantities, if only transiently (64).

In intact cells, lysophosphatidic acid can promote chemotaxis stimulated by a low concentration of FMLP (77). The relative importance of phosphatidic and lysophosphatidic acid is not yet definitely established. However, one or both could be important in the initiation of calcium flux in response to chemotactic agents, through a lipoxygenase-independent pathway.

C. Diglyceride

Diglyceride accumulates very early in the response of neutrophils to FMLP (63), as a result of phosphatidylinositol breakdown. As in platelets, the pathway could involve an initial breakdown of phosphatidylinositol-4,5-bisphosphate (see Ch. 6), with a secondary loss of phosphatidylinositol as it is rapidly converted to phosphatidylinositol-4,5-bisphosphate, but this has not been studied in neutrophils. The effects of diglycerides on neutrophils, if any, are unknown. If, as in platelets, they have effects similar to phorbol myristate acetate (see Chs. 3 and 6), they may be important effector substances. Phorbol myristate acetate stimulates neutrophil aggregation and selectively labilizes neutrophil-specific granules (78).

The presence of diglyceride-stimulatable protein kinase C in human granulocytes (79), and phosphorylation of a protein of similar molecular weight to P47 in platelets (see Ch. 6) during neutrophil secretion (80) are further evidence for the probable important role of the protein kinase C pathway and diglyceride in neutrophil function.

IX. SUMMARY AND OVERVIEW

While leukotriene B_4 appears to be critical in the neutrophil response to arachidonic acid, its role in neutrophil reactions to other agonists now appears to be relatively minor. It appears probable that neutrophil agonists such as FMLP and C5a, like ADP and thrombin with platelets, work largely independently of production of arachidonic acid metabolites. It may well turn out, as with ADP and thrombin in platelets, that there are some circumstances where 5-HETE and LTB_4 do enhance the overall response to the agonist.

With FMLP, the stimulation of phosphatidylinositol metabolism and formation of diglyceride, inositol trisphosphate, phosphatidic acid, and perhaps lysophosphatidic acid are likely to be important events in receptor-coupled stimulation leading to calcium flux, protein kinase activation, and other postreceptor events involved in cell stimulation.

A role of thromboxane A_2 produced by neutrophils in mediating cellular adhesion is consistent with current data.

PGE_2 and PGI_2 appear to be important physiologic neutrophil inhibitors, both acting by stimulating cellular adenylate cyclase to raise intracellular cAMP. Endothelial cell-derived PGI_2 could function locally to prevent neutrophils from adhering in their transit through the capillary wall. As discussed in Ch. 3, directed movement of neutrophils may occur best with a combination of the gradient of a chemotactic factor coupled with a small amount of PGE_2 or PGI_2 to prevent the cells from adhering too tightly.

REFERENCES

1a. R. T. Parmley, M. Takagi, J. C. Barton, L. A. Boxer, and R. L. Austin. *Am. J. Pathol. 109*:343 (1982).
1b. E. L. Gottfried. *Sem. Hematol. 9*:241 (1972).
2. G. V. Marinetti and K. Cattieu. *Chem. Phys. Lipids 31*:169 (1982).
3. C. N. Serhan, M. J. Broekman, H. M. Korchak, A. J. Marcus, and G. Weissman. *Biochem. Biophys. Res. Commun. 107*:951 (1982).
4. R. J. Mason, T. P. Stossel, and M. Vaughan. *J. Clin. Invest. 51*:2399 (1972).
5. J. E. Smolen and S. B. Shohet. *J. Clin. Invest. 53*:726 (1974).
6. D. F. Bainton. *J. Cell Biol. 58*:249 (1973).

7. P. Borgeat and B. Samuelsson. *Proc. Natl. Acad. Sci. USA 76:*2148 (1979).
8. W. F. Stenson and C. W. Parker. *J. Clin. Invest. 64*:1457 (1979).
9. E. J. Goetzl and F. F. Sun. *J. Exp. Med. 150*:406 (1979).
10. M. Waite, L. R. DeChatelet, L. King, and P. S. Shirley. *Biochem. Biophys. Res. Commun. 90*:984 (1979).
11. R. B. Zurier. *Adv. Prost. Thromboxane Res. 2*:815 (1976).
12. I. M. Goldstein, C. L. Malmsten, H. Kindahl, H. B. Kaplan, O. Radmark, B. Samuelsson and G. Weissmann. *J. Exp. Med. 148*:787 (1978).
13a. S. R. Turner, J. A. Campbell, and W. S. Lynn. *J. Exp. Med. 141*:1437 (1975).
13b. A. J. Marcus, L. B. Safier, H. L. Ullman, M. J. Broekman, N. Islam, T. D. Oglesby and R. R. Gorman. *Proc. Natl. Acad. Sci. 81*:903 (1984).
14a. P. Borgeat, M. Hamberg, and B. Samuelsson. *J. Biol. Chem. 251*:7816 (1976).
14b. W. Jubiz and G. Nolan. *Biochem. Biophys. Res. Commun. 114*:855 (1983).
15. J. J. O'Flaherty, H. J. Showell, P. A. Ward, and E. L. Becker. *Am. J. Pathol. 96*:799 (1979).
16. J. J. O'Flaherty, H. J. Showell, E. L. Becker, and P. A. Ward. *Prostaglandins 17*:915 (1979).
17. P. H. Naccache, H. J. Showell, E. L. Becker, and R. I. Sha'afi. *Biochem. Biophys. Res. Commun. 87*:292 (1979).
18. M. Volpi, P. H. Naccache, and R. I. Sha'afi. *Biochem. Biophys. Res. Commun. 92*:1231 (1980).
19. B. R. Andersen, H. J. Amirault, and G. C. LeBreton. *Prostaglandins 22*: 469 (1981).
20. C. J. Lammi-Keefe, D. E. Hammerschmidt, D. J. Weisdorf, and H. S. Jacob. *Inflammation 6*:227 (1982).
21. E. J. Goetzl and W. C. Pickett. *J. Exp. Med. 153*:482 (1981).
22. R. A. Lewis, E. J. Goetzl, J. M. Drazen, N. A. Soter, K. F. Austen, and E. J. Corey. *J. Exp. Med. 154*:1243 (1981).
23. A. W. Ford-Hutchinson, M. A. Bray, M. V. Doig, M. E. Shipley, and M. J. H. Smith. *Nature 286*:264 (1980).
24. I. Hafstrom, J. Palmblad, C. Malmsten, O. Radmark, and B. Samuelsson. *FEBS Lett. 130*:146 (1981).
25. H. J. Showell, P. J. Naccache, P. Borgeat, S. Picard, P. Vallerand, E. L. Becker, and R. Sha'afi. *J. Immunol. 128*:811 (1982).
26. C. N. Serhan, S. Raclin, J. E. Sonolen, H. Korchak, B. Samuelsson, and G. Weissman. *Biochem. Biophys. Res. Commun. 107*:1006 (1982).
27. C. N. Serhan, J. Fridovitch, E. J. Goetzl, P. B. Dunham, and G. Weissmann. *J. Biol. Chem. 257*:4746 (1982).
28. R. I. Sha'afi, P. H. Naccache, T. F. P. Molski, P. Borgeat, and E. J. Goetzl. *J. Cell. Phsyiol. 108*:401 (1981).

29. D. W. Goldman and E. J. Goetzl. *J. Immunol. 129*:1600 (1982).
30. E. J. Goetzl and W. C. Pickett. *J. Exp. Med. 153*:482 (1981).
31. P. H. Naccache, T. F. P. Molski, E. L. Becker, P. Borgeat, S. Picard, P. Vallerand, and R. I. Sha'afi. *J. Biol. Chem. 257*:8608 (1982).
32. W. Salzer, C. McCall, and J. O'Flaherty. *Fed. Proc. 42*:918 (1983).
33. E. J. Goetzl and F. F. Sun. *J. Exp. Med. 150*:406 (1979).
34. E. J. Goetzl, A. R. Brash, and A. I. Tauber. *Immunology 39*:491 (1980).
35. J. T. O'Flaherty, M. J. Thomas, C. E. McCall, and R. L. Wykle. *Res. Comm. Chem. Path. Pharm. 40*:475 (1983).
36. J. T. O'Flaherty, M. J. Thomas, M. J. Hammett, C. Carroll, C. E. McCall, and R. L. Wykle. *Biochem. Biophys. Res. Commun. 111*:1 (1983).
37a. E. A. Ham, D. D. Soderman, M. E. Zanetti, H. W. Dougherty, E. McCauley, and F. A. Kuehl, Jr. *Proc. Natl. Acad. Sci. USA 80*:4349 (1983).
37b. J. T. O'Flaherty, D. L. Kreutzer, and P. A. Ward. *Prostaglandins 17*:201 (1979).
38. G. Till, E. Kownatzki, M. Seitz, and D. Gemsa. *Clin. Immunol. Immunopathol. 12*:111 (1979).
39. I. Rivkin, J. Rosenblatt, and E. L. Becker. *J. Immunol. 115*:1126 (1975).
40. P. J. Spagnuolo, J. J. Ellner, A. Hassid, and M. J. Dunn. *J. Clin. Invest. 66*:406 (1980).
41. E. A. Kitchen, J. R. Boot, and W. Dawson. *Prostaglandins 16*:239 (1978).
42. J. L. Skosey, G. LeBreton, H. Lotsof, and D. C. Chow. *Fed. Proc. 42*: 695 (1983).
43. G. Weissmann, J. E. Smolen, and H. Korchak. *Adv. Prost. Thromboxane Res. 8*:1637 (1980).
44. J. E. Smolen, H. M. Korchak, and G. Weissmann. *Trends Pharmacol. Sci. 3*:483 (1982).
45. L. A. Boxer, J. M. Allen, M. Schmidt, M. Yoder, and R. L. Baehner, *J. Lab. Clin. Med. 95*:672 (1980).
46. J. McGillen, R. Patterson, and J. P. Phair. *J. Infect. Dis. 141*:382 (1980).
47. F. Bussolino and G. Camussi. *Prostaglandins 20*:781 (1980).
48a. H. E. Claesson, U. Lundberg, and C. Malmsten. *Biochem. Biophys. Res. Commun. 99*:1230 (1981).
48b. M. R. Buchanan, M. J. Vazquez, and M. A. Gimbrone. *Blood 62*:889 (1983).
48c. E. J. Goetzl, L. L. Brindley, and D. W. Goldman. *Immunology 50*:35 (1983).
48d. J. Maclouf, B. Fruteau de Laclos, and P. Borgeat. *Proc. Natl. Acad. Sci. USA 79*:6042 (1982).

49. W. Jubiz, O. Redmack, C. Malmsten, G. Hansson, J. Lindgren, J. Palmblad, A. Volen, and B. Samuelsson. *J. Biol. Chem. 257*:6106 (1982).
50. R. J. Smith, F. F. Sun, S. S. Iden, B. J. Bowman, H. Sprecher, and J. C. McGuire. *Clin. Immunol. Immunopathol. 20*:157 (1981).
51. R. M. J. Palmer and J. A. Salmon. *Immunology 50*:65 (1983).
52. F. Hirata, B. A. Corcoran, K. Venkatsubramanian, E. Schiffmann, and J. Axelrod. *Proc. Natl. Acad. Sci. USA 76*:2640 (1980).
53. G. M. Bokoch and P. W. Reed. *J. Biol. Chem. 255*:10223 (1980).
54. M. I. Siegel, R. T. McConnell, R. W. Bonser, and P. Cuatrecasas. *Biochem. Biophys. Res. Commun. 104*:874 (1982).
55. B. M. Waite, L. R. DeChatelet, L. King, and P. S. Shirley. *Biochem. Biochem. Biophys. Res. Commun. 90*:984 (1979).
56. A. W. Ford-Hutchinson. *Int. J. Immunopharmacol. 5*:17 (1983).
57. W. Salzer, C. McCall, and J. O'Flaherty. *Fed. Proc. 42*:918 (1983).
58. R. I. Sha'afi, P. H. Naccache, T. Alobaidi, T. F. P. Molski, and M. Volpi. *J. Cell. Physiol. 106*:215 (1981).
59. R. J. Smith, F. F. Sun, B. J. Bowman, S. S. Iden, H. W. Smith, and J. C. McGuire. *Biochem. Biophys. Res. Commun. 109*:943 (1982).
60. S. Cockcroft, J. P. Bennett, and B. D. Gomperts. *Biochem. J. 200*:501 (1981).
61. C. N. Serhan, H. M. Korchak, J. E. Smolen, M. J. Broekman, A. J. Marcus, and G. Weissmann. *Biochem. Biophys. Acta 762*:420 (1983).
62a. C. N. Serhan, M. J. Broekman, H. M. Korchak, A. J. Marcus, and G. Weissmann *Biochem. Biophys. Res. Commun. 107*:951 (1982).
62b. C. Lanni and E. L. Becker. *Am. J. Pathol. 113*:90 (1983).
62c. D. A. Peterson and J. M. Gerrard. *Med. Hypothesis* 7:1389 (1981).
62d. Y. Bromberg and E. Pick. *Cell. Immunol. 79*:240 (1983).
63. K. Yano, H. Hattori, A. Mai, and Y. Nozawa. *Biochim. Biophys. Acta. 752*:137 (1983).
64a. E. G. Lapentina, M. M. Billah, and P. Cuatrecasas. *J. Biol. Chem. 255*: 10966 (1980).
64b. B. J. Bormann, C. K. Huang, W. M. Macklin and E. L. Becker. *Proc. Natl. Acad. Sci. USA 81*:767 (1984).
65. R. F. O'Dea, O. H. Viveros, J. Axelrod, S. Aswinikaumar, E. Schiffman, and B. A. Corcoran. *Nature 272*:462 (1978).
66a. F. Hirata, B. A. Corcoran, K. Venkatasubramanian, E. Schiffman, and J. Axelrod. *Proc. Natl. Acad. Sci. USA 76*:2640 (1979).
66b. H. W. Mueller, J. T. O'Flaherty, D. G. Greene, M. P. Samuel, and R. C. Wykle. *J. Lipid Res. 25*:383 (1984).
67. F. Hirata. *J. Biol. chem. 256*:7730 (1981).
68. F. Hirata, E. Schiffman, K. Venkatasubramanian, D. Salomon, and J. Axelrod. *Proc. Natl. Acad. Sci. USA 77*:2533 (1980).
69. J. M. Lynch, G. Z. Lotner, S. Betz, and P. M. Henson. *J. Immunol. 123*: 1219 (1979).

70. G. Camussi, C. Tetta, F. Bussolino, F. Caligaris-Cappio, R. Coda, C. Masera, and G. P. Segoloni. *Int. Arch. Allergy Appl. Immunol. 64*:25 (1981).
71. J. O. Shaw, R. N. Pinckard, K. S. Ferrigni, L. McManus, and D. J. Hanahan. *J. Immunol. 123*:1847 (1981).
72. L. M. Ingraham, T. D. Coates, J. M. Allen, C. P. Higgins, R. L. Baehner, and L. A. Boxer. *Blood 59*:1259 (1982).
73a. J. T. O'Flaherty, R. L. Wykle, C. H. Miller, J. C. Lewis, M. Waite, D. A. Bass, C. E. McCall, and R. DeChatelet. *Am. J. Pathol. 103*:70 (1981).
73b. R. N. Pinckard, J. C. Ludwig, and L. M. McManus. *Fed. Proc. 42*:692 (1983).
74. R. N. Pinckard, R. S. Farr, and D. J. Hanahan. *J. Immunol. 123*:1847 (1979).
75. G. Camussi, C. Tetta, M. C. Deregibus, F. Bussolino, G. Spegoloni, and A. Vercellone. *J. Immunol. 128*:86 (1982).
76. G. Weissmann, C. Serhan, H. M. Korchak, J. E. Smolen, M. J. Broekman, and A. J. Marcus. *Trans. Assoc. Am. Physicians 94*:357 (1981).
77. J. M. Gerrard, C. C. Clawson, and J. G. White. *Am. J. Pathol. 100*:609 (1980).
78. J. G. White and R. D. Estensen. *Am. J. Pathol. 75*:45 (1974).
79. R. Minakuchi, Y. Takai, B. Yu, and Y. Nishizuka. *J. Biochem. 89*: 1651 (1981).
80. C. Schneider, M. Zanetti, and D. Romeo. *FEBS Lett. 127*:4 (1981).

BIBLIOGRAPHY

M. Bessis. *Blood Smears Reinterpreted.* Springer International, New York (1977).

P. Murphy. *The Neutrophil.* Plenum Press, New York (1976).

B. D. Cheson, J. T. Curnutte, and B. M. Babior. *Prog. Clin. Immunol. 3*:1 (1977).

M. C. Pike and R. Snyderman. *Adv. Inflammation Res. 4*:109 (1982).

B. Wolach, R. L. Baehner, and L. A. Boxer. *Israel J. Med. Sci. 18*:897 (1982).

9

Basophils

Basophils are the least numerous of the circulating granulocytes. They are discussed before eosinophils since certain functions of the latter are antagonistic to the effects of basophils, and a discussion of the basophil first will facilitate understanding of eosinophil function. Some of what we know about blood basophils and prostaglandins is by inference only as a result of studies on leukemic basophils or on tissue mast cells. Since basophils and mast cells are probably related, this section will mention data on mast cells as well as from basophils. It is already evident that there are differences as well as similarities between these cells.

I. ANATOMY OF THE BASOPHIL

The general morphology of the basophil is similar to that of the neutrophil except that, instead of specific and azurophilic granules, basophils contain basophil granules (Fig. 9-1). Ultrastructurally these granules have a typical grainy appearance. Chemically these granules contain heparin and histamine.

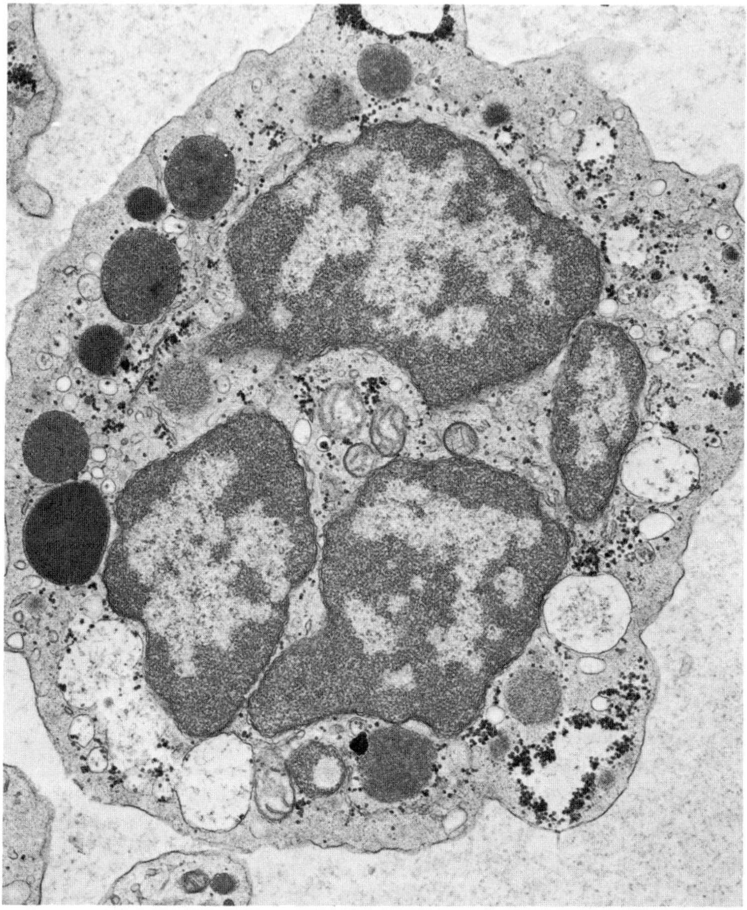

Fig. 9-1 A human blood basophil with its characteristic granules. (X16,500.) (Figure courtesy of Dr. J. G. White.)

II. THE FUNCTION OF THE BASOPHIL

Basophils can move in an ameboid fashion, although slower than other granulocytes. Accumulation of basophils in certain conditions (i.e., the Jones-Mote reaction) suggests there may be specific basophil chemoattractants. Basophils show very little, if any, phagocytic ability. Their most notable function is the degranulation stimulated by IgE antibodies and immune complexes.

The ability of basophils to react to very small doses of stimuli may be important for host defense against small concentrations of bacteria, viruses, or foreign protein. In other conditions (i.e., allergies) the hypersensitivity is detrimental to the host as the basophil discharges histamine and various other chemicals to contribute to allergic and anaphylactic reactions. The secretion of heparin, stimulated by postprandial lipemia, may contribute significantly to clearing of serum lipids.

III. METABOLISM OF ARACHIDONIC ACID AND EICOSAPENTEANOIC ACID IN BASOPHILS

A. Arachidonic Acid

Arachidonic acid is converted by the cyclooxygenase pathway primarily to PGD_2 in mast cells (human and rat) (1,2) and in leukemic basophils (rat) (3). Small amounts of PGE_2, $PGF_{2\alpha}$, thromboxane B_2, and 6-keto-$PGF_{1\alpha}$ are

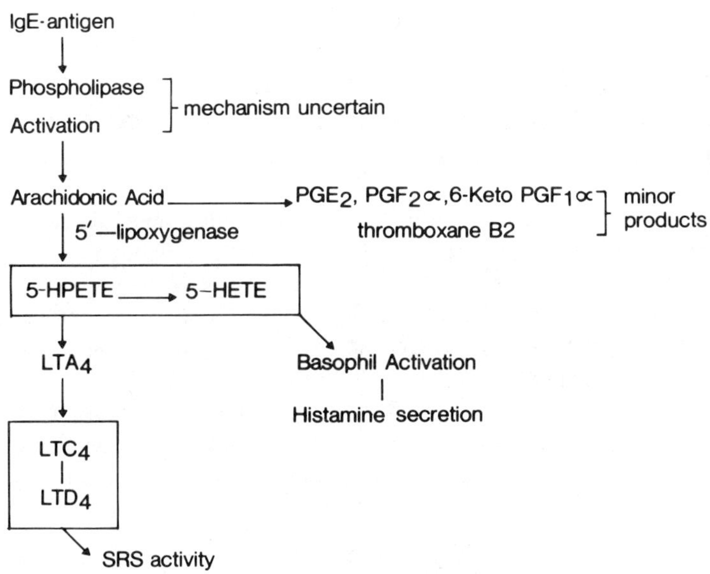

Fig. 9-2 Metabolism of arachidonic acid in human basophils. Note: Human mast cells make a significant amount of PGD_2 in contrast to human basophils shown in the figure, which do not appear to produce PGD_2.

also formed (1,2). *In human basophils, however, no detectable PGD_2 appears to be produced and only a small amount of thromboxane B_2* (2) (Fig. 9-2).

The lipoxygenase pathway is active in mast cells and leukemic basophils with production of 5-HETE and several leukotrienes (LT), including LTC_4 and LTD_4. The precise mixture of these leukotrienes may depend on the species. For murine mastocytoma cells, LTC_4 is a major product (4,5), whereas for rat basophil leukemic cells it is LTD_4 (6,7). Human mast cells and leukemic basophils have been shown to produce significant quantities of 5-HETE, LTB_4, and LTC_4 or LTD_4 (8-10a). However, normal human blood basophils appear to produce much less LTD_4 (about 1×10^{-17} LTD mole equivalent per basophil) than human mast cells (average 28×10^{-17} LTD mole equivalents per mast cell) in response to anti-IgE antibody (2).

B. Eicosapentaenoic Acid

Studies using murine mastocytoma cells show that these cells can efficiently convert eicosapentaenoic acid to LTB_5, but form comparatively little LTC_5 compared with their production of LTC_4 from arachidonic acid (10b).

IV. EFFECTS OF ARACHIDONIC ACID AND ENDOGENOUSLY DERIVED METABOLITES ON BASOPHILS

Arachidonic acid can enhance antigen-induced basophil histamine release (11). Cyclooxygenase inhibitors also enhance such release, whereas a variety of lipoxygenase inhibitors decrease it (11,12). The addition of two lipoxygenase products (5-HPETE and 5-HETE) to human basophils will enhance antigen-induced histamine release, whereas several other lipoxygenase products (LTB_4, LTC_4, LTD_4, 11-HPETE, 12-HPETE, and 15-HPETE) and the cyclooxygenase product, PGD_2, are ineffective (13,14). In the presence of cytochalasin B, LTB_4 is, however, effective (15). These findings provide evidence that 5-HPETE and 5-HETE (and to a lesser extent LTB_4) are the active products in basophils. Differences in species or in cell type (mast cell versus basophil) may occur. With rat mast cells, 12-HETE and 5-HETE are both effective (16), whereas with the isolated guinea pig lung 15-HPETE and 13-hydroperoxylinoleic acid are effective (17). In human mast cells in airway tissue, indomethacin enhances histamine release, but one report suggests neither indomethacin, 5-HPETE, nor PGD_2 is active on purified human mast cells (2).

V. THE EFFECT ON BASOPHILS OF PROSTAGLANDINS WHICH STIMULATE PRODUCTION OF cAMP

A. Prostaglandins E_1 and E_2

PGE_1 and PGE_2 both inhibit histamine release from human peripheral blood basophils (18,19). Both also raise cAMP levels (19). Other prostaglandins have been studied and the order of potency $PGE_1 = PGE_2 > PGA_2 = PGA_1 > PGB_2 > PGF_{1\alpha} = PGF_{2\alpha}$ is the same as their order of potency in raising cAMP levels (20). These studies were done in a mixed population of leukocytes, so it is not absolutely certain that the cAMP was basophil derived. Since cAMP does not readily pass across the cell membrane, it can be presumed that the effective cAMP was that produced inside the basophil. Studies with other agents are consistent with a general inhibition of basophil secretion being produced by an elevated cAMP. PGE_1 and the cAMP analogue, dibutyryl cAMP, have also been shown to inhibit basophil adhesion to glass capillary tubes (21).

VI. THE RELEASE OF ARACHIDONIC ACID FROM BASOPHIL AND MAST CELL PHOSPHOLIPIDS

When radiolabeled arachidonic acid is incubated with rat basophil leukemia cells, it is incorporated primarily into phosphatidylcholine (66%) and to a lesser extent into phosphatidylethanolamine (17%), phosphatidylinositol (8%), phosphatidylserine (2%), or neutral lipids (5%) (22). Whether release of arachidonic acid occurs primarily through the phospholipase C or the phospholipase A_2 pathway or both is not clearly established. The evidence to date is presented below.

A. The Phospholipase C Pathway

After stimulation of rat mast cells with various agonists, including anti-IgE and compound 48/80 (a histamine-releasing agent), there is a selectively increased incorporation of $^{32}PO_4$ into phosphatidic acid, phosphatidylcholine, and phosphatidylinositol (23,24). Using compound 48/80 increased incorporation of arachidonic acid into diglyceride associated with increased diglyceride production shortly after the stimulus has been shown (25). An active diglyceride lipase has also been demonstrated in these mast cells (26).

B. The Phospholipase A_2 Pathway

Crews et al. reported that stimulation of IgE receptors on rat basophilic leukemia cells is associated with a transient rise and fall of methylated phospholipids, calcium influx, release of arachidonic acid from phosphatidylcholine, and secretion of histamine (22). Evidence was presented that these events are linked and occur in sequence. The phosphatidylcholine which is methylated using (methyl-^{3}H) methionine is selectively enriched in arachidonic acid. 3-Diazaadenosine and homocysteine, thiolactone inhibitors of phospholipid methylation, also blocked calcium influx, the release of arachidonic acid, and the secretion of histamine (22,26).

The loss of arachidonic acid following cell stimulation by antigen-IgE was primarily from phosphatidylcholine, suggesting the phospholipase A_2 pathway was primarily involved, since little loss was seen from phosphatidylinositol (22). However, these results were obtained measuring loss of radioactivity, not absolute amounts. If, as the authors suggest, phosphatidylethanolamine (PE) is first methylated to phosphatidylcholine (PC) and then the arachidonic acid is released from the PC, there should be an apparent loss of labeled arachidonic acid from PE. The fact that this was not seen suggests that the synthesis of PC from PE could serve primarily to replenish a depleted pool of PC, or that the newly synthesized PC is only a small fraction of the localized pool of PC from which the arachidonic acid is released and the methylation serves primarily to influence membrane viscosity in the vicinity of the phospholipase A_2 enzyme.

Cells washed three times in buffer without calcium to deplete external calcium and perhaps intracellular stores do not show release of arachidonic acid from rat basophil leukemia cell phospholipids unless calcium is added, showing such release requires calcium (presumably for phospholipase activation) (27), consistent with studies in other cells. Addition of the calcium ionophore A23187 to these cells activates phospholipases, but in a less specific fashion than with antigen-IgE (arachidonic acid is lost from PE as well as PC). This suggests that the basophil, as with other cells, has both a specific receptor-coupled pathway as well as a nonspecific lipase pathway. Dexamethasone, which induces synthesis of a phospholipase A_2 inhibitor protein, has been shown to inhibit IgE-mediated histamine release from human basophils (28), but fails to inhibit the release of histamine, PGD_2, or leukotrienes from purified human lung mast cells (29). The reason for this difference is not clear.

VII. OTHER LIPID MEDIATORS

A. Platelet-Activating Factor [Acetyl Glycerylether Phosphorylcholine (AGEPC)

AGEPC is synthesized by antigen-stimulated IgE-sensitized rabbit basophils (27,30,31), but either not at all or in very small amounts by human basophils (32-36a). Human mast cells, do, however, synthesize significant amounts of AGEPC, approximately 30-150 times more than human neutrophils (2).

B. Phosphatidic Acid (PA) Lysophosphatidic (LPA) Acid

Increased incorporation of $^{32}PO_4$ into phosphatidic acid and lysophosphatidic acid occurs in stimulated basophils (36b). Effects of PA and LPA on basophils or mast cells have not been assessed.

C. Lysophosphatidylserine (LPS)

LPS will enhance histamine release from rat mast cells (37a).

D. Diglyceride

Studies of the effect of diglyceride on basophils or mast cells have not yet been reported. However, phorbol myristate acetate which activates protein kinase C, similar to diglyceride in other cells, does cause secretion of histamine from mast cells and considerably potentiates secretion induced by a low concentration of the calcium ionophore A23187 (37a). This suggests diglyceride activated protein kinase C is present in mast cells as in other blood cells.

VIII. OVERVIEW OF HUMAN BASOPHIL RESPONSES

A. Activation Pathway

Studies with inhibitors suggest that a lipoxygenase product produced by basophils is involved in secretion of histamine. The primary active compound appears to be 5-HPETE or 5-HETE. Production of diglycerides, phosphatidic acid, and possibly lysophosphatidic acid could represent an alternative activation pathway.

B. Inhibitory Pathway

PGE_2 (or PGI_2 ?), perhaps produced by basophils in small amounts or produced by other cells, notably monocytes, can activate basophil adenylate cyclase to raise cellular cAMP and inhibit histamine secretion.

C. Relation of Basophils and Mast Cells

Tissue mast cells possess a much larger capacity for synthesizing prostaglandins and leukotrienes than blood basophils. If the tissue mast cells are derived from blood basophils, there must be substantial production or activation of the enzymes responsible for prostaglandin and leukotriene synthesis during this transformation process.

APPENDIX 9-1 IMPORTANT SPECIES DIFFERENCES

Rat serosal mast cells generate mono-HETEs and LTB_4, but no LTC_4 or LTD_4 (38). Mouse bone marrow-derived mast cells and mouse mastocytoma cells produce LTC_4 without any significant LTD_4 (4,10b,39). Rat leukemic basophils and human leukemic basophils generate LTD_4 and LTB_4 with only small amounts of LTC_4 after the first few minutes (6,40). Dog mastocytoma cells produce LTB_4, LTC_4, and LTD_4 in a ratio of about 3:7:2 (40).

REFERENCES

1. L. J. Roberts, R. A. Lewis, J. A. Lawson, B. J. Sweetman, K. F. Austen, and J. A. Oates. *Prostaglandins 15*:717 (1978).

2. D. W. MacGlashan, Jr., R. P. Schleimer, S. P. Peters, E. S. Schulman, G. K. Adams, A. K. Sobotka, H. H. Newball, and L. M. Lichtenstein. *Fed. Proc. 42*:2504 (1983).
3. S. F. Falkenhein, H. MacDonald, M. M. Huber, D. Koch, and C. W. Parker. *J. Immunol. 125*:163 (1980).
4. R. C. Murphy, S. Hammarstrom, and B. Samuelsson. *Proc. Natl. Acad. Sci. USA 76*:4275 (1979).
5. S. Hammarstrom, R. C. Murphy, B. Samuelsson, D. A. Clark, C. Mioskowski, and E. J. Corey. *Biochem. Biophys. Res. Commun. 91*:1266 (1979).
6. C. W. Parker, M. M. Huber, M. K. Hoffman, and S. F. Faulkenhein. *Prostaglandins 18*:673 (1979).
7. H. R. Morris, G. W. Taylor, P. J. Piper, M. N. Samhoun, and J. R. Tippins. *Prostaglandins 19*:185 (1980).
8. L. D. Yecies, H. J. Wedner, and C. W. Parker. *J. Immunol. 123*:2814 (1979).
9. D. W. MacGlashan, Jr., R. P. Schleimer, S. P. Peters, E. S. Schulman, G. K. Adams, III, H. H. Newball, and L. L. Lichtenstein. *J. Clin. Invest. 70*:747 (1982).

10a. S. P. Peters. D. W. MacGlashan, Jr., E. S. Schulman, R. P. Schleimer, and L. M. Lichtenstein. *Fed. Proc. 42*:1375 (1983).

10b. R. C. Murphy, W. C. Pickett, B. R. Culp, and W. E. M. Lands. *Prostaglandins 22*:613 (1981).

11. G. Marone, A. Kagey-Sobotka, and L. M. Lichtenstein. *J. Immunol. 123*:1669 (1979).
12. G. Marone, S. Hammarstrom, and L. N. Lichtenstein. *Clin. Immunol. Immunolpathol. 17*:177 (1980).
13. S. P. Peters, M. I. Siegel, A. Kagey-Sobotka, and L. M. Lichtenstein. *Nature 292*:455 (1981).
14. S. P. Peters, A. Kagey-Sobotka, D. W. MacGlashan, Jr., M. I. Siegel, and L. M. Lichtenstein. *J. Immunol. 129*:797 (1982).
15. A. Kagey-Sobotka, R. P. Schleimer, S. P. Peters, and L. M. Lichenstein. *Fed. Proc. 42*:1342 (1983).
16. W. F. Stenson, C. W. Parker, and J. J. Sullivan. *Biochem. Biophys. Res. Commun. 96*:1045 (1980).
17. J. J. Adcock, L. G. Garland, S. Moncada, and J. A. Salmon. *Prostaglandins 16*:163 (1978).
18. L. M. Lichtenstein and R. DeBernardo. *J. Immunol. 107*:1131 (1971).
19. H. R. Bourne, L. M. Lichtenstein, and K. L. Melmon. *J. Immunol. 108*: 695 (1972).
20. J. M. Lichtenstein, E. Gillespie, H. R. Bourne, and C. S. Henney. *Prostaglandins 2*:519 (1972).
21. R. E. Bryant and M. C. Sutcliffe. *J. Clin. Invest. 54*:1241 (1974).

22. F. T. Crews, Y. Morita, A. McGivney, F. Hirata, R. P. Siraganian, and J. Axelrod. *Arch. Biochem. Biophys. 212*:561 (1981).
23. D. A. Kennerly, T. J. Sullivan, and C. W. Parker. *J. Immunol. 122*:152 (1979).
24. D. A. Kennerly, C. J. Secosan, C. W. Parker, and T. J. Sullivan. *J. Immunol. 123*:1519.
25. D. A. Kennedy, T. J. Sullivan, P. Sylwester, and C. W. Parker. *J. Exp. Med. 150*:1039 (1979).
26. F. T. Crews, Y. Morita, F. Hirata, J. Axelrod, and R. P. Siraganian. *Biochem. Biophys. Res. Commun. 90*:42 (1980).
27. P. M. Henson. *J. Exp. Med. 131*:287 (1970).
28. R. P. Schleimer, L. M. Lichtenstein, and E. Gillespie. *Nature 292*:454 (1981).
29. R. P. Schleimer, D. W. MacGlashan, E. S. Schulman, S. S. Peters, N. F. Adkinson, H. H. Newball, G. K. Adams, L. M. Lichtenstein, and E. Gillespie. *Fed. Proc. 41*:487 (1983).
30. J. Benveniste, P. M. Henson, and C. G. Cochrane. *J. Exp. Med. 136*: 1356 (1977).
31. P. M. Henson. *J. Clin. Invest. 60*:481 (1977).
32. S. J. Betz, G. Z. Lotner, and P. M. Henson. *J. Immunol. 125*:2749 (1980).
33. R. A. F. Clark, J. I. Galin, and A. P. Kaplan. *J. Allergy Clin. Immunol. 58*:623 (1976).
34. R. A. Lewis, E. J. Goetzl, S. I. Wasserman, F. H. Valone, R. H. Rubin, and K. F. Austen. *J. Immunol. 114*:87 (1975).
35. G. Camussi, F. Bussolino, C. Tetta, J. Benveniste, and A. Vercellone. In *Hemostasis, Prostaglandins and Renal Disease*. G. Remuzzi, G. Mecca, G. deGaetano (eds). Raven Press, New York, (1980).
36a. Sanchez-Martin and D. Lagnuoff. *Nature 279*:250 (1979).
36b D. L. Fagan and T. J. Sullivan. *Fed. Proc. 42*:1083 (1983).
37a. T. W. Martin and D. Lagunoff. *Nature 279*:250 (1979).
37b. A. S. Heinman and F. T. Crews. *Fed. Proc. 43*:974 (1984).
38. R. A. Lewis, J. Mencia-Huerta, R. J. Soberman, D. Hoover, A. Marfat, E. J. Corey, and K. F. Austen. *Proc. Natl. Acad. Sci. USA 79*:7904 (1982).
39. E. Razin, J. M. Mencia-Huerta, R. A. Lewis, E. J. Corey, and K. F. Austen. *Proc. Natl. Acad. Sci. USA 79*:4665 (1982).
40. M. J. Phillips, W. M. Gold, and E. J. Goetzl. *J. Immunol. 131*:906 (1983).

10
Eosinophils

The eosinophil, a cell with a particular role in allergic and parasitic disorders, has chemotactic responses similar to neutrophils, although sometimes to different stimuli, but has important functions–inhibition of some mast cell activities and attacks on parasites–which are quite different.

I. THE ANATOMY OF THE EOSINOPHIL

Similar to the neutrophil, the eosinophil has a central centrosome (a well-developed golgi complex, centrioles, and radiating microtubules). The eosinophil usually has a bilobed nucleus. Surrounding the nucleus in the periphery of the cell are the characteristic eosinophil granules (Fig. 10-1). Inside the limiting membrane, in human eosinophils, there is a homogeneous matrix, and in most granules an opaque crystal. The periodicity of the crystal is about 3 nm in human eosinophils. These granules contain eosinophil peroxidase. Eosinophils also possess small specific microgranules believed to be the site of arylsulfatase B activity. Glycogen is plentiful. Mitochondria are more numerous and larger than in neutrophils, and ribosomes and endoplasmic reticulum persist longer than in neutrophils.

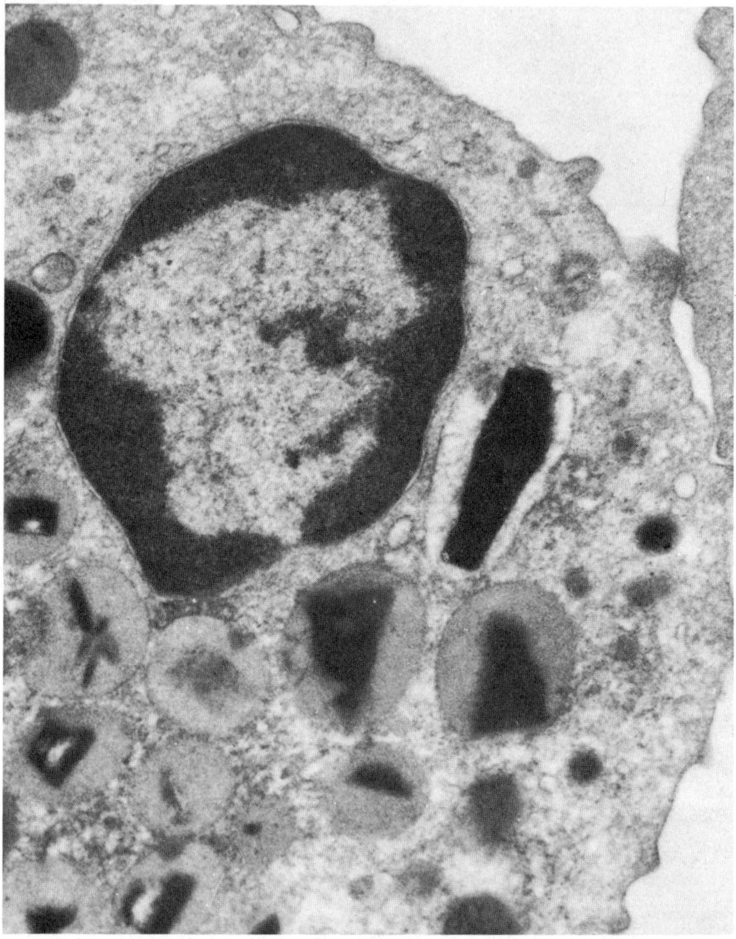

Fig. 10-1 A human eosinophil showing the characteristic granules. (×19,800).

II. THE FUNCTION OF THE EOSINOPHIL

A. Chemotaxis

Eosinophils show selective chemotaxis toward two tetrapeptides, termed the eosinophil chemotactic factor of anaphylaxis. C5a and the C567 complex are chemotactic for eosinophils, as are the HETEs (discussed later).

B. Inhibition of Basophil Activitors

Eosinophils possess a number of components which have specific inhibitory or destructive effects toward basophil and neutrophil activators released during allergic reactions. Eosinophil peroxidase will convert leukotriene C_4 to isomers of leukotriene B_4, thus abolishing the slow-reacting substance activity of LTC_4 (1). Phospholipase D present in eosinophils can inactivate platelet-activating factor. Lysophospholipase, probably localized in the eosinophil plasma membrane, can degrade lysophospholipids. Eosinophil histaminase degrades histamine released from basophils or mast cells. 15-HETE, produced by eosinophils, inhibits the 5-lipoxygenase of neutrophils, thus inhibiting neutrophil 5-HETE and LTB_4 production (2). 15-HETE would therefore be expected to inhibit basophil and mast cell production of leukotrienes but this is not certain since 15-HETE stimulated 5-HETE and LTB_4 synthesis in one mast/basophil cell line. (Of interest, 15-HETE also inhibits platelet and thymic lymphocyte lipoxygenases.)

C. Antiparasite and Antitumor Effects

Eosinophils appear to have a specific antiparasite property. In particular, they can induce antibody-dependent or complement-dependent damage to the larval-tissue stages of some helminth parasites. In addition, the secretion of eosinophil peroxidase has been shown to enhance macrophage-mediated tumor cell killing (3).

III. THE METABOLISM OF ARACHIDONIC ACID IN EOSINOPHILS

Arachidonic acid metabolism in eosinophils has been investigated by several laboratories, and further clarification is needed in view of considerable apparent differences from species to species. In human eosinophils, the predominant metabolites of arachidonic acid are products of the 15-lipoxygenase enzymes (4), with 15-HETE being the major metabolite (Fig. 10-2). Evidence that 11-HETE is the major metabolite has not been confirmed (5). Leukotrienes derived from 15-HPETE are also formed (4). In murine eosinophils, 12-HETE is the predominant product, with 15-HETE being only slightly less plentiful (6). Small amounts of LTB_4, LTC_4, and LTD_4, were found to be produced by horse eosinophils (7). Small amounts of PGEs have been reported to be synthesized by eosinophils (8,9a), however, more recent studies have not been able to confirm this.

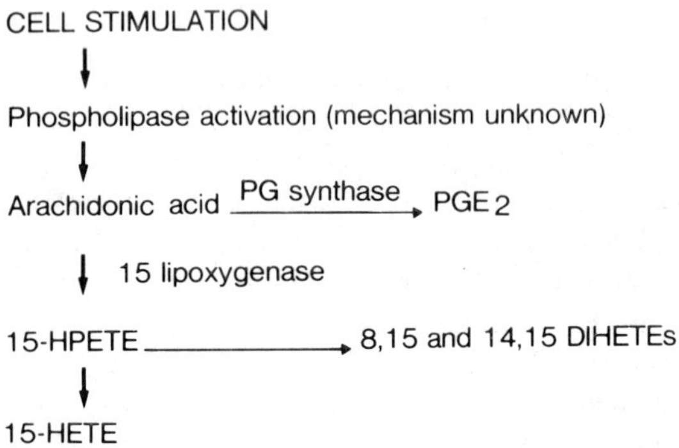

Fig. 10-2 The pathways of arachidonic acid metabolism in human eosinophils. Leukotriene B_4 (LTB_4), LTC_4, 5, 15-di-HETE and two isomers of LTB_4, (5(S), 12(R)-6-trans-LTB_4 and 5(S), 12(S)-b-trans-LTB_4), may also be produced (see text), but it will be important to confirm that these were not produced by small amounts of contaminating neutrophils or basophils. 15-HPETE = 15-hydroperoxyeicosatetraenoic acid; 15-HETE = 15-hydroxyeicosatetraenoic acid.

One recent investigation suggests 15-HETE is the predominant product only when external arachidonic acid is added. When human eosinophils were stimulated by the calcium ionophore A23187 in the absence of external arachidonic acid, roughly equivalent amounts of 15-HETE, 5,15-di-HETE, LTB_4, LTC_4 and two isomers of LTB_4 were formed (9b).

IV. EFFECT OF ARACHIDONIC ACID METABOLITES ON EOSINOPHILS

A. Effect of Endogenous Arachidonic Acid Metabolites on Eosinophils

LTB_4, 5-HPETE, and 5-HETE have been shown to be chemotactic for human eosinophils (10). 15-HPETE and 15-HETE have not yet been evaluated as to their possible effects on eosinophil chemotaxis. Murine eosinophils respond chemotactically to 12-HETE, the predominant product from these cells (11). Murine eosinophil chemotaxis stimulated by eosinophil-stimulation promoter is inhibited by lipoxygenase inhibitors, providing evidence that the 12-HETE or perhaps LTB_4 generated endogenously play a role in the eosinophil chemotaxis (10).

LTB_4 also promotes eosinophil-mediated complement-dependent killing of the schistosomula of *Schistosoma mansoni* (12).

B. Exogenously Derived Arachidonic Acid Metabolites

Eosinophil chemotactic factor from neutrophils, mast cells, and macrophages is derived from arachidonic acid through a lipoxygenase pathway and may be identical to LTB_4.

HHT and 12-HETE from platelets are both chemotactic for human eosinophils (13). PGD_2 from mast cells shows potent and selective enhancement of eosinophil movement (14).

PGE_1 inhibits eosinophil adhesion to glass capillary tubes (15). This effect is probably mediated by a PGE_1-stimulated rise in eosinophil cAMP, as dibutyryl cAMP has a similar effect. PGE_1 and PGE_2 both inhibit eosinophil chemotaxis stimulated by C5a (13).

V. RELEASE OF ARACHIDONIC ACID FROM EOSINOPHIL PHOSPHOLIPIDS

Murine eosinophils produce 12-HETE in response to eosinophil-stimulation promoter (ESP), implicating ESP in the release of the arachidonic acid precursor from eosinophil phospholipids (5).

VI. SUMMARY AND OVERVIEW

Knowledge of the role of arachidonic acid metabolites in eosinophil function is expanding rapidly but is still incomplete. It is beginning to look as if a lipoxygenase product (15-HPETE, 15-HETE, or LTB_4) might be an endogenous metabolite produced in response to eosinophil activators which mediate cell activation. Eosinophil interaction with mast cells is intriguing. The mast cell product PGD_2 selectively promotes eosinophil movement. Mono-HETES and LTB_4 produced by mast cells attract eosinophils although probably not selectively. Eosinophils attracted to the site of a hypersensitivity reaction, where mast cells are activated, may then produce a number of products including 15-HETE which inhibits the 5-lipoxygenase responsible for producing mast cell leukotrienes. However, recent evidence of LPC_4 production by eosinophils raised the possibility that eosinophils may, under some conditions, promote bronchoconstriction or other symptoms associated with allergies, rather than be just a mast cell/basophil inhibitor.

APPENDIX 10-1 IMPORTANT SPECIES DIFFERENCES

Whereas human and porcine eosinophils produce primarily 15-lipoxygenase products, particularly 15-HETE, guinea pig and mouse eosinophils produce primarily 12-lipoxygenase products. In the case of guinea pig eosinophils, very little 15-HETE is produced (16).

REFERENCES

1. E. J. Goetzl. *Biochem. Biophys. Res. Commun. 106*:270 (1982).
2. J. Y. Vanderhoek, N. S. Tare, J. M. Bailey, A. L. Goldstein, and D. H. Pluznik. *J. Biol. Chem. 257*:12191 (1982).
3. C. F. Nathan and S. J. Klebanoff. *J. Exp. Med. 155*:1291 (1982).
4. J. Turk, R. L. Maas, A. R. Brash, L. J. Roberts, II, and J. A. Oates. *J. Biol. Chem. 257*:7068 (1982).
5. F. Goetzl, P. F. Weller, and F. F. Sun. *J. Immunol. 124*:926 (1980).
6. J. Turk, T. H. Rand, R. L. Maas, J. A. Lawson, A. R. Brash, L. J. Roberts, II. D. G. Colley, and J. A. Oates. *Biochim. Biophys. Acta 750*:78 (1983).
7. A. Jorg, W. R. Henderson, R. C. Murphy, and S. J. Klebanoff. *J. Exp. Med. 155*:390 (1982).
8. T. Hubscher. *J. Immunol. 114*:1379 (1975).
9. T. Hubscher. *J. Immunol. 114*:1389 (1975).

9a. W. R. Henderson, J. B. Harley, and A. S. Fauchi. *Immunology 51*: 679 (1984).

10. L. Nagy, T. H. Lee, E. J. Goetzl, W. C. Pickett, and A. B. Kay. *Clin. Exp. Immunol. 47*:541 (1982).
11. T. H. Rand, J. Turk, R. L. Maas, and D. G. Colley. *J. Immunol. 129*: 1239 (1982).
12. R. Moqbel, P. Suzanne, E. Sass-Kuhn, E. J. Goetzl, and A. B. Kay. *Clin. Exp. Immunol. 52*:519 (1983).
13. E. J. Goetzl and R. R. Gorman. *J. Immunol. 120*:526 (1978).
14. E. J. Goetzl, P. F. Weller, and F. H. Valone. *Adv. Inflammation Res. 1*:157 (1979).
15. R. E. Bryant and M. C. Sutcliffe. *J. Clin. Invest. 54*:1241 (1974).
16. D. M. Smith, L. Boies, E. Haus, M. Makooi-Moorehead, and J. G. White. *Fed. Proc. 42*:917 (1983).

11
Monocytes

The blood monocyte can enter tissues to become a tissue macrophage. Since macrophages and monocytes are related, this section will mention some data obtained using macrophages, as well as data from monocytes.

I. THE ANATOMY OF THE MONOCYTE

The monocyte contains a single, large, irregular, kidney-shaped or multi-lobed nucleus (Fig. 11-1). Within the nucleus are one or two small nucleoli, usually visible only by electron microscopy. An eccentrically located centrosome (golgi, centromeres with emanating microtubules) is present. Two populations of granules are distributed randomly in the cytoplasm, one peroxidase positive containing lysosomal enzymes and one peroxidase negative. Mitochondria, rough endoplasmic reticulum, ribosomes, and polysomes are scattered in the cytoplasm. Small numbers of glycogen particles are present. A non-specific esterase present diffusely in monocytes is frequently used as a marker for cells of the monocyte/macrophage lineage.

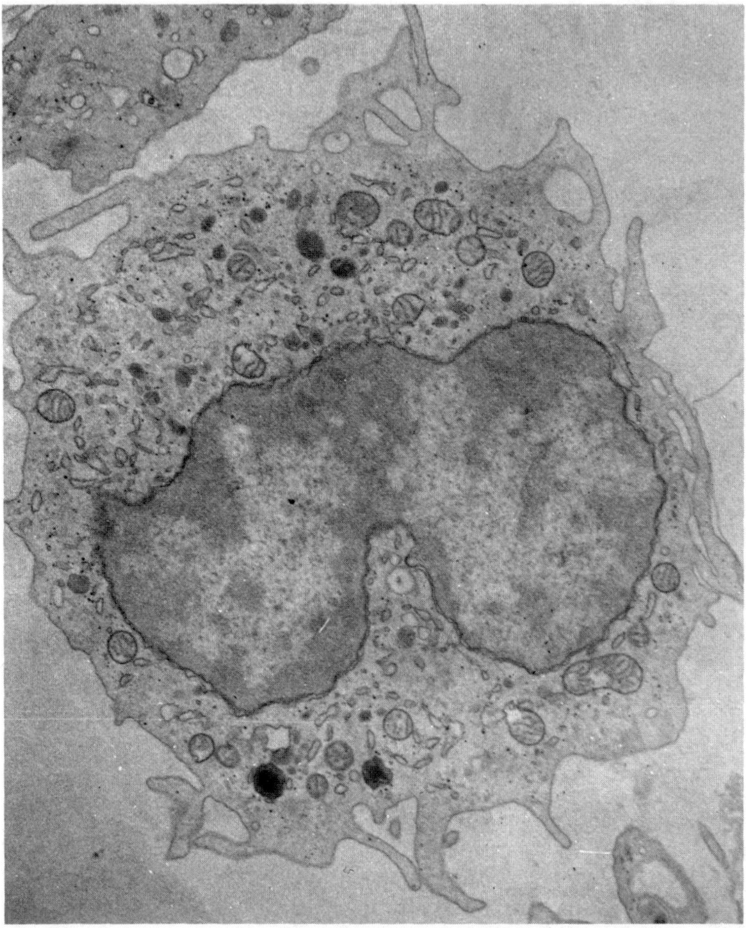

Fig. 11-1 An electron micrograph of a human blood monocyte. (×10,900.)

II. THE LIPIDS OF MONOCYTES

Phosphatidylcholine (46%) is the principal phospholipid of human monocytes, with phosphatidylethanolamine (29%), sphingomyelin (9%), phosphatidylinositol and lysophosphatidylcholine (7%), and phosphatidylserine (5%) present to a lesser extent (1). These proportions are similar to those in lymphocytes, but compared with other human blood cells, phosphatidylcholine is relatively increased and sphingomyelin relatively decreased. Arachidonic acid constitutes about 20 mol% of all fatty acids in human monocyte phospholipids (1,2). This percentage is much higher than that in granulocytes, but similar to that in lymphocytes (1). Alkylacylglycerol phosphorylcholine represents a substantial proportion of choline glycerophospholipids in guinea pig peritoneal macrophages (14%) and rat alveolar macrophages (35%) (3,4). Since this form of phosphatidylcholine is important as a precursor of platelet-activating factor, the finding is consistent with the relatively high production of platelet-activating factor by macrophages. Monocytes respond to C5a or to bacterial products in a similar fashion to neutrophils. Consistent with their slower movement however, monocyte/macrophages generally arrive at sites of infection or inflammation in vivo considerably after neutrophils.

III. THE FUNCTION OF THE MONOCYTE

A. Chemotaxis

Monocytes can show significant chemotaxis although their movement is slower than granulocytes.

B. Adherence and Spreading

Monocytes will readily adhere to surfaces such as a glass slide and will spread out on the surface.

C. Phagocytosis and Killing

Monocytes are very actively phagocytic. Phagocytosis and killing of microorganisms is facilitated by the prior attachment of opsonins such as IgG antibodies for the complement component C3b to the microorganisms. Receptors for the Fc portion of the IgG or for C3b on the macrophage surface are important for these processes.

D. Regulation of and Interaction with Lymphocyte Function

For many antigens, processing by monocytes/macrophages is essential for lymphocyte recognition of and response to the antigen. Monocytes also produce chemicals, including prostaglandins, that modulate lymphocyte responsiveness.

E. Transformation

An important property of monocytes is their ability to transform into cells with altered and/or enhanced activities. The full range of transformations possible and the precise characteristic of cells in each state are only partly understood. Monocytes entering tissues may settle in the liver as Kupfer cells (slightly more than half), may enter the lung to become pulmonary macrophages (about 15%), may reside in the peritoneum (about 8%) or may travel to diverse sites including bone (ie. as osteoclasts). Cells at such sites may remain relatively quiescent or be further transformed into activated cells with particular characteristics, whose nature may depend in part on the specific stimulus. Exposure to lipopolysaccharide and adherence to a surface are two examples of stimuli which alter the properties of monocytes/macrophages.

IV. ARACHIDONIC ACID METABOLISM BY MONOCYTES/MACROPHAGES

A. Peripheral Blood Monocytes

Human peripheral blood monocytes synthesize both cyclooxygenase and lipoxygenase metabolites (Fig. 11-2) (5-11). The relative proportion of metabolites from the two pathways varies with the stimulus. When opsonized zymosan or immunoglobin G complex-coated Sephadex beads were used, cyclooxygenase metabolites predominated (11a). In contrast, with A23187 as the stimulus, lipoxygenase products were the major metabolites (about 70%). The major cyclooxygenase metabolite of human monocytes is thromboxane B_2. HHT (12L-hydroxy-5,8,10-heptadecatrienoic acid) is also produced concomitant with thromboxane as in platelets. PGE_2, $PGF_{2\alpha}$, and 6-keto $PGF_{1\alpha}$ are produced in lesser amounts. The ratio of

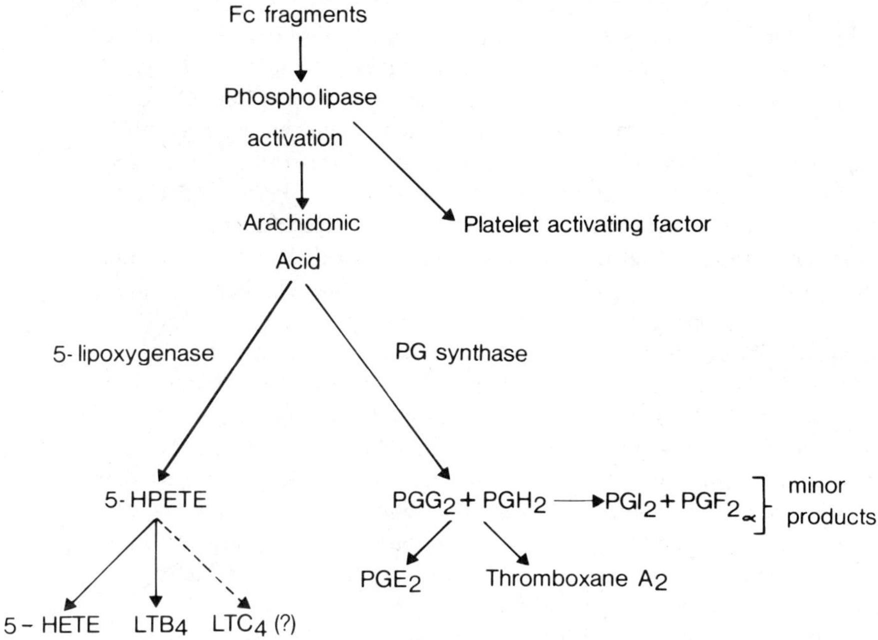

Fig. 11-2. Pathways of arachidonic acid metabolism in human monocytes. PGE_2 and thromboxane A_2 are the major cyclooxygenase-derived products.

thromboxane B_2 to PGE_2 has varied from 2.7 to 12, depending on the experiment, in three separate reports (6,9,11a). One study using gas chromatography-mass spectrometry failed to detect any $PGF_{2\alpha}$ or 6-keto $PGF_{1\alpha}$ (6). Pawlowski et al., who do report their presence, show them as very small peaks on their HPLC tracings (11a). Further confirmation of their identity is desirable.

The principal lipoxygenase metabolite of human monocytes is 5-HETE (11a). Significant amounts of LTB_4 and LTC_4 are also produced in response to A23187, but less so with zymosan (11b). 12-HETE was present to a small extent, but its production was in proportion to the number of contaminating platelets. With almost all platelets removed, the production of 12-HETE was barely detectable.

Some evidence suggests PGE_2 production occurs primarily in a subgroup of low-density monocytes (10). Since thromboxane B_2 was not assessed in the study, it remains for further investigation to clarify whether both thromboxane and PGE_2 production are increased in this subgroup or whether there is a monocyte subpopulation which can synthesize primarily PGE_2. This would be important to know for better understanding of monocyte regulation of lymphocyte function (see Chs. 12 and 17).

Studies with peritoneal macrophages in mice and guinea pigs raise the possibility that the relative production of thromboxane B_2 and PGE_2 may vary dramatically, depending on how the cells were obtained. In one study resident mouse peritoneal macrophages produced less PGE_2 than BCG-induced cells (Table 11-1) (12). In another study, resident guinea pig macrophages produced less PGE_2 than adherent starch-induced macrophages (4). It is tempting to speculate that certain stimuli may redirect monocyte/macrophage prostaglandin and thromboxane synthesis. This could require synthesis of new proteins by the macrophages or might just require some change in regulatory cofactor. The conversion of BCG-induced peritoneal macrophages from predominant PGE_2 production to predominant thromboxane B_2 production by changing from McCoy's 5A culture medium to Dulbecco's modified Eagles's medium (12) suggests relatively subtle factors could be important. The importance of these studies for human monocytes/macrophages is that it is premature to conclude that the human cells always produce primarily thromboxane B_2. There

Table 11-1 Variation in the Ratio of PGE_2/TxB_2 Production by Macrophages

Species	Type of peritoneal macrophages	PGE_2 (pg/10^6 cells)	TxB_2 (pg/10^6 cells)	Ratio of $PGE_2 TxB_2$
Mouse	Resident	243	269	0.9
	Peptone-induced	123	345	0.4
	BCG-induced	510	322	1.6
Guinea pig	Resident	4,700	12,000	0.4
	Starch-induced	9,200	11,600	0.8
	Starch-induced and Adherent	21,000	2,300	9.5

are likely to be conditions where PGE_2 production is predominant, and this has important implications for monocyte/macrophage regulation of lymphocytes through production of PGE_2.

B. Alveolar Macrophage

Synthesis of PGE_2 by human alveolar macrophages was 10-fold higher than that of peripheral blood monocytes, whereas synthesis of thromboxane B_2 was about 25-fold increased (6). Further studies are necessary to understand whether tissue macrophages generally have a greater synthetic capacity than blood monocytes. Human alveolar macrophages also produce significant amounts of leukotriene B_4 (up to 200 ng/10^6 cells in response to A23187 and 80 ng/10^6 cells in response to opsonized zymosan), as well as a small amount of LTC_4 (10 ng/10^6 cells in response to A23187) (13a,13b).

V. EFFECTS OF ARACHIDONIC ACID AND METABOLITES ON MONOCYTE FUNCTION

An evaluation of the influence of arachidonic acid and metabolites on monocyte function must first address two separate types of monocyte/macrophage stimulation. First, there is the relatively quick "activation" which occurs when macrophages are exposed to A23187, platelet-activating factor, leukotriene C, zymosan particles, Fc fragments, and so on. This is an immediate reaction of monocytes or macrophages which can be assessed by evaluating the production of reactive oxygen species, including superoxide and H_2O_2, and is important for phagocytosis and killing. There is also a "transformation" which macrophages can undergo from a relatively dormant cell to a much more active one. The second type of activation appears particularly important for macrophage tumoricidal activity. Present data can be best explained by a promoting effect of PGE_2 on conversion of the "resting" monocyte/macrophage to the "transformed-active" state, but there is also an inhibitory effect of PGE_2 on the end activity whether adhesion, spreading, chemiluminescence, or tumor killing (see below). Throughout this section, I have chosen to use the terms "immediate" activation and "transformed-active" state to facilitate discussion of these separate types of processes. Much of the present literature uses the single term "activated" to describe both processes, and this confuses the issue.

A. Conversion of Monocytes/Macrophages from Basal to the Transformed-Active State

1. PGE_2 and $PGF_{2\alpha}$

Lipopolysaccharide transforms resident mouse peritoneal macrophages into cells with a high capacity to kill tumor cells. Indomethacin blocks this effect of lipopolysaccharide (12,14a). The effect of lipopolysaccharide can be mimicked by addition of PGE_2 or $PGF_{2\alpha}$ (12). Since lipopolysaccharide induces PGE_2 synthesis in these macrophages, the results have been used to indicate that PGE_2 is the active mediator stimulated by lipopolysaccharide which converts macrophages from the resting to transformed-active state (Fig. 11-3). Whether other types of monocytes/macrophages respond similarly and whether other factors in addition to PGE_2 may be important need to be assessed.

It is possible that some of the other positive effects of PGE_2 to enhance macrophage function may be similarly associated with PGE_2-enhanced macrophage transformation. For example PGE_1 and PGE_2 were found to en-

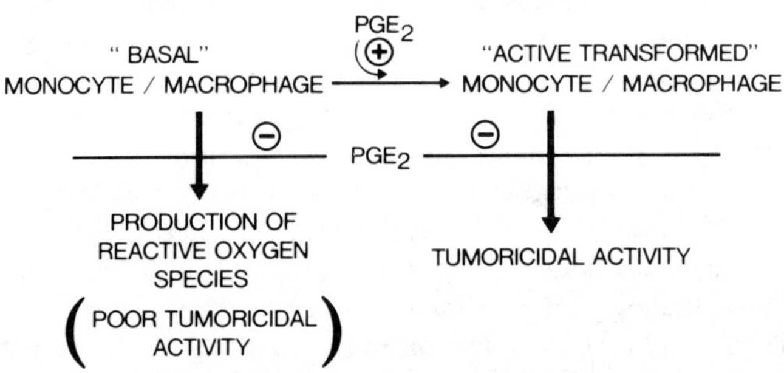

Fig. 11-3 PGE_2 promotes the conversion of mouse peritoneal macrophages to a cell which I call here a transformed-active cell which has the new property of being able to kill tumor cells. Paradoxically, PGE_2 appears to inhibit the more immediate activation events of either the resting cell (i.e., superoxide production) or the transformed-active cell. The longer time frame needed for the positive effects suggests that PGE_2 might promote synthesis of new proteins. The inhibitory effect of PGE_2 on immediate activation events could well result from the action of PGE_2 to raise cellular cyclic AMP to inhibit monocyte/macrophage phospholipases and to inhibit the secretion of already synthesized granule proteins.

hance the collagenase production by endotoxin-stimulated cultured guinea pig peritoneal macrophages (14b). Inhibition of endotoxin-mediated collagenase production by indomethacin suggests this effect is mediated by PGE_2 produced by macrophages in response to endotoxin. Similarly, PGE_1 and PGE_2 augment the procoagulant activity of lipopolysaccharide stimulated rabbit alveolar macrophages, and can overcome inhibition of this process by indomethacin (14c). In the latter reaction PGE_2 was not effective unless the macrophages were also stimulated by lipopolysaccharide suggesting other components of the cellular response in addition to PGE_2 were important.

Phagocytosis of sheep erythrocytes by mouse peritoneal macrophages was enhanced up to 30% by PGE_2, $PGF_{1\alpha}$, $PGF_{1\beta}$, and PGA_1 (15). $PGF_{2\alpha}$ was the most active, suggesting this is not related to effects of prostaglandins on macrophage cAMP. The mechanism of the effect is unknown.

Neither PGEs, PGFs, nor PGBs are directly chemotactic for monocytes. However, PGE_2 can significantly enhance the chemotaxis of human monocytes in response to complement-activated human serum (16). PGE_1, in contrast, had no effect.

2. Thromboxane A_2

The effect of thromboxane A_2 on monocytes is unknown. This is an important question in view of the considerable thromboxane A_2 production by monocytes and macrophages. Studies with thromboxane synthetase inhibitors might provide helpful information to answer this question.

3. Leukotrienes B_4 and C_4

It is possible that the inhibition of monocyte generation of leukocyte inhibitory factor by leukotrienes B_4 and C_4 might be related to inhibition of the conversion of monocytes/macrophages to the transformed-active state (17). Leukotriene C_4 appears to promote more immediate events such as the macrophage oxidative burst (see below).

B. Immediate Activation of Monocytes

1. Activating Lipids

Arachidonic acid. Arachidonic acid has been shown to induce chemiluminescence of phagocytosing monocytes (30).

15-HPETE. 15-HPETE stimulates chemiluminescence of unstimulated or phagocytosing macrophages (30). These results implicate a lipoxygenase metabolite as important in monocyte activation.

Leukotriene C_4. Leukotriene C_4 excites superoxide and hydrogen peroxide production in guinea pig peritoneal macrophages (18), and could be an important endogenously produced activator. Support for this idea comes from studies showing inhibition of the A23187-induced production of reactive oxygen species by lipoxygenase inhibitors (19a). However, since macrophages produce other lipoxygenase products in addition to LTC_4, these may also be important.

Leukotriene D_4. Leukotriene D_4, but not LTC_4 or LTE_4 promote the adhesiveness of pig pulmonary alveolar macrophages (19b).

Platelet-Activating factor. Platelet-activating factor will stimulate chemiluminescence and hydrogen peroxide production in guinea pig peritoneal macrophages (20). Since it is produced in considerable quantities by monocytes, it might be an endogenous activator. Studies with inhibitors of the production or effects of platelet-activating factor are needed to properly assess this possibility.

2. Inhibitory Prostaglandins

PGE_1, PGE_2, and PGI_2. PGE_1 and PGE_2 both inhibit zymosan stimulation of macrophage chemiluminescence (21). PGE_1 and PGI_2 also inhibit the monocyte production of platelet-activating factor in response to Fc, C3b, C3d, and A23187 (22). Since a phospholipase activity appears to be necessary for platelet-activating factor production, and may be important for the production of the activated oxygen species, it is likely that PGE_1, PGE_2, and PGI_2 exert their inhibitory effects on these immediate activation processes through their established action to stimulate macrophage adenylate cyclase levels to raise cell cAMP levels (23-26).

The inhibitory effect of PGE_1 and PGE_2 on the tumoricidal activity of interferon-activated (transformed-active) macrophages of mice (24), and of transformed-active macrophages of mice pretreated with BCG (27), may also be related to inhibition by prostaglandins of the immediate activation process involved in the generation of active oxygen radicals.

Taffet et al. (26) have used the lesser effectiveness of PGI_2 in inhibiting the tumor cell killing of lipopolysaccharide transformed-active macrophages to argue against a direct relationship between the effect of inhibitory prostaglandins and cell cAMP. However, the instability of PGI_2 relative to PGE_2 makes this comparison difficult.

PGE_1 and PGE_2 inhibit the adhesion and spreading properties of mouse peritoneal macrophages (23). PGA_2 and PGB_2 were much less effective, while $PGF_{2\alpha}$ had no effect. This inhibition may also be related to a cAMP-mediated effect to inhibit cellular adhesion and spreading.

VI. THE RELEASE OF ARACHIDONIC ACID FROM MONOCYTES/MACROPHAGES

For arachidonic acid metabolites to be important in monocyte/macrophage physiology, they must be produced in response to physiologic stimuli. This is indeed the case. Arachidonic acid release and synthesis of prostaglandins and related products from monocytes/macrophages can be stimulated by lymphokines, zymosan, antibody-coated erythrocytes, *Corynebacterium parvum,* endotoxin, antigen-antibody complexes including IgE-immune complexes, Fc fragments, aggregated IgG, and the calcium ionophore A23187 (7,9,10,17,21-25,28a). The pathway for release of arachidonic acid from monocytes has not been well studied although evidence for involvement of both a phospholipase C acting on polyphosphoinositides, and phospholipase A_2 acting on phosphatidylinositol have been presented, with the specific pathway utilized depending on the stimulus (28b). Work of Albert and Snider suggests that arachidonic acid may be preferentially released from alkyl-20:4: glycerol phosphoryl choline, providing both arachidonic acid and 1-alkyl-glycerol phosphoryl choline, the precursor of platelet-activating factor (3).

A. Effect of Cyclic AMP

Analogues of cyclic AMP including dibutyryl cyclic AMP and 8-Bromo-cyclic AMP have been shown to inhibit the zymosan-induced release of arachidonic acid from the mouse resident peritoneal macrophages (29a). These findings suggest that raised cellular cyclic AMP levels in monocytes/macrophages, as in platelets (see Chs. 4 and 6) inhibit cell phospholipases involved in arachidonic acid release.

B. Effect of Interferon

Using resident peritoneal macrophages from mice, it has been shown that fibroblast interferon beta (IFN-β) can exert a substantial inhibition of the release of arachidonic acid from macrophage phospholipids (29a). IFN-β appeared to exert its effect by raising the level of cyclic AMP in the cells. The lowered PGE_2 production by these macrophages as a result of IFN-β was associated with a significant decrease in the ability of the macrophages to suppress lymphocyte proliferation and lymphokine production. A similar phenomenon appears to occur in human monocytes where IFN-β has been shown to produce marked inhibition of PGE production (29a).

C. Adherent Versus Non-Adherent Cells

Major differences exist between adherent macrophages and those in suspension. In general adherent cells are functionally more active—for example, being able to express Ia antigen and produce interleukin I in response to lymphokine challenge, or to show enhanced superoxide production. Using thioglycollate elicited peritoneal macrophages from mice, Kunkel and Duque showed that these cells showed high basal PGE_2 production (29c). They speculated that the high PGE_2 levels kept the cells in a less responsive state. Within 2 hours of these cells adhering to plastic dishes, PGE_2 production fell dramatically. The lower PGE_2 production of adherent macrophages was associated with increased superoxide formation by these cells in response to zymosan or phorbol myristate acetate. The biochemical step influenced by adherence was not determined but might well be the release of arachidonic acid, usually the rate-limiting step in cellular prostaglandin formation. Further studies are clearly needed to assess this possibility and to determine whether the adherence of other types of monocytes/macrophages is associated with similar changes in arachidonic acid metabolism.

VII. STUDIES USING INHIBITORS

Studies using inhibitors of the conversion of macrophages from the resting to transformed-active state have been discussed earlier. Here, we are concerned only with the immediate activation process. Inhibitors of prostaglandin synthesis (aspirin and indomethacin) have been found to have no effect on macrophage chemiluminescence stimulated by A23187 or during phagocytosis of zymosan (19a,30). In contrast, lipoxygenase inhibitors, including nordihydroguiaretic acid and eicosatetraynoic acid, were effective inhibitors. The results provide support for a lipoxygenase product being an endogenous activator of monocytes, but more data are needed in this respect.

VIII. OTHER LIPID MEDIATORS

A. Platelet-Activating Factor

Human monocytes secrete significant amounts of platelet-activating factor in response to receptor-specific activation involving Fc, C3b, and C3d receptors, and in response to A23187 (22,31).

IX. OVERVIEW

Present data are most consistent with monocytes/macrophages existing in two forms, a basal and a transformed-active form. Both basal and transformed-active cells can undergo an immediate form of stimulation with production of reactive oxygen species, including superoxide and hydrogen peroxide. A monocyte/macrophage lipoxygenase product is implicated as an endogenous activator produced in response to activating agents such as A23187 and zymosan particles. Prostaglandins which raise cAMP levels in monocytes/macrophages, including PGE_2, PGE_1, and PGI_2, are effective inhibitors of the production of reactive oxygen species, and cAMP appears to have as a major action, as in other cell types, inhibition of cellular phospholipases.

However, studies of the effect of PGE_2 on monocytes/macrophages suggest that there are clearly instances where PGE_2 can promote positive changes in macrophages. In one example, PGE_2 clearly promotes the conversion of resident mouse peritoneal macrophages to cells which I have termed transformed-active macrophages which have a particular role in tumor cell killing. It is paradoxical that while PGE_2 promotes the conversion of the resting to the transformed-active cell, it nevertheless can inhibit the effect of this cell to kill tumor cells. Clearly, much more work needs to be done to better understand how PGE_2 can have both positive and negative effects on cellular function. The role of macrophage prostaglandin and leukotriene production in modulating functional changes associated with macrophage adherence to surfaces also needs further study.

A considerable literature has focused on PGE_2 production by monocytes/macrophages being an important negative regulator of lymphocyte function. Recent studies show human blood monocytes ordinarily produce primarily thromboxane A_2 and very little PGE_2. Whether there are conditions where human monocyte/macrophage PGE_2 production is augmented relative to thromboxane A_2 is an area requiring further investigation. Certainly, many studies are consistent with monocyte/macrophage PGE_2 production, when it does occur, as being important in suppressing lymphocyte proliferation. A role of interferon to inhibit monocyte/macrophage synthesis of PGE_2 and the associated suppression of lymphocyte activity may be one mechanism whereby interferon can promote immune responsiveness.

APPENDIX 11-1 IMPORTANT SPECIES DIFFERENCES

1. Guinea pig macrophages have a much higher content of sphingomyelin (19%) than human blood monocytes (31).
2. Mouse peritoneal macrophages have been reported to synthesize predominantly PGE_2 and PGI_2 (32), in contrast to guinea pig peritoneal cells which make primarily thromboxane A_2 and PGE_2, and human blood monocytes which make primarily thromboxane A_2 (as assessed by production of its metabolite—thromboxane B_2). It is possible that these differences may relate more to conditions used to obtain and culture the cells rather than to real species differences.

REFERENCES

1. G. V. Marinetti and K. Cattieu. *Chem. Phys. Lipids 31*:169 (1982).
2. T. P. Stossel, R. J. Mason, and A. L. Smith. *J. Clin. Invest. 54*:638 (1974).
3. T. Sugiura, Y. Onuma, N. Sekiguchi, and K. Waku. *Biochim. Biophys. Acta 712*:515 (1982).
4. D. H. Albert and F. Snyder. *Fed. Proc. 42*:710 (1983).
5. J. I. Kurland and R. Bockman. *J. Exp. Med. 147*:952 (1978).
6. J. Morley, M. A. Bray, R. W. Jones, D. H. Nugteren, and D. A. van Dorp. *Prostaglandins 17*:730 (1979).
7. J. H. Passwell, J-M. Dayer and E. Merler. *J. Immunol. 123*:115, (1979).
8. M. S. Kennedy, J. D. Stobo, and M. E. Goldyne. *Prostaglandins 20*: 135 (1980).
9. M. E. Goldyne and J. D. Stobo. *Prostaglandins. 24*:623 (1982).
10. K. Brune, M. Glatt, H. Kalin, and B. A. Peskar. *Nature. 274*:261 (1978).
11a. N. A. Pawlowski, G. Kaplan, A. L. Hamill, Z. A. Cohn, and W. A. Scott. *J. Exp. Med. 158*:393 (1983).
11b. R. A. Lewis and K. F. Austen. *J. Clin. Invest. 73*:889 (1984).
12. M. E. Snider, R. H. Fertel, and B. S. Zwilling. *Cell Immunol. 74*:234 (1982).

13a. A. O. S. Fels, N. A. Pawlowski, E. B. Cramer, T. K. C. King, Z. A. Cohn and W. A. Scott. *Proc. Natl. Acad. Sci. U.S.A. 79*:7866 (1982).
13b. P. Godard, M. Damon, F. B. Michel, E. J. Corey, K. F. Austen and R. A. Lewis. *Clin. Res. 31*:549A (1983).
14a. B-E. Drysdale and H. S. Shin. *J. Immunol. 127*:760 (1981).
14b. L. M. Wahl, C. E. Olsen, A. L. Sandberg, and S. E. Mergenhagen. *Proc. Natl. Acad. Sci. U.S.A. 74*:4955 (1977).
14c. R. G. Sitrin, H. B. Kaltreider, and M. E. Goldyne. *J. Immunol. 132*: 867 (1984).
15. E. Razin, S. Bauminger, and A. Globerson. *J. Reticuloendothel. Sco. 23*:237 (1978).
16. W. McClatchey and R. Snyderman. *Prostaglandins 12*:415 (1976).
17. D. G. Payan, F. H. Valone, and E. J. Goetzl. *Fed. Proc. 42*:444 (1983).
18. H. P. Harting. *Eur. J. Pharmacol. 91*:159 (1983).
19a. L. K. Lim, N. H. Hunt, and M. J. Weideman. *Biochem. Biophys. Res. Commun. 114*:549 (1983).
19b. D. J. L. McIver, N. A. M. Paterson and S. Schurch. Prostaglandins and Leukotrienes '84, May 8-11, Washington, D.C., Abstract 142 (1984).
20. H-D. Harting, M. J. Parnham, J. Winkelmann, W. Englberger, and U. Hadding. *Int. J. Immunopharmacol. 5*:115 (1983).
21. M. J. Weidemann, B. A. Peskar, K. Wrogemann, E. T. Rietschel, H. Staudinger, and H. Fischer. *FEBS Lett. 89*:136 (1978).
22. G. Camussi, F. Bussolino, C. Tetta, W. Piacibello, and M. Aglietta. *Int. Arch. Allergy Appl. Immunol. 70*:245 (1983).
23. W. D. Cantarow, H. T. Cheung, and G. Sundharadas. *Prostaglandins 16*: 39 (1978).
24. R. M. Schultz, N. A. Pavlidis, W. A. Stylos, and M. A. Chirigos. *Science 202*:320 (1978).
25. D. Gemsa, L. Steggeman, J. Menzel, and G. Till. *J. Immunol. 114*: 1422 (1975).
26. S. M. Taffet, T. E. Eurell, and S. W. Russell. *Prostaglandins 24*:763 (1982).
27. M. E. Snider, R. H. Fertel, and B. S. Zwilling. *Cell Immunol. 74*:234 (1982).
28a. J. L. Humes, R. J. Bonney, L. Pelus, M. E. Dahlgren, S. J. Sadowski, F. A. Kuehl, Jr., and P. Davies. *Nature 269*:149 (1977).
28b. A. Emilsson and R. Sundler. *J. Biol. Chem. 259*:3111 (1984).
29a. D. Boraschi, S. Censini, M. Bartalini, G. Scapigliati, G. Barbarulli, E. Vicenzi, M. B. Donati and A. Tabliabue. *J. Immunol. 132*:1987 (1984).
29b. P. Dore-Duffy, W. Perry and H. H. Kuo. *Cell. Immunol. 79*:232 (1983).
29c. S. L. Kunkel and R. E. Duque. *Prostaglandins. 26*:893 (1983).

30. R. L. Smith and M. J. Weidemann. *Biochem. Biophys. Res. Commun.* *97*:973 (1980).
31. G. Camussi, M. Aglietta, R. Coda, F. Bussolino, W. Piacibello and C. Tetta. *Immunology 42*:191 (1981).

BIBLIOGRAPHY

R. Van Furth. *Birth Defects. 19*:3 (1983).

R. Van Furth and W. Slutter. *Trans. Roy. Soc. Trop. Med. Hygeine. 77*: 614 (1983).

12

Lymphocytes

I. ANATOMY

Circulating lymphocytes vary in size from small to large. All have a round to kidney-shaped nucleus with a nucleolus (not ordinarily visible on smears because of the perinucleolar dense chromatin) (Fig. 12-1). A small golgi complex is present. Within the cytoplasm mitochondria are prominent, whereas only small amounts of dispersed glycogen are present. Some smooth and rough endoplasmic reticulum is present, as are a few lysosomes and the occasional Gall body. The lymphocyte surface almost always has microvillosities important for micropinocytosis.

II. LIPIDS

Compared with other blood cells, lymphocyte phosphatidylcholine content (about 44% of cell phospholipid) is increased, and the sphingomyelin content (about 10%) is decreased (1). Phosphatidylethanolamine (29%) and phosphatidylserine plus phosphatidylinositol (13%) are similar to other blood cells. Cardiolipin (3.2%) is much higher than in other blood cells. Arachidonic

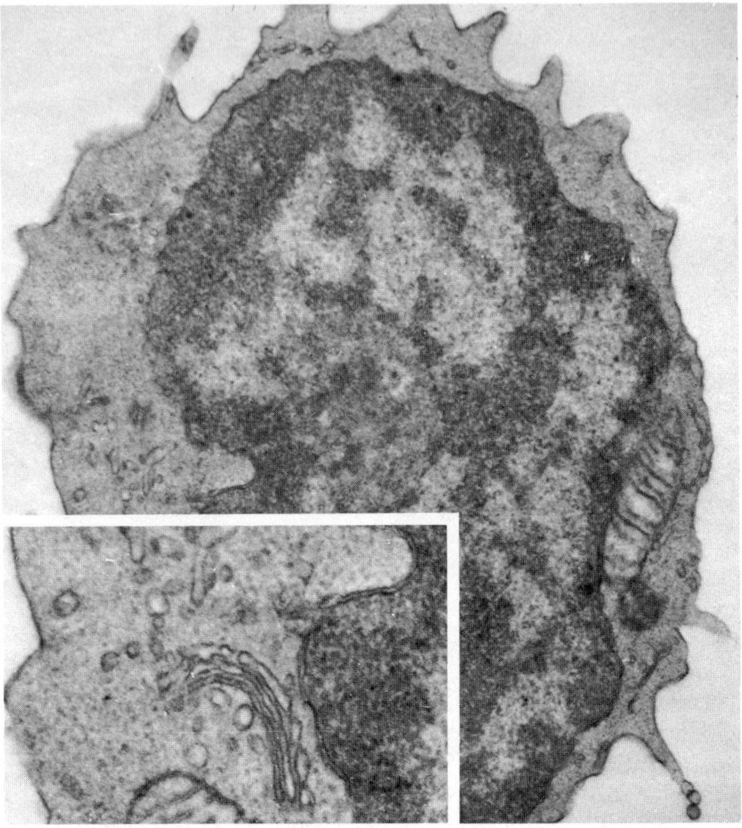

Fig. 12-1 A small lymphocyte with a kidney-shaped nucleus. A golgi region is present in the region where the nucleus is indented (enlarged, bottom left). (×20,700, insert ×36,000.)

acid constitutes about 20 mol% of all fatty acids in human lymphocyte phospholipids, a proportion similar to monocytes (2).

III. FUNCTIONS OF LYMPHOCYTES

There are several classes of lymphocytes with different functional properties.

A. T Cells

T lymphocytes have an important role in cellular immunity. They show mitogenic responses to lectins such as phytohemagglutinin (PHA) and concanavalin A.

B. B Cells

B lymphocytes are the lymphocytes responsible for production of immunoglobulins. Peripheral blood B cells differentiate into antibody forming and secreting plasma cells.

C. Suppressor and Helper Cells

Cells which produce soluble mediators that inhibit all T- and B-cell responses are called suppressor cells. Helper cells, in contrast, promote such responses.

D. Natural Killer Cells

Natural killer (NK) cells are large granular lymphocytes that possess the capacity to destroy tumor cells and some normal cells without previous exposure to the target cell. NK cells, which are selectively deficient in the Chediak-Higashi syndrome (3), have physical and functional characteristics similar to cytolytic T lymphocytes, but contain some lysosomal granules similar to myeloid cells (4). NK cells can be found at sites of tumors in animal models and may possess migratory and motile capabilities. NK cell cytotoxic activity is inhibited by agents which raise cellular cAMP or interfere with microtubules and is enhanced by cGMP analogues and agents which raise cellular cGMP levels (5-7). In some studies the effects of modulating cGMP levels was small, and whether this is really an effector substance must be questioned.

IV. PRODUCTION OF PROSTAGLANDINS AND RELATED CHEMICALS BY LYMPHOCYTES

Lymphocytes produce very little in the way of prostaglandins and related arachidonic acid metabolites compared with platelets, monocytes, and neutrophils. In mixed populations of lymphocytes and monocytes or macrophages, almost all of the prostaglandins produced are monocyte or macrophage derived (8-11). Initial evidence suggested the production of small amounts of 5-HETE, 12-HETE, PGE_2, $PGF_{2\alpha}$, and thromboxane A_2 by lymphocytes (10-13). More recent studies using purified human T lymphocytes have established that 15-HETE is the major arachidonate metabolite of these cells, with considerable amounts of 11-HETE and 5-HETE and small amounts of LTB_4 and all trans-5,12-diHETE (14). Additional studies are needed, however, to better define any variations in different T-lymphocyte subpopulations (helper, suppressor etc.) and to learn whether the pattern of arachidonic acid metabolism can change with the conditions of cell stimulation.

V. EFFECTS OF PROSTAGLANDIN PRECURSORS ON LYMPHOCYTE FUNCTION

A. Arachidonic Acid

Low doses (0.3-3 μM) of arachidonic acid added to cells cultured in lipid-free or lipid-poor media can result in substantial increases in thymidine uptake in response to phytohemagglutinin or concanavalin A (15). Linoleic and linolenic acids are less effective.

Exogenous arachidonate at 8 μM was shown to stimulate human T-lymphocyte chemokinesis (16).

High doses (30-100 μM) of arachidonic acid and other long-chain fatty acids inhibit lectin-induced mitogenesis (17,18). This effect could be due to a toxic effect of these fatty acids since the media used contained low levels of albumin.

Arachidonic acid incubated with NK cells inhibits cytotoxicity (19).

VI. EFFECTS OF PROSTAGLANDINS AND RELATED CHEMICALS ON LYMPHOCYTE FUNCTION

A. Inhibitory Effects

Inhibitory effects are dealt with first as they are better understood and more completely characterized. PGE_1 and PGE_2 both inhibit lymphocyte activation by T-cell mitogens such as phytohemagglutin and concanavalin A (20-23). Pokeweed mitogen responses (B cells) are not affected (24); however, antibody formation is inhibited (25). The inhibitory effects of added PGE_1

and PGE_2 can be most clearly demonstrated using T-cell-enriched and monocyte-depleted preparations, perhaps because endogenous monocyte PGE production masks the effects of added prostaglandins (26).

PGE_1 and PGE_2 inhibit NK cell cytotoxicity against tumor target cells (27,28). PGA_1 and PGA_2 also have some inhibitory activity whereas PGB_1, PGB_2, $PGF_{1\alpha}$, and $PGF_{2\alpha}$ are not effective.

The inhibitory effects of these prostaglandins are mediated by a rise in cellular cAMP due to PGE stimulation of lymphocyte adenylate cyclase. The inhibitory effect of cAMP occurs very early on in the mitogen response as shown by PGE_1 and PGE_2 inhibition of PHA and PPD-tuberculin-induced inositol incorporation into phosphatidylinositol (29).

Leukotriene B_4, but not leukotriene C_4, has been found to inhibit T-lymphocyte proliferation and production of leukocyte-inhibitory factor (30a). However, these effects of LTB_4 require relatively high concentrations (10^{-7}-10^{-6} M) and are of relatively small magnitude (maximum effect about 20% inhibition). Studies by others have failed to show any significant effect of either LTB_4 or LTD_4 on the response of a mixed population of peripheral blood lymphocytes to phytohaemagglutinin, concanavalin A or pokeweed mitogen (30a).

15-HETE, itself an arachidonic acid metabolite produced by T lymphocytes and an inhibitor of the 5-lipoxygenase, produces a progressive inhibition of the mitogenic response of mouse spleen cells to the T-cell mitogen PHA. 15-HETE has no effect on the response to the B-cell mitogen-lipopolysaccharide (31).

B. Stimulatory Effects

Kelly and co-workers using inhibitors (see below) have suggested that thromboxane A_2 may stimulate lymphocyte mitogenesis (32). No direct effect of thromboxane A_2 has yet been demonstrated; and indeed this may be difficult since the mitogenic response is evaluated over many hours while thromboxane A_2 has a half-life of about 30 sec, and prolonged exposure to small amounts generated continuously might be important.

LTB_4 and 5-HETE enhance the migration of human T lymphocytes in vitro (33). 5-HETE has also been shown to mimic the effect of PHA in elevating lymphocyte cGMP levels (34).

Leukotriene B_4 augments natural killer cell-mediated cytotoxicity against herpes simplex virus infected and uninfected target cells (35). The maximal effect is seen at very low concentrations of LTB_4 (10^{-10} M), but is of relatively small magnitude.

15-HPETE and LTB_4 can activate T-lymphocytes to become suppressor T-cells (36a,36b,36c). In these studies, OKT_4(+) T-cells incubated with 15-HPETE or LTB_4 resulted in the conversion of these cells to radiation sensitive OKT8(+) suppressor T-cells which inhibit the IgG production of lymphocytes in response to pokeweed mitogen (36b,36c). An alternate mechanism for LTB_4 induced suppression may be via a direct or indirect stimulation of PGE_2 production by monocytes (36a).

In the absence of monocytes, LTB_4 may enhance lymphocyte proliferation in response to mitogens (36d).

LTB_4, LTC_4 and LTD_4 can all promote γ-interferon production of mouse splenic lymphocytes, overcoming, in part, the requirement for the presence of helper cells (36e).

In cyclophosphamide treated mice, PGE_2 has been reported to promote NK cell activity, quite opposite in its effect to inhibit NK cells in normal mice (36f).

C. Studies Using Inhibitors

The use of cyclooxygenase inhibitors has produced varied effects on lymphocyte mitogenesis, perhaps reflecting the conditions used and the balance of stimulatory and inhibitory prostaglandins and thromboxanes (32,37-43). Inhibition has, however, been found in several studies using aspirin and indomethacin (37-39,43a). Since prostaglandins are inhibitory, and thromboxane synthetase inhibitors were also effective inhibitors of lymphocyte mitogenesis, this suggests that the active product might be thromboxane A_2 (32). However, this effect of thromboxane synthetase inhibition could be due to increased PGE_2 resulting from diversion of PGH_2 toward prostaglandin rather than thromboxane synthesis. Similar data using lipoxygenase inhibitors have been used to suggest that a lipoxygenase product may also stimulate lymphocyte mitogenesis and the associated PHA-stimulated rise in cGMP (30b).

With NK cells the addition of indomethacin has been reported to enhance activity (19,43b), although this might have reflected inhibition of PGE_2 production by contaminating monocytes rather than a direct effect of indomethacin on NK cells.

D. Lymphocyte Differentiation

PGE_1 and other agents which elevate lymphocyte cAMP induce the development of early maturation antigens in both T and B cells (44,45). Stimulation by early addition of agents which raise cellular cAMP of antigen-induced antibody production might be explained by the effect of cAMP to induce B-cell differentiation (46).

VII. THE RELEASE OF ARACHIDONIC ACID FROM LYMPHOCYTE PHOSPHOLIPIDS

One of the first changes to occur in lymphocytes following addition of phytohemagglutinin (PHA) is the turnover of membrane phosphatidylinositol (47, 48). Breakdown of phosphatidylinositol through the action of phospholipase C is in other cells associated with the release of arachidonic acid (see Ch. 4), and it is likely that this occurs also in lymphocytes. Studies of Parker et al. (49) show that stimulation of human lymphocytes by PHA is associated with a release of arachidonic acid within 1 min, consistent with this concept. Pure populations of T cells do not produce significant PGE_2 or thromboxane B_2 in response to PHA. This, however, may be due to the paucity or absence of cyclooxygenase in these lymphocytes. Combined T cells and monocytes do produce more thromboxane B_2 in response to PHA than monocytes alone, and Goldyne and Stobo suggest this is because arachidonic acid released from the T cells is used by the monocytes (50). Their culture conditions were long (40 h) and had low levels of albumin, and whether a similar effect occurs in vivo is not certain.

Studies of Hoffman et al. (51) have provided evidence that enhanced methylation of phosphatidylcholine to phosphatidylethanolamine occurs when NK cells are exposed to susceptible tumor targets. Inhibition of the methylation reaction inhibited NK cell cytotoxicity, suggesting this process, as in neutrophils, may be an early event in NK cell stimulation, perhaps leading to phospholipase A_2 activation. A phospholipase A_2-like activity was demonstrated in the NK cells with loss of arachidonic acid from phosphatydylcholine. The use of inhibitors suggested the phospholipase A_2 activity was required for cytotoxicity. Whether arachidonic acid released and converted to an active metabolite or lysophosphatidylcholine or perhaps another active lipid is responsible for NK cell activation and/or killing is not yet clear. Lipomodulin, a phospholipase-inhibitory protein, has recently been found to inhibit NK cell activity (52). This provides additional support for a role of a phospholipase, but whether the active phospholipase is phospholipase A_2 or C will require further research.

VIII. OTHER LIPID ACTIVATORS

A. Phosphatidic Acid/Lysophospatidic Acid

Attempts to stimulate lymphocyte mitogenesis using lysophosphatidic acid have not been successful (L. Filipovitch, personal communication), but perhaps this results from the need to have the stimulus present for some time. Lysophosphatidic acid is probably rapidly metabolized by cells.

B. Diglyceride

The influence of diglycerides on lymphocyte function is unknown. If they function in a similar fashion to phorbol myristate acetate, which promotes mitogenesis, and can act different from, yet synergistically (as a comitogen) with the calcium ionophore (53), they could be important endogenous mediators produced on initial breakdown of phosphoinositides. The similarity of this effect to the interaction of agents which raise intracellular calcium and agents which stimulate protein kinase C in lymphocyte activation to the role of these processes in platelet activation (see Chs. 3 and 6) suggests the synergistic effect of processes which raise cytoplasmic calcium and other interactive processes should be further explored in lymphocytes.

IX. OVERVIEW

A. Lymphocyte Activation

Stimulation of lymphocyte mitogenesis by the calcium ionophore A23187 (54) suggests that lymphocytes, like other blood cells, are stimulated by a receptor-coupled stimulus leading to a rise in cytoplasmic calcium and cell activation. The mechanism for stimulating calcium flux is unknown. Stimulation of phosphatidylinositol turnover by PHA and partial inhibition of the response to PHA by thromboxane synthetase inhibitors and lipoxygenase inhibitors suggest that diglycerides, phosphatidic acid (or lysophosphatidic acid), thromboxane A_2, or lipoxygenase products could be involved. Thromboxane A_2 production in response to PHA appears to need monocytes, and is therefore not likely to be a purely internal cell activation mechanism. One or more of the lipoxygenase products are possible candidates for the internal activation mechanism; however, as with platelets and neutrophils, it may turn out that the essential mechanism is related to the initial phosphatidylinositol metabolism and its immediate products, and that the arachidonic acid metabolites are ancillary and supportive but not essential components. It is possible that different subpopulations of lymphocytes are activated by different products. Of particular interest in this regard are studies showing the 5-lipoxygenase inhibitor 15-HETE blocks T- but not B-cell mitogenesis.

B. Inhibition of Lymphocytes

Prostaglandin E production by other blood cells, probably particularly monocytes, provides an inhibitory or suppressor activity toward T-cell mitogenesis. The effect appears to work through an elevation of lymphocyte cAMP. This mechanism appears to account for diminished T-cell responsiveness in Hodgkin's disease (55). 15-HETE may function as an endogenous T-lymphocyte-produced feedback inhibitor.

In mouse spleen cells, Webb and co-workers have identified an alternate suppressor pathway, in which it appears that lymphocyte-synthesized PGE regulates a suppressor cell population which responds to the prostaglandin by secreting a heat-stable 38,000-dalton protein with suppressor activity (56,57).

LTB_4 produced through the 5-lipoxygenase pathway may promote lymphocyte activation, but in a normal mitogen assay stimulation of suppressor T-cells as well as other subsets could result in an apparent overall neutral effect. Resolution of current conflicting data will clearly require sophisticated biochemical and functional analysis of these individual lymphocyte subsets.

APPENDIX 12-1 IMPORTANT SPECIES DIFFERENCES

The transformation of mice lymphocytes can be inhibited by LTD_4 and LTE_4 (58), whereas these are ineffective as inhibitors of human lymphocyte mitogenesis (30b).

REFERENCES

1. E. L. Gottfried. *J. Lipid Res.* *8*:321 (1967).
2. T. P. Stossel, R. J. Mason, and A. L. Smith. *J. Clin Invest.* *54*:638 (1974).

3. T. Haliotis, J. Roder, M. Klein, J. Ortlado, A. S. Fauci, and R. B. Herberman. *J. Exp. Med. 151*:1039 (1980).
4. T. Timonen, J. R. Ortaldo, and R. B. Herberman. *J. Exp. Med. 153*:569 (1981).
5. P. Katz and A. M. Zaytown. Quoted in P. Katz, J. C. Roder, A. M. Zaytown, R. B. Herberman, and A. S. Fauci. *J. Immunol. 129*:297 (1982).
6. J. C. Roder and M. Klein. *J. Immunol. 123*:2785 (1979).
7. P. Katz, A. M. Zaytown, and A. S. Fauci. *J. Immunol. 129*:287 (1982).
8. V. A. Ferraris and F. R. DeRubertis. *J. Clin. Invest. 54*:378 (1974).
9. D. Gordon, M. A. Bray, and J. Morley. *Nature 262*:401 (1976).
10. M. S. Kennedy, J. D. Stobo, and M. E. Goldyn. *Prostaglandins 20*: 135 (1980).
11. A. D. Bankhurst, E. Hastain, J. S. Goodwin, and G. T. Peake. *J. Lab. Clin. Med. 97*:179 (1981).
12. C. W. Parker, W. F. Stenson, M. G. Huber, and J. P. Kelly. *J. Immunol. 122*:1572 (1979).
13. S. Bauminger. *Prostaglandins 16*:351 (1978).
14. E. J. Goetzl. *Biochem. Biophys. Res. Commun. 101*:344 (1981).
15. J. P. Kelly and C. W. Parker. *J. Immunol. 122*:1556 (1979).
16. J. McCarty and E. J. Goetzl. *Cell Immunol. 43*:103 (1979).
17. J. Mertin and D. Hughes. *Int. Arch. Allergy Appl. Immunol. 48*: 203 (1975).
18. A. A. Mihas, R. G. Gibson, and B. I. Hirchowitz. *Proc. Soc. Exp. Biol. Med. 149*:1026 (1975).
19. R. Bray, S. Abrams, and Z. Brahmi. *Cell Immunol. 78*:100 (1983).
20. J. S. Goodwin, A. D. Bankhurst, and R. P. Messner. *J. Exp. Med. 146*:1719 (1977).
21. A. Novogrodsky, A. L. Rubin, and K. H. Stenzel. *J. Immunol. 122*: 1 (1979).
22. T. Sims, J. A. Clagett, and R. C. Page. *Clin. Immunol. Immunopathol. 33*:150 (1979).
23. J. W. Smith, A. L. Steiner, W. M. Newberry, Jr., and C. W. Parker. *J. Clin. Invest. 50*:432 (1971).
24. G. D. Stockman and D. M. Mumford. *Exp. Hematol. 2*:65 (1974).
25. O. J. Plescia, A. H. Smith, and K. Grinwich. *Proc. Natl. Acad. Sci. U.S.A. 72*:1848 (1975).
26. J. S. Goodwin, R. P. Messner, and G. T. Peake. *J. Clin. Invest. 62*:753 (1978).
27. M. J. Brunda, R. B. Herberman, and H. T. Holden. *J. Immunol. 124*:2682 (1980).
28. M. J. Droller, M. U. Schneider, and P. Perlmann. *Cell. Immunol. 39*:165 (1978).

29. H. Offner and J. Clausen. *Lancet 2*:400 (1974).
30a. J. E. Guttery, A. Tilden, D. K. Herron, P. Gallagher, S. R. Baker and E. A. Ades. *J. Clin. Lab. Immunol. 13*:151 (1984).
30b. D. G. Payan and E. J. Goetzl. *J. Immunol. 131*:551 (1983).
31. J. M. Bailey, R. W. Bryant, C. E. Low, M. B. Pupillo, and J. Y. Vanderhoek. *Cell. Immunol. 67*:112 (1982).
32. J. P. Kelly, M. C. Johnson, and C. W. Parker. *J. Immunol. 122*:1563 (1979).
33. D. G. Payan and E. J. Goetzl. *J. Clin. Immunol. 1*:266 (1981).
34. R. Coffee. *Int. J. Pharmacol. 2*:240 (1980).
35. M. Rola-Pleszczynski, L. Gagnon, and P. Sirois. *Biochem. Biophys. Res. Commun. 113*:531 (1983).
36a. M. Rola-Pleszczynski, P. Borgeat, and P. Sirois. *Biochem. Biophys. Res. Commun. 108*:1531 (1982).
36b. N. Gualde, M. Riguad and J. S. Goodwin. *Clin. Res. 31*:490A (1983).
36c. J. S. Goodwin and R. Atluru. Conference on Prostaglandins and Leukotrienes '84, May 8-11, Washington, D.C., Abstract 49 (1984).
36d. M. Rola-Pleszczynski, L. Gagnon, E. J. Corey, C. Pouliot and V. Radoux Conference on Prostaglandins and Leukotrienes '84, May 8-11, Washington, D.C., Abstract 75 (1984).
36e. H. M. Johnson and B. A. Torres. *J. Immunol. 132*:413 (1984).
36f. C. Favalli, T. Jezzi, C. Rinaldi-Garaci, A. Mastino, A. T. Palamara and E. Garaci. Conference on Prostaglandins and Leukotrienes, May 8-11, Washington, D.C., Abstract 131 (1984).
37. J. E. Crout, B. Hepburn, and R. E. Ritts, Jr. *N. Engl. J. Med. 292*: 221 (1975).
38. J. S. Goodwin, D. S. Selinger, R. P. Messner, and W. P. Reed. *Infect. Immunol. 19*:430 (1978).
39. G. Opelz, P. I. Terasaki, and A. A. Hirata. *Lancet 2*:478 (1973).
40. L. M. Pachman, N. B. Esterly, and R. D. A. Peterson. *J. Clin. Invest. 50*:226 (1971).
41. G. S. Panayi and A. Rix. *Rheumatol. Rehab. 13*:179 (1974).
42. R. S. Panosh and C. R. Anthony. *Clin. Exp. Immunol. 12*:114 (1976).
43a. M. J. Smith, M. Hoth, and K. Davis. *Ann. Intern. Med. 83*:509 (1975).
43b. H. S. Koren, S. J. Anderson, D. G. Fischer, C. S. Copeland, and P. J. Jensen. *J. Immunol. 127*:2007 (1981).
44. M. P. Sheid, G. Goldstein, U. Hammerling, and E. A. Boyse. *Ann. N.Y. Acad. Sci. 249*:531 (1975).
45. M. P. Sheid, G. Goldstein, and E. A. Boyse. *J. Exp. Med. 147*:1727 (1978).
46. T. Kishimoto and K. Ishizaka. *J. Immunol. 116*:534 (1976).
47. D. B. Fisher and G. C. Mueller. *Biochim. Biophys. Acta 248*:434 (1971).

48. D. O. Lucas, S. B. Shohet, and E. Miller. *Immunology 106*:768 (1971).
49. C. W. Parker, J. P. Kelly, S. F. Falkenhein, and M. G. Huber. *J. Exp. Med. 149*:1487 (1979).
50. Goldyn and Stobo. *Prostaglandins 24*:623 (1982).
51. T. Hoffman, F. Hirata, P. Bougnoux, B. A. Fraser, R. H. Goldfarb, R. B. Herberman, and J. Axelrod. *Proc. Natl. Acad. Sci. USA 78*:3839 (1981).
52. T. Hattori, F. Hirata, T. Hoffman, A. Hizuta, and R. B. Herberman. *J. Immunol. 131*:662 (1983).
53. A. M. Mastro and M. C. Smith. *J. Cell. Physiol. 116*:51 (1983).
54. J. R. Luckasen, J. G. White, and J. H. Kersey. *Proc. Natl. Acad. Sci. USA 71*:5088 (1974).
55. J. S. Goodwin, R. P. Messner, A. D. Bankhurst, G. T. Peake, J. H. Saiki, and R. C. Williams, Jr. *N. Engl. J. Med. 297*:963 (1977).
56. D. R. Webb and A. T. Jamieson. *Cell. Immunol. 24*:45 (1976).
57. D. R. Webb and I. Nowowiejski. *Cell. Immunol. 41*:72 (1978).
58. D. R. Webb, I. Nowowiejski, C. Healy, and T. J. Rogers. *Biochem. Biophys. Res. Commun. 104*:1617 (1982).

BIBLIOGRAPHY

W. F. Stenson and C. W. Parker. *In Prostaglandins*. J. B. Lee (ed.). Elsevier, New York (1982).

13

The Endothelial Cell

I. CELLULAR ANATOMY

A. Morphology

Endothelial cells line the blood vessels and capillaries throughout the circulation. In vivo, large vessel endothelial cells are flattened cells, with their undersurface attached to the basement membrane covering the subendothelial matrix of the blood vessel (Fig. 13-1). In contrast, capillary endothelial cells exist as tubelike structures covering the lining basement membrane. Endothelial cells contain an oval or flattened nucleus and a perinuclear region containing the Golgi complex. Small areas of rough endoplasmic reticulum and mitochondria are more frequent in the region near the nucleus. The peripheral zone of the endothelial cell has many vesicles. These are particularly numerous adjacent to the luminal and abluminal plasma membranes. Many, but not all types of endothelial cells, have characteristic granules, Weibel-Palade bodies, which contain von Willebrand protein (1). These granules are elongated and contain tubular structures. Arterial and venous endothelial cells form a continuous surface with close-fitting junctions between cells. Some visceral capillaries have a fenestrated endothelium.

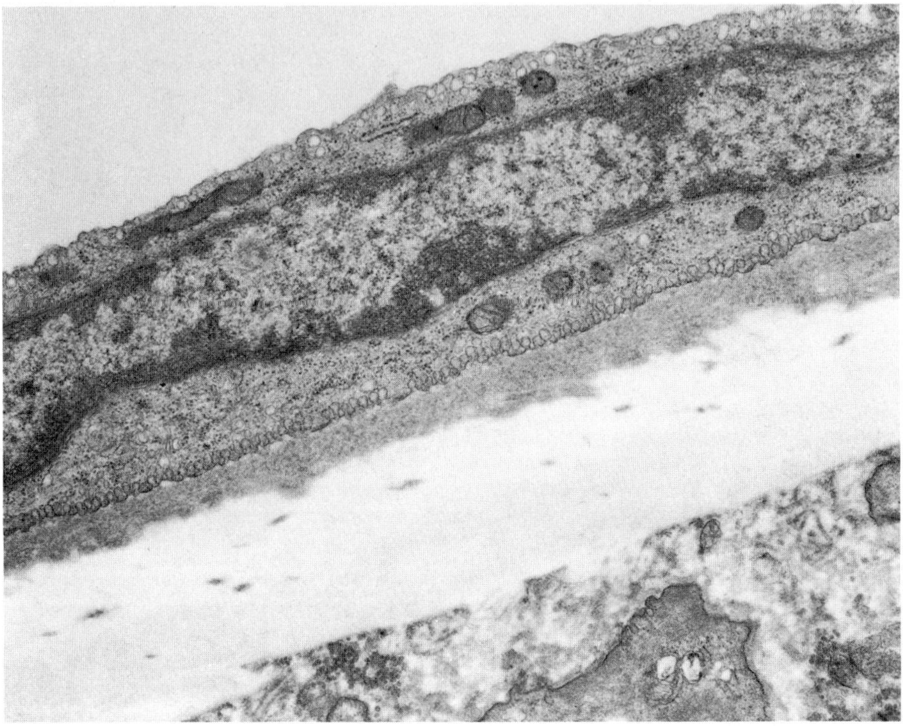

Fig. 13-1 A cross section of an endothelial cell from an intact perfused aorta. The lumen of the vessel is above the cell, the basement membrane, beneath. (X13,000.) (Photo courtesy of Dr. J. G. White.)

B. Lipids

The principal phospholipid of endothelial cells is phosphatidylcholine (variously reported as 32-51% of lipid phosphorus) (2,3a). The content of sphingomyelin is lower than that in platelets in one report (8% of lipid phosphorus) (3a), but not in a second (17-21% of lipid phosphorus) (2). The discrepancies between these findings have not yet been explained.

Phosphatidylinositol (PI) (6.3% of lipid phosphorus) contains primarily arachidonic acid (33.5% by weight), stearic acid (40%), and oleic acid (13.4%). Dihomo-γ-linolenic acid is present in relatively high amounts (3.5%

of the fatty acids in PI and 9.2% of the fatty acids in phosphatidylserine). Eicosapentaenoic acid appears to be incorporated into endothelial cell lipids in a fashion similar to arachidonic acid.

II. ENDOTHELIAL CELL FUNCTION

Endothelial cells serve to line the inner surface of blood vessels forming a nonthrombogenic surface. Several properties of endothelial cells render them antithrombotic. Thrombin is formed in the bloodstream as a result of activation of coagulation; it binds to a receptor, a protein called thrombomodulin, located on the endothelial cell surface. Thrombin, when complexed to thrombomodulin, is inactivated with respect to initiating the cleavage of fibrinogen or stimulating platelet aggregation, but is activated in terms of its ability to cleave protein C to form the anticoagulant protein, activated protein C. At the same time as the endothelial cell protein thrombomodulin thus reverses the activity of thrombin (from procoagulant to anticoagulant), the thrombin stimulates secretion of PGI_2 and plasminogen activator from the endothelial cell. The antithrombotic action of PGI_2 is discussed in Chs. 6 and 16. Plasminogen activator from endothelial cells seeks out and binds to clots where it promotes clot lysis through cleavage of plasminogen to form plasmin.

When there is vessel injury and the endothelial cell lining is lost, endothelial cells proliferate and migrate into the region of injury to restore the original surface. Such migration is significantly affected by the nature of the underlying surface. When exposed to interstitial collagens (types I and III), as would occur with a deep injury where the basement membrane is lost, endothelial cells proliferate much faster than when exposed only to basement membrane collagens (types IV and V), as would occur if only the endothelial cells are lost during the injury. This, presumably, reflects the greater need to restore an endothelial cell surface with a deeper injury. Endothelial cells also synthesize and secrete collagens—the proportion of the various types being appropriate to the situation (3b).

The formation and maintenance of an antithrombotic surface is not the only function of endothelial cells. They form a barrier to the movement of leukocytes out of the bloodstream, and yet will under some circumstances contract to allow the egress of these cells and the increased vascular permeability associated with an inflammatory reaction. Under conditions of stress, endothelial cells secrete von Willebrand factor to enhance coagulation.

III. METABOLISM OF ARACHIDONIC ACID AND RELATED FATTY ACIDS BY ENDOTHELIAL CELLS

A. Arachidonic Acid

The major product of arachidonic acid metabolism in endothelial cells is prostaglandin I_2 or prostacyclin (4). Smaller but potentially significant quantities of prostaglandin E_2, prostaglandin $F_{2\alpha}$, and thromboxane A_2 are also produced (5-7). Studies using pig endothelial cells suggest that subcultured cells produce a relatively higher proportion of PGE_2, such that PGE_2 production equals or exceeds PGI_2 production (7). 11-HETE and 15-HETE are produced through the cyclooxygenase pathway in fetal calf aorta and human umbilical artery endothelial cells (8a,8b). Lipoxygenase products may also be produced by endothelial cells (9). In fetal calf aorta (perhaps representing endothelial cell activity) 12-HETE production was prominent when cyclooxygenase activity was inhibited (8a). In pig coronary and pulmonary arteries production of a LTD_4-like substance has been shown, but it has not been clearly demonstrated that the cells involved were endothelial cells (10). The full spectrum of lipoxygenase metabolites has not yet been reported.

Endothelial cell synthesis of PGI_2 from arachidonic acid can be inhibited by aspirin and indomethacin. Inhibition of prostaglandin synthesis appears to occur with similar concentrations of aspirin as found in platelets (11). Endothelial cells, at least in culture, are actively synthesizing new proteins so that the duration of inhibition is shorter than with platelets. In vivo, endothelial cells may be much more dormant and the inhibition may last for a longer interval.

B. Dihomo-γ-linolenic Acid

Bovine aorta will convert dihomo-γ-linolenic acid to a variety of cyclooxygenase-derived products, including primarily 12h-17:2, 11h-20:3, and 15h-20:3, with small amounts of 12-oxo-8,10-heptadecadienoic acid (12o-17:2), 10,11,12-trihydroxy-8-heptadecenoic acid, 8,11,12-trihydroxy-9-heptadecenoic acid, PGE_1, and $PGF_{1\alpha}$ (12). 12h-17:2 is produced through the action of prostacyclin synthetase as PGI_2 cannot be formed due to the absence of the 5,6-double bond. Small amounts of the lipoxygenase metabolite 12h-20:3 are also formed.

C. Eicosapentaenoic Acid

Rat aorta will not convert eicosapentaenoic acid to PGI_3 (13). However, with human umbilical vessels, and bovine endothelial cells, some conversion of eicosapentaenoic acid to PGI_3 is seen, although to a lesser degree than the conversion of arachidonic acid to PGI_2 (14,15). With the studies performed in intact vessels, smooth muscle cells as well as endothelial cells could have been responsible for the conversion.

IV. EFFECTS OF ENDOGENOUS ARACHIDONIC ACID METABOLITES ON ENDOTHELIAL CELLS

A. Prostacyclin

So far there has been very little done in the way of studies of the effect of prostacyclin on endothelial cell function. Important questions could be asked in terms of the effects of prostacyclin on the tightness of the bond between the endothelial cell and subendothelial cell lining and on the contractility, permeability, and various other functions of the endothelial cells.

B. 15-HETE

15-HETE will modestly stimulate endothelial cell migration (15b).

V. EFFECTS OF EXOGENOUS PROSTAGLANDINS AND RELATED LIPID MEDIATORS ON ENDOTHELIAL CELLS

A. Platelet-Activating Factor (AGEPC)

Injection of AGEPC intracutaneously increased the permeability of small venules. This effect appears due to an action of AGEPC to produce gaps between endothelial cells, perhaps by stimulating contraction of the endothelial cells (16a). Consistent with this, platelet activating factor stimulates a flux of calcium in endothelial cells (16b).

B. 12-HETE

12-HETE significantly reduces the migration of endothelial cells in response to bovine retinal extact.

VI. RELEASE OF ARACHIDONIC ACID FROM ENDOTHELIAL CELLS

Release of arachidonic acid for synthesis of prostacylin from endothelial cell phospholipids occurs in response of the endothelial cell to thrombin, melittin, nitroglycerin (17-19), leukotriene C (20), 1-des-amino-8-D-arginine vasopressin (DDAVP) (21), bradykinin (22,23a), histamine (23a), substance P (23b), thromboxane A_2 (23c), and by a factor or factors from monocytes (23d). An unidentified factor in plasma also promotes endothelial cell PGI_2 synthesis (24). Estrogens have been shown to increase PGI_2 production by female endothelial cells (25). The latter effect takes some time to develop and probably results from induction of new protein synthesis by the endothelial cell. Some evidence supports the idea that endothelial cell PGI_2 production is increased when the cells are in a contact cell monolayer (26). Hypoxia appears to stimulate PGI_2 synthesis by vascular tissue, but to a relatively small degree (27). Angiotensin II stimulates PGI_2 production in bovine but not piglet or human endothelial cells (28).

The release of arachidonic acid from endothelial cell phospholipids is inhibited in the presence of raised intracellular cAMP levels, as occurs with other blood cells. In the presence of a phosphodiesterase inhibitor, PGI_2 itself can significantly raise endothelial cell cAMP levels (29).

Endothelial cells cannot convert linoleic acid to arachidonic acid, and are therefore dependent on arachidonic acid in plasma to maintain the arachidonic acid in their phospholipids. Linoleic acid and eicosapentaenoic acid can reduce the incorporation of arachidonic acid into cellular phospholipids (30). In the presence of high levels of linoleic acid, endothelial cell prostacyclin production is therefore reduced (31). Endothelial cells, as with other cells, can release arachidonic acid and synthesize prostaglandin in response to cell injury. This has been well demonstrated in response to high concentrations of acetyl glyceryl ether phosphorylcholine and its lyso derivative (2).

VI. OVERVIEW

At the present time it would appear that synthesis of prostacyclin by endothelial cells in response to thrombin in particular may have an important role in preventing propagation of clots, inhibiting platelet aggregation, and maintaining the vessel in a dilated form. There has been some consideration that the prostacyclin may diffuse primarily into the smooth muscle cell where its role to dilate the vessel wall is more important than its role in platelets. However, it is apparent that in the interaction of endothelial cells with platelets there must be enough diffusion that the endothelial cells may have significant influence on platelet behavior at the endothelial cell blood vessel junction. The prostacyclin and PGE_2 produced by endothelial cells may also have effects to inhibit the chemotaxis of neutrophils and the stimulation of lymphocytes. However, elevation of cAMP does not inhibit random neutrophil migration, and this probably would allow the cells to migrate through the endothelial cell lining.

APPENDIX 13-1 SPECIES DIFFERENCES IN ENDOTHELIAL CELL PROSTAGLANDIN PRODUCTION

Pig aorta endothelial cells may make more PGE_2 than PGI_2 (22), whereas bovine (5) and human endothelial cells appear to make more PGI_2 than PGE_2. It is possible that these reported species differences reflect differences in the culture media and other conditions of the assays, or differences in the vascular site of origin of the endothelial cells rather than real species differences.

Human vasculature (endothelial cells) and bovine endothelial cells can convert eicosapentaenoic acid to PGI_3 whereas rat blood vessels do not (13-15a).

REFERENCES

1. D. D. Wagner, J. B. Olmsted, and V. J. Marder. *J. Cell. Biol. 95*: 355, (1982).
2. A. N. Siakotos and G. Rouser. *Lipids 4*:234 (1969).
3a. A. J. Marcus, M. J. Broekman, B. B. Weksler, E. A. Jaffe, L. B. Safier, H. L. Ullman, N. Islam, and K. Tack-Goldman. *Ann. N.Y. Acad. Sci. Sci. 401*:195 (1982).
3b. J. A. Madri and S. K. Williams. *J. Cell. Biol. 97*:153 (1983).
4. A. J. Marcus, B. B. Weksler, and E. A. Jaffe. *J. Biol. Chem. 253*: 7138 (1978).
5. A. E. Ali, J. C. Barrett, and T. E. Eling. *Prostaglandins 20*:667 (1980).
6. C. Ingerman-Wojenski, M. J. Silver, J. B. Smith, and E. Macarak. *J. Clin. Invest. 67*:1292 (1981).
7. C. N. Chesterman, A. Ager, and J. L. Gordon. *J. Cell Physiol. 116*: 45 (1983).

8a. W. S. Powell. *J. Biol. Chem. 257*:9457 (1982).
8b. B. N. Y. Setty, M. J. Stuart and R. W. Walenga. *Fed Proc. 43*:757 (1984).
9. J. E. Greenwald, J. R. B. Bianchine, and L. K. Wong. *Nature 281*:588 (1979).
10. P. J. Piper, L. G. Letts, and S. A. Galton. *Prostaglandins 25*:591 (1983).
11. E. A. Jaffe and B. B. Weksler. *J. Clin. Invest. 63*:532 (1979).
12. W. S. Powell. *J. Biol. Chem. 257*:9465 (1982).
13. G. Horsnstra, E. Christ-Hazelhof, E. Haddeman, F. Ten Hoor, and D. H. Nugteren. *Prostaglandins 21*:727 (1981).
14. J. Dyerberg, K. A. Jorgensen, and T. Arnfred. *Prostaglandins 22*:857 (1982).
15a. I. Morita, R. Takahashi, Y. Saito, and S. Murota. *Thromb. Res. 31*:211 (1983).
15b. J. E. Graeber, R. W. Wallenga, T. B. Conner, M. J. Stuart and B. M. Glaser. *Fed. Proc. 43*:588 (1984).
16a. D. M. Humphrey, L. M. McManus, D. J. Hanahan, and R. N. Pinckard. *Fed. Proc. 42*:1376 (1983).
16b. T. A. Brock, R. W. Alexander and M. A. Gimbrone, Jr. *Fed. Proc. 43*: 460 (1984).
17. R. I. Levin, E. A. Jaffe, B. B. Weksler, and K. Tack-Goldman. *J. Clin. Invest. 67*:672 (1981).
18. K. Schror, L. Grodzinska, and H. Darius. *Thromb. Res. 23*:59 (1981).
19. J. Mehta, P. Mehta, and N. Ostrowski. *J. Lab. Clin. Med. 102*:116 (1983).
20. E. B. Cramer, L. Pologe, N. A. Pawlowski, Z. A. Cohn, and W. A. Scott. *Proc. Natl. Acad. Sci. USA 80*:4109 (1983).
21. J. J. F. Belch, M. Small, F. McKenzie, P. A. Hill, G. D. O. Lowe, D. E. McIntyre, C. D. Forbes, and C. R. M. Prentice. *Thromb. Haemost. 47*: 122 (1982).
22. P. J. Jose, D. A. Page, B. E. Wolstenholme, T. J. Williams, and D. C. Dumonde. *Inflammation 5*:363 (1981).
23a. F. Alhenc-Gelas, S. J. Tsai, K. S. Callahan, W. B. Campbell, and A. R. Johnson. *Prostaglandins 24*:743 (1982).
23b. P. A. Barley, C. K. Derian and M. A. Moskowitz. *Fred. Proc. 43*:359 (1984).
23c. L. S. Olanoff, P. J. Kochel, J. A. Cook, W. C. Wise, and P. V. Halushka. *Fed. Proc. 43*:758 (1984).
23d. C. R. Albrightson, N. L. Baenzinger, and P. Needleman. *Fed. Proc. 43*: 933 (1984).
24. J. M. Seid, P. B. B. Jones, and R. C. G. Russell. *Clin. Sci. 64*:387 (1983).

25. C. Seillan, C. Ody, F. Rosso-Marie, and D. Duval. *Prostaglandins 26*:3 (1983).
26. A. Eldor, I. Vlodavsk, E. Hyam, R. Atzmon, B. B. Weksler, A. Raz, and Z. Fuks. *J. Cell Physiol 114*:179 (1983).
27. A. Edlund, B. B. Fredholm, P. Patrignani, C. Patrono, A. Wennmalm, and M. Wennmalm. *J. Physiol. 340*:487 (1983).
28. C. Ody, C. Seillan, F. Russo-Marie, and D. Duval. *Thrombosis. Res. 31*: 219 (1983).
29. A. F. A. Brotherton and J. C. Hoak. *Proc. Natl. Acad. Sci. USA 79*:495 (1982).
30. A. A. Spector, T. L. Kaduce, J. C. Hoak, and G. L. Fry. *J. Clin. Invest. 68*:1003 (1981).
31. A. Nordoy, B. Svensson, and J. C. Hoak. *Eur. J. Clin. Invest. 9*:5 (1979).

BIBLIOGRAPHY

A. P. Fishman (ed.). *Endothelium*. Ann. N.Y. Acad. Sci. Vol. 401, 1982.
J. A. Madri. *Prog. Hemostas. Thromb. 6*:1 (1982).

14

Vascular Smooth Muscle Cells

I. ANATOMY

Smooth muscle cells are found in the walls of arteries and veins, beneath the endothelium lining the lumen of the vessel. The precise arrangement of smooth muscle cells varies with the blood vessel studied. In the aorta, smooth muscle cells exist in layers with intervening elastic lamellae. In veins, only a small amount of collagen may separate smooth muscle cells. Moreover, the angle of orientation of the smooth muscle cells within the vessel wall may vary from nearly circular (i.e., perpendicular to the direction of blood flow) to spiral (for example—an angle of 75° relative to the long axis of the vessel).

Adjacent to the nucleus, at the nuclear poles, in the center of the cell is a zone with the golgi, some mitochondria, and rough endoplasmic reticulum (Fig. 14-1). The majority of the space between the nucleus and the cell wall is composed of filaments (Fig. 14-2) with occasional lysosomal bodies, lipid droplets and glycogen. Thin filaments, actin, are much more frequent than the thick filaments, believed to be myosin (ratio about 12-15:1) (1,2). Ashton et al. (3) have provided electron micrographs suggesting actin filaments may be arrayed around the myosin filaments. Intermediate

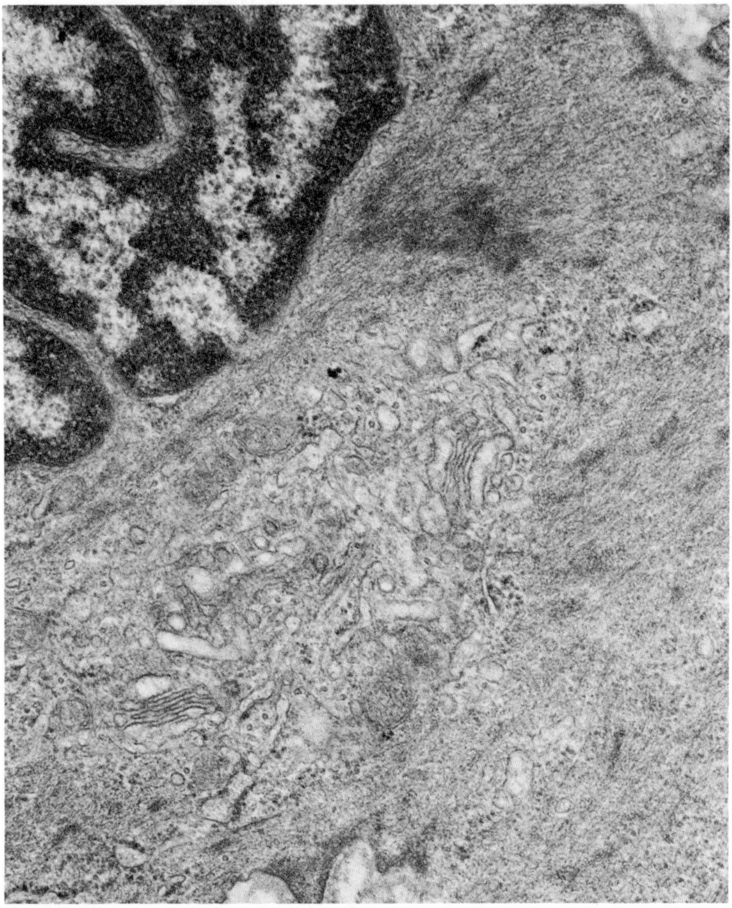

Fig. 14-1 A view of the perinuclear region of a smooth muscle cell from a rabbit aorta. (X33,000.)

filaments and dense bodies are present in the cell interior, together with the thin and thick filaments. The dense bodies are sites of attachment of the actin filaments and appear to act similar to the Z-disk of skeletal muscle to anchor and orient these filaments during contraction.

Adjacent to the cell membrane, at the periphery of the smooth muscle cell, is a zone enriched in smooth endoplasmic reticulum and caveolae.

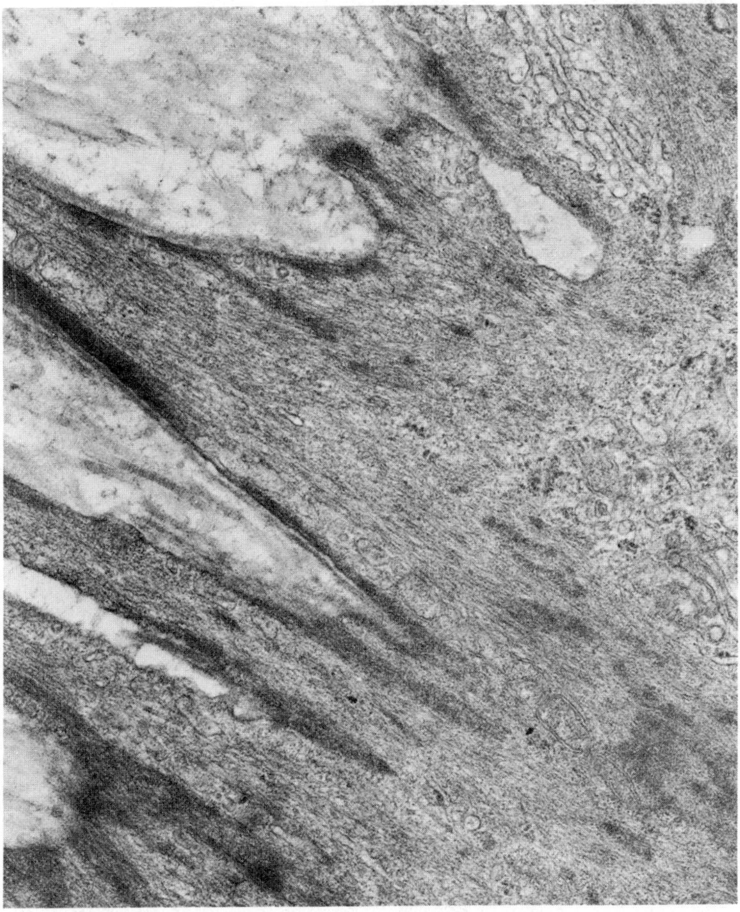

Fig. 14-2 A view of the peripheral region of a smooth muscle cell from the rabbit aorta. This region is rich in microfilaments. There are several collagen fibers in the interstitial region outside the smooth muscle cell. (×25,000.)

The smooth endoplasmic reticulum appears to function similar to the dense tubular system of platelets and the sarcotubules of skeletal muscle to sequester and release calcium to control the contractile activity of the cell. The caveolae are invaginations of the plasma membrane. Their function is uncertain, but they may function, in part, in a fashion analogous to the t-tubules of skeletal muscle and the surface-connected canalicular system of platelets in the transmission of messages from the cell exterior into the endoplasmic reticulum. The sacs of endoplasmic reticulum and the caveolae are frequently found in close association.

Smooth muscle cells in large arteries appear to differ from those in veins and arterioles in that they contain relatively more sarcoplasmic reticulum (i.e., 5% of the cell cytoplasm compared with 2% in the portal anterior mesenteric vein) (4a). Large artery smooth muscle can also maintain significant contractile responses in calcium-free media, presumably because of the extra capacity for internal calcium storage. These differences between large arteries and arterioles and veins have been related to the fact that the former are generally of multi-unit character with each cell individually innervated while the latter are generally 'single-unit' in nature (i.e., many gap junctions between cells and the ability of the cells to be spontaneously active) (4b).

An important consideration with vascular smooth muscle cells relative to other blood cells is that potential dependent (i.e., depolarization) stimulation of calcium flux is of major importance (4c). Consistent with this, calcium channel blocking drugs (i.e., verapamil, diltiazam, nefedipine) which are generally more effective inhibitors of potential dependent than receptor operated pathways of calcium flux, tend to be more effective at inhibiting vascular smooth muscle contraction that in inhibiting the function of other blood cells (i.e., platelets).

II. FUNCTION

A. Contraction

The state of the smooth muscle cell (i.e., contracted or relaxed) controls the size of the blood vessel lumen. The major function of the smooth muscles are to control the amount of resistance to flow through the lumen. Additionally, in some vessels, such as the aorta, pulse synchronized contraction occurs (4d). The latter may function primarily to reduce the extent of increase in vessel wall diameter at times of sudden increases in pressure in order to prevent injury to the vessel wall and to facilitate flow. Constriction or narrowing of a vessel may also be important to achieve hemostasis at a site of vessel injury. Undesirable degrees of contraction or vasospasm can lead to tissue ischemia. Relaxation of a vessel may be associated with enhanced permeability and increased movement of plasma or cells from the blood into the tissues and edema. The extent to which the latter occurs may depend on various factors including, for example, a differential in the effect on arteries and veins (i.e., more edema would be expected if arterial dilation occurred without a concomitant venous dilation or if venoconstriction occurred by itself).

Contraction of vascular smooth muscle cells appears critically controlled by the level of cytoplasmic calcium. Endo et al. (5), using chemically skinned pulmonary artery, found half-maximal tension at 5×10^{-7} M calcium. Calcium regulation of contractile activity appears to occur primarily through calcium binding to calmodulin. The calcium-calmodulin complex has high affinity for the calatylic subunit of a protein kinase which phosphorylates the 20,000 dalton myosin light chain with activation of actomyosin ATPase to general tension. Evidence for calcium acting on a protein associated with native tropomyosin which activates actomyosin ATPase has also been put forward but appears less important (6).

Recent studies suggest that two calcium-dependent regulatory processes interact to produce the usual pattern of contraction and relaxation. Myosin phosphorylation appears important for the initial shortening velocity of the vascular smooth muscle which is subserved by normally cycling actin-myosin cross-bridges. However, muscle tension (stress) appears to be maintained in part through an alternate regulatory mechanism subserved by slowly cycling or latch bridges which require calcium, but at lower concentrations than myosin phosphorylation (7).

B. Relaxation

Relaxation of smooth muscle cells can be achieved by removing the agonist stimulating contraction or by removing calcium from the system. Relaxation, under these conditions, shows an initial rapid phase which appears to result from myosin dephosphorylation as a result of the action of myosin light chain phosphatase, and a later slow phase which appears due to a slow inactivation of nonphosphorylated cross bridges (8).

cAMP decreases the Ca^{2+}-induced force in skinned smooth muscles (9). A mechanism for this effect has been proposed—cAMP activation of a protein kinase which phosphorylates myosin light-chain kinase so that it is ineffective in producing phosphorylation of myosin (10-14). This mechanism is based on studies of the isolated proteins. Prostaglandins and other agents which stimulate the synthesis of vascular smooth muscle cAMP and produce relaxation may act through this, or perhaps through other mechanisms (i.e., protein kinase-mediated enhancement of calcium uptake by the sarcoplasmic reticulum, extrusion of calcium across the sarcolemmal membrane, or inhibition of calcium influx) (15).

C. Lipid Metabolism

Hydrolysis of cholesterol esters through the activity of cholesterol ester hydrolase, an enzyme in smooth muscle lysosomes, is an important mechanism for the metabolism of cholesterol esters in the vascular wall (16).

III. METABOLISM OF ARACHIDONIC ACID BY VASCULAR SMOOTH MUSCLE

PGI_2 (prostacyclin) is the major product of arachidonic acid metabolism in vascular tissue (17). Some thromboxane B_2 and lipoxygenase metabolites may also be formed. In cultured vascular smooth muscle cells from rat mesenteric arteries, the ratio of $PGI_2/PGE_2/PGF_{2\alpha}$ was found to be approximately 100:5:2.5 (18).

The production of PGI_2 by smooth muscle cells has been compared with that of endothelial cells. In the normal rabbit aorta, Eldor et al. (19) suggest almost all the PGI_2 production at the luminal surface originates in the endothelial cells. Following deendothelialization, PGI_2 production at the luminal surface was virtually absent; however, a neointima of smooth muscle cells formed gradually and synthesized increasing quantities of PGI_2 with time after injury. However, they also noted, using punch biopsies of the entire vessel wall, that the total PGI_2 production of the vessel wall showed very little change after deendothelializing injury. Cells other than endothelial cells, located deep in the vessel wall, must be able to synthesize a substantial amount of PGI_2. An alternate explanation for the findings of Eldor et al. is that deendothelialization results in exposure of the cells on the luminal surface to an inhibitor of PGI_2 production, perhaps hydroperoxy forms of arachidonic acid generated when the endothelial cells are damaged, or by platelets and neutrophils interacting with the injured vessel wall. The finding of an increase in PGI_2 synthesis following recovery might then be due to a gradual decrease of inhibitor at the luminal surface rather than a selective acquisition of prostacyclin-synthesizing enzymes by neointima smooth muscle cells.

IV. INFLUENCE OF ARACHIDONIC ACID AND ENDOGENOUSLY PRODUCED DERIVATIVES ON SMOOTH MUSCLE CELLS

A. Contractile Properties

Care must be taken in the interpretation of studies of vascular smooth muscle since in vivo responses are not always identical to effects on isolated vessel strips. In this discussion, I shall refer primarily to in vivo data. Although a variety of indirect effects might come into play in vivo, I believe understanding in vivo effects is more important, at the present time, to an overall evaluation of the effects of prostaglandins and related chemicals on vascular smooth muscle. In a sense, therefore, this chapter is a bridge between the in vitro studies emphasized in earlier chapters and the in vivo studies emphasized in the last five chapters. In general, as can be seen from the discussion of specific vascular beds, PGI_2, PGE_1 and PGE_2 are vasodilators whereas thromboxane A_2, $PGF_{2\alpha}$, and leukotrienes C_4 and D_4 are vasconstrictors, but there are many important exceptions.

1. The Mesenteric Vasculature

Infusion of arachidonic acid into the mesenteric artery causes vasodilation. This response is associated with increased formation of 6-keto-$PGF_{1\alpha}$, and it is blocked by the PGI_2 synthetase inhibitor tranylcypromine (20). These results strongly suggest the vasodilation is due to PGI_2 formed from arachidonic acid. In contrast to PGI_2 which dilates the mesenteric vasculature (due to relaxation of the smooth muscle cells), thromboxane A_2 and prostaglandin endoperoxide analogues are vasoconstrictors. Effects of endogenous production of thromboxane A_2 can be seen in some circumstances. For example, 32 days after unilateral renal artery compression, the response to an infusion of arachidonic acid is now vasoconstriction. This response is accompanied by increased thromboxane B_2 formation and is blocked by the thromboxane synthetase inhibitor imidazole, strongly suggesting it is due to the formation of thromboxane A_2 (20). Whether the thromboxane A_2 is platelet, macrophage, or smooth muscle derived is not established. A decrease in PGI_2 production in response to arachidonic acid 32 days after unilateral renal artery compression may play a role in unmasking the effect of the thromboxane A_2.

Leukotrienes C_4 and D_4 exert potent vasconstrictor action on the mesenteric vascular bed in the dog and cat (21-23). Leukotriene E_4 is also a vasoconstrictor, but is much less potent. As vasoconstrictors in the mesenteric bed, LTC_4 and LTD_4 are of similar activity to PGD_2 and about 10 times more active than $PGF_{2\alpha}$ (23,24).

2. The Renal Vascular Bed

Arachidonic acid infused into the renal artery produced vasodilation and an increase in renal blood flow (25). These effects are probably mediated principally by conversion of arachidonic acid to the vasodilator PGE_2 in the kidney (26).

Renal PGE_2 production and the vasodilator effect of PGE_2 appear to be particularly important to balance the effect of renal vasoconstrictor influences to maintain renal blood flow. For example, in human subjects with volume depletion, congestive heart failure, the nephrotic syndrome, or cirrhosis of the liver with ascites, the administration of a prostaglandin synthase inhibitor results in reduced renal perfusion (27-30). Increased PGE_2 synthesis in the kidney in these circumstances may be secondary to production of angiotension II or kinins.

Thromboxane A_2 produces renal vasoconstriction, and production of this substance may have a role in reduced renal perfusion in some patients with the hepatorenal syndrome (31).

Leukotrienes C_4 and D_4 exert a very weak vasodilator effect on the renal vascular bed. LTE_4 has no effect on renal perfusion (23).

3. The Pulmonary Vasculature

Arachidonic acid. When arachidonic acid is injected as a bolus, the response is pulmonary vasoconstriction in a variety of species (32-35). However, when pulmonary vascular resistance is first increased and the arachidonic acid is then given more slowly as an infusion, the response in the cat and the dog is decreased pulmonary vascular resistance (vasodilation) (33,36, 37). Studies using porcine vessels show that arachidonic acid relaxes intralobar arteries, associated with production of PGI_2 by these vessels, but constricts intralobar veins which produce predominantly thromboxane A_2 (38). This differential effect on arteries and veins could explain the variation in the effect of arachidonic acid on the overall pulmonary vascular resistance.

Prostaglandins, thromboxanes, and leukotrienes. In both the cat and the dog lung a number of prostaglandins and thromboxanes are vasoconstrictors in the following order of potency: PGH_2 analogue $>$ $PGF_{2\alpha}$

$>$ $PGD_2 > PGE_2 >$ thromboxane B_2 (39). Leukotriene D_4 also constricts the pulmonary artery (40). The effect of leukotriene D_4 on pulmonary vasoconstriction in the sheep can be blocked by indomethacin and may be secondary to production of thromboxane A_2 (41). PGI_2, in contrast, has pulmonary vasodilator activity (42-44). The vasodilator activity of leukotriene E_4, however, appears secondary to PGI_2 production, and when PGI_2 synthesis is blocked, LTE_4 has some vasoconstrictor activity (44). Leukotriene B_4 increased pulmonary lymph flow without a change in pulmonary vacular resistance (40).

Clinical relevance. Recent studies suggest that activated-complement-, endotoxin-, and oxidant-induced pulmonary vasoconstriction may be secondary to production of thromboxane A_2 (45-47), whereas hypoxia-induced pulmonary vasoconstriction may be secondary to leukotriene production (48). The former may be important in the genesis of pulmonary edema in shock states (38). The latter may be important in neonates with hypoxemia and pulmonary hypertension (persistent pulmonary hypertension of the newborn) (49). Treatment with cyclooxygenase inhibitors or thromboxane synthase inhibitors protects against many of the adverse hemodynamic consequences of endotoxic shock and improves survival but does not prevent lung permeability changes (46,50,51).

4. The Cerebral Vasculature

The slow intracerebral infusion of arachidonic acid will cause brain edema (rats) which can be inhibited by dexamethasone but not by indomethacin (52).

The effects of prostaglandins on cerebral vessels vary to some extent on the method of administration. In dogs, cats, mice, and monkeys $PGF_{2\alpha}$ will cause vasoconstriction by any route (53,54). $PGF_{1\alpha}$ is similarly a vasoconstrictor although less potent. PGE_2 and PGA_1 given intravenously in the basilar artery cause vasodilation, whereas when applied topically to the artery they cause vasoconstriction (53). Variable results have been reported with PGE_1, with vasodilator responses more likely when the drug was given intravascularly to animals with intact skulls, and vasoconstriction more frequent when it was given to animals who had received craniotomy (54). One study of PGE_1 in humans gave equivocal results (55a). Thromboxane A_2 is a vasoconstrictor in the cerebral vasculature, while PGI_2 is a vasodilator (55b).

Infusion of PGE_1 and PGI_2-analogues into humans has been associated with headaches which have been suggested to result from vasodilator effects of these compounds on the cerebral circulation (56).

5. The Coronary Vascular Bed

Arachidonic acid. Injection of arachidonic acid into the coronary artery causes vasodilation, which can be blocked by the cyclooxygenase inhibitor indomethacin (57,58). The effect of arachidonic acid is due to its conversion to PGI_2 (see below) (59).

Prostaglandins, thromboxane, and leukotrienes

Vasodilation. PGI_2 is a potent coronary vasodilator, effective whether injected into the coronary artery or applied directly to the surface of the left ventricle (59). PGH_2 is also a vasodilator, but its effect can be inhibited by blocking prostacyclin synthetase, showing that its effect is secondary to its intracoronary conversion to PGI_2 (59). PGE_1 also is a coronary vasodilator (62). PGE_2 is a weak coronary vasodilator in rabbits and dogs but a vasoconstrictor in several other species (57,60,62,63).
Vasoconstriction. Studies with thromboxane A_2 analogues have provided good evidence that thromboxane A_2 is a potent coronary vasoconstrictor (64). Leukotrienes C_4 and D_4 and platelet-activating factor are also coronary vasoconstrictors (65,66a,66b). The effect of platelet-activating factor, at least in the pig, may result from secondary production of thromboxane A_2 (66c).

6. The Cutaneous Vasculature

PGE_1, PGE_2, $PGF_{2\alpha}$, PGD_2, and PGI_2 produce vasodilation when injected into the skin (67,68). LTC_4 and LTD_4 also increase microcirculatory flow in the skin (69).

7. Edema and Transcapillary Fluid Flux

In the dog forelimb, PGE_1 produces potent arteriolar dilation (70,71). PGE_1 does not produce edema, in contrast to other vasodilators, including bradykinin or histamine which produce in addition to vasodilation a large increase in the permeability of the microvascular membranes to plasma proteins. Some increase in lymph flow and lymph protein content may be seen with PGE_1. However, even with very high rates of infusion of PGE_1, small vein and capillary hydrostatic pressures do not increase despite considerable arteriolar dilation, presumably because the veins dilate proportionately.

Whereas prostaglandins used alone are poor producers of edema, prostaglandin synthetase inhibitors are potent inhibitors of edema in many situations where there is inflammation (68,73). The reason for the effectiveness of cyclooxygenase inhibitors appears to be that vasodilatory prostaglandins produce a marked potentiation of the effect of histamine and bradykinin on edema (73-76). There is a strong correlation between the ability of prostaglandins to induce vasodilation and their ability to potentiate edema formation (68,77,78), and the former effect may explain the latter. Mediator synergism independent of vasodilation may also occur (79).

B. Lipid Metabolism

PGI_2, 6-keto $PGF_{1\alpha}$, and 6-keto PGE_1 all enhance acid cholesterol ester hydrolase activity in smooth muscle cells from rabbit thoracic aorta (80a). These effects appear to result from the effect of these agents to stimulate adenylate cyclase and raise intracellular cAMP levels. PGE_1 and PGE_2 were not effective. PGI_2-mediated activation of this enzyme may be important to vascular metabolism of cholesterol esters, preventing the buildup in the vessel wall of free and esterified cholesterol, one of the hallmarks of degenerative arterial disease.

C. DNA Synthesis

PGI_2 and PGE_2 have been shown to inhibit the serum stimulated synthesis of DNA in embryonic rat thoracic aorta smooth muscle cells (80b). In the presence of indomethacin used to inhibit endogenous PGI_2 formation, serum stimulated DNA synthesis is enhanced suggesting that endogenously produced PGI_2 may play a role in the control of smooth muscle cell proliferation.

V. THE RELEASE OF ARACHIDONIC ACID FROM SMOOTH MUSCLE CELL PHOSPHOLIPIDS

Norepinephrine incubated with cultured rabbit aorta smooth muscle cells increased ^{32}P-orthophosphate labeling of phosphatidylinositol (81), a response associated in other tissues with release of arachidonic acid (see Ch. 4). Metabolism of arachidonic acid was not studied, however. Using vascular smooth muscle cells derived from rat mesenteric arteries, vasopressin and angiotensin II were found to increase PGI_2 synthesis (82). The effect of vasopressin, presumably mediated by stimulating arachidonic acid release from cell phospholipids, was little affected by changing the extracellular calcium, but was blocked by TMB-8, an intracellular calcium antagonist, suggesting intracellular calcium was required (83a).

VI. STUDIES USING INHIBITORS

Various experiments using inhibitors of the synthesis of prostaglandins and thromboxanes have so far not conclusively shown a role for prostaglandins in the agonist activity of substances other than arachidonic acid (20), though modulation (slight inhibition or enhancement) of the effects of norepinephrine or angiotensin II to contract some vessels has been demonstrated (83b). However, cold-induced forearm vasoconstriction was found to be inhibited by the thromboxane synthetase inhibitor dazoxiben in individuals whose arachidonic acid induced platelet aggregation was also inhibited by dazoxiben (83c). Furthermore, it has been suggested that the action of hydralazine as an antihypertensive may be related to its ability to inhibit thromboxane synthesis by platelets and vascular smooth muscle (84). Chronic treatment of hypertensive animals with clonidine and α-methyldopa appears to inhibit thromboxane formation associated with increased prostacyclin formation and a rise in cAMP (20,85a). Thromboxane synthetase inhibitors may be effective in improving blood flow following artificially induced cerebral vasospasm (85b).

VII. OTHER ACTIVE LIPIDS

A. Platelet-Activating Factor

Platelet-activating factor is a vasoconstrictor of the coronary circulation (66a). It will also increase vascular permeability in the skin (86).

B. Lysophosphatidic Acid

Lysophosphatidic acid causes contraction of smooth muscle from rabbit duodenum and rat uterus, but its action on vascular smooth muscle has not been well studied. The fact that it produces hypertension in rats and guinea pigs and hypotension in cats and rabbits has suggested it may have actions on vascular smooth muscle (87-90). In cats the hypotension is preceded by a marked increase in pulmonary vascular resistance, possibly secondary to the effects of this agent on platelets.

VIII. OVERVIEW

A review of the role of prostaglandins, thromboxanes, and leukotrienes in smooth muscle cell function is complicated by the variety of responses of these cells, depending of their site of origin. In vivo cellular responses may depend on the associated cells in the organ of interest, their pattern of arachidonic acid metabolism, and their response to metabolites. Contractile and relaxant responses of smooth muscle cells to arachidonic acid metabolites may be direct or indirect. Sorting out the mechanism of the effect of these agents in all vascular beds may take some time. Already, it is apparent that effects of these agents to produce vasoconstriction or vasodilation or to potentiate edema formation are important in a number of clinical circumstances. Better understanding of both beneficial and undesirable effects of these agents should facilitate treatment in a wide variety of disorders.

REFERENCES

1. A. P. Somlyo, C. E. Devine, A. V. Somlyo, and R. V. Rice. *Phil. Trans. Roy. Soc. Lond. B. 265*:223 (1973).
2. R. A. Murphy, J. T. Herlihy, and J. Megerman. *J. Gen Physiol. 64*:691 (1974).
3. F. T. Ashton, A. V. Somlyo, and A. P. Somlyo. *J. Mol. Biol. 98*:17 (1975).

4a. C. E. Devine, A. V. Somlyo, and A. P. Somlyo. *J. Cell. Biol. 52*:690 (1972).

4b. G. Burnstock. In Smooth Muscle. E. Bulbring, A. E. Brading, A. W. Jones and T. Tomita (eds.). Edward Arnold, London. (1970).

4c. S. F. Flaim and R. Zelis (eds.). Calcium Blockers Mechanisms of Action and Clinical Applications. Urban and Schwarzenberg, Baltimore/Munich (1982).

4d. A. Mangel, M. Fahim, C. Van Breemen. *Science. 215*:1627 (1982).

5. M. Endo, T. Kitazawa, S. Yagi, M. Iino, and Y. Kakuta. In *Excitation-Contraction Coupling in Smooth Muscle*, R. Casteels, T. Godfraind, and J. C. Ruegg (eds.). Elsevier/North Holland, Amsterdam (1977).
6. R. Casteels, R. Godfraind, and J. C. Ruegg. *Excitation-Contraction Coupling in Smooth Muscle*. Elsevier/North Holland, Amsterdam (1977).
7. M. O. Aksoy, S. Mras, K. E. Kamm, and R. A. Murphy. *Am. J. Physiol. 245*:C255 (1983).
8. W. T. Gerthoffer and R. A. Murphy. *Am. J. Physiol. 245*:C271 (1983).
9. W. G. L. Kerrick and P. E. Hoar. *Nature 292*:253 (1981).

10. R. S. Adelstein, M. A. Conti, D. R. Hathaway, and C. B. Klee. *J. Biol. Chem 253*:8347 (1978).
11. M. A. Conti and R. S. Adelstein. *J. Biol. Chem. 256*:3178 (1981).
12. U. Mrwa, M. Troschka, and J. C. Ruegg. *FEBS Lett. 107*:371 (1979).
13. P. J. Silver and J. DiSalvo. *J. Biol. Chem. 254*:9951 (1979).
14. B. Vallet, A. Molla, and J. G. Demaille. *Biochim. Biophys. Acta 674*: 256 (1981).
15. W. R. Kukovetz, G. Poch, and S. Holzmann. In *Vasodilation*, P. M. Vanhoutte and I. Luesen (eds.). Raven Press, New York (1981).
16. T. Takano, W. J. Black, T. J. Peters, and C. deDuve. *J. Biol. Chem. 249*:6732 (1974).
17. S. Moncada, R. Gryglewski, S. Bunting, and J. R. Vane. *Nature 263*: 663 (1976).
18. A. Hassid and C. Williams. *Am. J. Physiol. 245*:C279 (1983).
19. A. Eldor, D. J. Falcone, D. P. Hajjar, C. R. Minick, and B. B. Weksler. *J. Clin. Invest. 67*:735 (1981).
20. S. Greenberg. In *Prostaglandins: Organ and Tissue Specific Actions*, S. Greenberg, P. J. Kadowitz, and T. F. Burks (eds.). Marcel Dekker, Inc., New York. (1982).
21. W. M. Armstead, H. L. Lippton, A. L. Hyman, and P. J. Kadowitz. *Fed. Proc. 42*:500 (1983).
22. B. M. Chapnick and K. J. Smart. *Fed. Proc. 42*:639 (1983).
23. L. P. Feigen. *J. Pharmacol. Exp. Ther. 225*:682 (1983).
24. B. M. Chapnick, L. P. Feigen, A. L. Hyman, and P. J. Kadowitz, *Am. J. Physiol. 235*:H326 (1978).
25. L. P. Feigen, B. M. Chapnick, J. E. Flemming, and P. J. Kadowitz. *Am. J. Physiol. 233*:H573 (1977).
26. D. J. Levenson, C. E. Simmons, Jr. and B. M. Brenner. *Am. J. Med. 72*: 354 (1982).
27. J. J. Walshe and R. C. Venuto. *Ann. Int. Med. 91*:47 (1979).
28. R. S. Muther, D. M. Potter, and W. M. Bennett. *Ann. Int. Med. 94*:317 (1981).
29. L. Arisz, A. J. Donker, J. R. Brentjens, and G. K. Vanderhelm. *Acta Med. Scand. 199*:121 (1976).
30. T. D. Boyer, P. Zia, and T. B. Reynolds. *Gastroenterology 77*:215 (1979).
31. R. D. Zipser, G. Ravdan, R. Duke, and T. E. Little. *Clin. Res. 30*:468A (1982).
32. C. A. Gruetter, D. V. McNamara, A. L. Hyman, and P. J. Kadowitz. *Can. J. Physiol. Pharmacol. 56*:206 (1978).
33. A. L. Hyman, E. W. Spannhake, and P. J. Kadowitz. *Am. J. Physiol. 239*:H40 (1980).
34. P. J. Kadowitz, E. W. Spannhake, L. P. Feigen, S. Greenberg, and A. L. Hyman. *Can. J. Physiol. Pharmacol. 55*:1369 (1977).

35. T. C. Wicks, J. C. Rose, M. Johnson, P. W. Ramwell, and P. A. Kot. *Circ. Res. 38*:167 (1976).
36. A. L. Hyman, P. J. Kadowitz, W. E. M. Lands, C. G. Crawford, J. Fried, and J. Barton. *Proc. Natl. Acad. Sci. USA 75*:3522 (1978).
37. E. W. Spannhake, A. L. Hyman, and P. J. Kadowitz. *J. Pharmacol. Exp. Ther. 212*:584 (1980).
38. S. Greenberg, C. McGowan, and T. M. Glenn. *Am. J. Physiol. 241*: H34 (1981).
39. P. J. Kadowitz, A. L. Hyman, C. A. Gruetter, E. W. Spannhake, and S. Greenberg. In *Prostaglandins: Organ and Tissue-Specific Actions*, S. Greenberg, P. J. Kadowitz, and T. F. Burks (eds.). Marcel Dekker, Inc., New York. (1982).
40. T. C. Noonan, R. R. Garcia-Szabo, and A. B. Malik. *Fed. Proc. 42*: 2573 (1983).
41. T. Ahmed, L. Yerger, A. Wanner, and B. Marchette. *Fed. Proc. 42*: 302 (1983).
42. A. L. Hyman and P. J. Kadowitz. *Circ. Res. 45*:404 (1979).
43. P. J. Kadowitz, B. M. Chapnick, L. P. Feigen, A. L. Hyman, P. K. Nelson, and E. W. Spannhake. *J. Appl. Physiol. 45*:408 (1978).
44. O. C. Feddersen, R. C. Murphy, and N. F. Voelkel. *Fed. Proc. 42*: 302 (1983).
45. J. D. Cooper, J. W. McDonald, M. Ali, E. Menkes, J. Masterson, and P. Klement. *Surgery 88*:215 (1980).
46. R. Winn, J. Harlan, B. Nadir, L. Harker, and J. Hildebrandt. *J. Clin. Invest. 72*:911 (1983).
47. G. H. Gurtner, A. Knoblauch, P. L. Smith, H. Sies, and N. F. Adkinson. *J. Appl. Physiol. 55*:949 (1983).
48. M. L. Morganroth, R. C. Murphy, and N. F. Voelkel. *Fed. Proc. 42*: 303 (1983).
49. K. R. Stenmark, S. L. James, N. F. Voelkel, W. H. Toews, J. T. Reeves, and R. C. Murphy. *N. Engl. J. Med. 309*:77 (1983).
50. J. R. Fletcher and P. W. Ramwell. *Adv. Prostaglandin Thromboxane Res. 7*:821 (1980).
51. W. C. Wise, J. A. Cook, T. Eller, and P. V. Halushka. *J. Pharmacol. Exp. Ther. 215*:160 (1980).
52. P. H. Chan, R. A. Fishman, J. Caronna, J. W. Schmidley, G. Prioleau, and J. Lee. *Ann. Neurol. 13*:625 (1983).
53. J. Handa, S. Yoneda, M. Matsuda, and H. Handa. *Surg. Neurol. 2*:251 (1974).
54. R. P. White. In *Prostaglandins: Organ and Tissue-Specific Actions*, S. Greenberg, P. J. Kadowitz, and T. F. Burks (eds). Marcel Dekker, Inc., New York. (1982).
55a. L. Steiner, D. M. C. Forster, V. Bergual, and L. A. Carbon. *Neuroradiology 4*:20 (1972).

55b. K. S. Paul, E. T. Whalley, C. Forster, R. Lye and J. Dutton. *J. Neurosurg. 57*:334 (1982).
56. J. Parantainen and H. Vagaatalo. *Trends Pharm. Sci. 4*:379 (1983).
57. P. S. Kulkarni, R. Roberts, and P. Needleman. *Prostaglandins 12*: 337 (1976).
58. T. H. Hinze and G. Kaley. *Circ. Res. 40*:313 (1977).
59. G. J. Dusting, S. Moncada, and J. R. Vane. *Prostaglandins 13*:3 (1977).
60. G. J. Dusting, D. J. Chapple, R. Hughes, S. Moncada, and J. R. Vane. *Cardiovasc. Res. 12*:720 (1978).
61. W. W. Nichols and J. Mehta. In *Platelets and Prostaglandins in Cardiovascular Disease*. J. Mehta and P. Mehta (eds.). Futura Publishing Co., Mount Kisco, N.Y. (1981).
62. E. J. Cornish, R. G. Goldie, E. V. Krstew, and R. C. Miller. *Clin. Exp. Pharmacol. Physiol. 10*:171 (1983).
63. M. L. Ogletree, J. B. Smith, and A. M. Lefer. *Am. J. Physiol. 235*: H400 (1978).
64. A. M. Lefer, E. F. Smith, III, H. Araki, J. B. Smith, D. Aharony, D. A. Claremon, R. L. Magolda, and K. C. Nicolaou. *Proc. Natl. Acad. Sci. USA 77*:1706 (1980).
65. M. J. Panzenbeck, A. Baez, and G. Kaley. *Fed. Proc. 42*:639 (1983).
66a. J. Benveniste, C. Boullet, C. Brink, and C. Labat. *Br. J. Pharmacol. 80*:81 (1983).
66b. S. R. Jolly. *Fed. Proc. 43*:335 (1984).
66c. G. Feuerstein, D. Ezra, L. M. Boyd, E. Hayes, P. W. Ramwell and R. E. Goldstein. Conference on Prostaglandins and Leukotrienes '84. May 8-11, Washington, D.C., Abstract 39 (1984).
67. T. J. Williams. *J. Physiol. 254*:4P (1976).
68. T. J. Williams, and M. J. Peck. *Nature (Lond.) 270*:530 (1977).
69. H. Bisgaard, J. Kristensen, and J. Sondergaard. *Br. J. Dermatol (Suppl. 25) 109*:124 (1983).
70. R. M. Daugherty, Jr., J. M. Schwinghamer, S. Surndall, and F. J. Haddy. *J. Lab. Clin. Med. 72*:869 (1968).
71. R. M. Daugherty, Jr. *Am. J. Physiol. 216*:567 (1971).
72. J. J. Maciejko, A. N. Gorman, and G. J. Grega. *Microvasc. Res. 17*: S146 (1979).
73. T. J. Williams and J. Morley. *Nature (Lond.) 246*:215 (1973).
74. S. Moncada, S. H. Ferreira, and J. R. Vane. *Nature (Lond.) 246*:217 (1973).
75. G. Thomas and G. B. West. *J. Pharm. Pharmacol. 25*:747 (1973).
76. A. J. Lewis, D. J. Nelson, and M. F. Sugrue. *Br. J. Pharmacol. 55*:51 (1975).
77. M. G. Johnson, J. B. Hay, and H. Z. Movat. *Agents Actions 6*:705 (1976).
78. M. M. Kopaniak, J. B. Hay, and H. Z. Movat. *Microvasc. Res. 15*:77 (1978).

79. E. Amelang, C. M. Prasad, R. M. Raymond, and G. J. Grega. *Circ. Res. 49*:298 (1981).
80a. D. P. Hajjar, B. B. Weksler, D. J. Falcone, J. M. Hefton, K. Tack-Goldman, and C. R. Minick. *J. Clin. Invest. 70*:479 (1982).
80b. N. E. Owen. *Fed. Proc. 43*:387 (1984).
81. P. O. Hagen, J. E. Wikberg, M. L. Akers, and M. G. Caron. *Thromb. Haematol. 50*:394 (1983).
82. A. Hassid, C. Williams, and J. Ruffier. *Fed. Proc. 42*:500 (1983).
83a. J. P. Oudinet and A. Hassid. *Fed. Proc. 42*:501 (1983).
83b. U. Frostermann, G. Hertting, and B. Neufang. *Br. J. Pharmacol. 81*: 623 (1984).
83c. A. J. Cowley and S. Heptinstall. Conference on Prostaglandins and Leukotrienes '84. May 8-11, Washington, D. C., Abstract 229 (1984).
84. B. J. Woolley, H. W. Mendenhall, Y. Sakane and T. M. Glenn. *Fed. Proc. 40*:713 (1981).
85a. S. Greenberg. *Methods Findings Exp. Clin. Pharmacol. 3*:233 (1981).
85b. T. Fukumori, E. Tami, Y. Maeda and A. Scikenaga. *Stroke. 15*:306 (1984).
86. M. O'Donnell, B. Yaremko, H. Crowley, and A. F. Welton. *Fed. Proc. 42*:442 (1983).
87. A. Tokumura, K. Fukuzawa, and H. Tsukatani. *Lipids* 7:572 (1978).
88. A. Tokumura, K. Fukuzawa, Y. Akamatsu, S. Yamada, T. Suzuki, and H. Tsukatani. *Lipids 7*:468 (1978).
89. K. A. Schumacher, H. G. Classen, and M. Spath. *Thromb. Hemostas. 42*:631 (1979).
90. A. Tokumura, T. Kume, K. Fukuzawa, and H. Tsukatani. *J. Pharmacol. Exp. Ther. 219*:219 (1981).
91. P. Hedqvist. In *Prostaglandins Synthetase Inhibitors*, H. J. Robinson and J. R. Vane (eds.). Raven Press, N.Y. (1974).

BIBLIOGRAPHY

E. Bulbring, A. F. Brading, A. W. Jones, and T. Tomita (eds.). *Smooth Muscle: An Assessment of Current Knowledge*. Edward Arnold, London (1981).

A. P. Somlyo and A. V. Somlyo. *Pharmacol. Rev. 20*:197 (1968) and *22*:249 (1970).

A. P. Somlyo and A. V. Somlyo. *Meth. Pharmacol. 3*:3 (1975).

III

THE ROLE OF PROSTAGLANDINS AND RELATED CHEMICALS IN VIVO IN CELL-CELL INTERACTIONS INVOLVING BLOOD CELLS

15

Assessment of the Production of Prostaglandins and Related Chemicals In Vivo

There are many pitfalls in trying to measure in vivo production of prostaglandins and related chemicals. The low levels and the rapid degradation of prostaglandins in vivo, coupled with the potential, as a result of activation of platelets or blood vessel injury, for artifactual production of some of these compounds during blood sampling, means that great caution must be exercised in measurement of the compounds in vivo.

I. PLASMA LEVELS

A. PGE_2, $PGF_{2\alpha}$

These two prostaglandins are present in plasma in extremely low levels, and are rapidly metabolized in the lung. Furthermore, any platelet activation during blood sampling will produce spuriously high levels. At the present time the levels of these prostaglandins in plasma must be considered unmeasurable unless a specific condition causing a marked elevation of the prostaglandin is present. It may be possible, however, to get a realistic assessment of their production by using assays of their metabolites.

1. Prostaglandin E_2

PGE_2 is rapidly metabolized following intravenous injection into humans, with only 3% remaining as PGE_2 after 90 seconds. The major metabolite found in plasma in the first few minutes is 15-keto-13,14-dehydro PGE_2. This metabolite has a half-life of about 8 min in blood (1a). However this metabolite is unstable, and it may be best to induce the formation of a single stable bicyclic degradation product (11-deoxy-15-keto-13,14-dihydro-11,16-cyclo-PGE_2) and to assay this compound (1b). Longer-lived plasma metabolites probably exist but are not well studied.

2. Prostaglandin $F_{2\alpha}$

$PGF_{2\alpha}$ is metabolized very quickly to 15-keto-13,14,dihydro $PGF_{2\alpha}$. For the first few minutes after infusion of $PGF_{2\alpha}$ into humans, this is the major plasma metabolite (2). In this initial period, the plasma levels of this metabolite reached higher concentrations than any later-formed metabolite. However, after the first few minutes 5_α, 7_α-dihydroxy-11-ketotetranorprostane-1,16-dioic acid was the major metabolite in plasma. This compound, also the major urinary metabolite of $PGF_{2\alpha}$, could be detected in plasma for several hours after the $PGF_{2\alpha}$ infusion. Based on present evidence, it would seem best to measure 15-keto-13,14-dihydro $PGF_{2\alpha}$ under circumstances where slow, continual formation of $PGF_{2\alpha}$ is expected, or where sampling can be frequent, but to assay the tetranor metabolite where sampling is infrequent and where the pattern of synthesis is unknown. A further complication in assessing in vivo $PGF_{2\alpha}$ in man is that $PGF_{2\alpha}$ metabolites may form from degradation of PGE_2 and PGD_2 (2-4). Variations in animal species are discussed in App. 15-1.

B. Prostaglandin D_2

The metabolism of PGD_2 in man has not yet been well studied. In the monkey, a variety of urinary metabolites have been identified (3). The pattern of these metabolites suggests that the major route of PGD_2 metabolism may not be via the 15-OH-prostaglandin dehydrogenase, consistent with other evidence that PGD_2 is not a good substrate for this enzyme (5,6). Rather, a considerable proportion of PGD_2 appears to be metabolized to $PGF_{2\alpha}$ or $PGF_{2\alpha}$ metabolites. At the present time, it is likely that PGD_2 will have a very short half-life in vivo, but the major plasma metabolite in humans is not yet established. Recently, it has been found that incubating PGD_2 with human plasma in vitro results in its conversion to 9-deoxy-Δ^9,Δ^{12}-13,13-dihydro-prostaglandin D_2, but whether this metabolite is significant in vivo is not certain (7b).

C. Prostaglandin I_2

The concentration of PGI_2 plus 6-keto $PGF_{1\alpha}$ in human peripheral plasma has been found to be less than 0.5 pg/ml in healthy male subjects (8). Other recent estimates, while not sensitive to quite such low concentrations, have not found detectable 6-keto $PGF_{1\alpha}$ (i.e., less than 40 pg/ml and less than 10 pg/ml) (9,10). Using a bioassay, Haslam found the level of PGI_2 in rabbit blood to be 0.06 pmol/ml (11). Whereas there may be some debate about the precise levels of PGI_2 and 6-keto $PGF_{1\alpha}$ in human plasma, it is clear they are very low due to their short half-lives (12a). Based on estimates of total body production from measurement of urinary metabolites, and a maximum plasma half-life for 6-keto $PGF_{1\alpha}$ of 30 min, Frolich and Rosenkranz have calculated that true plasma levels of 6-keto $PGF_{1\alpha}$ in normals must be less than 27 pg/ml (12b). PGI_2 is certainly not the circulating hormone it was originally suggested to be. Although PGI_2 escapes inactivation by lung prostaglandin dehydrogenase, it is bound and inactivated by red blood cells (13).

Two metabolites, 2,3-dinor-6,15-diketo-13,14-dihydro-$PGF_{1\alpha}$ and 2,3-dinor-6,15-diketo-13,14-dihydro-$PGF_{1\alpha}$-1,20 dicarboxylic acid, have been detected in plasma (14).

D. Thromboxane A_2

The immediate degradation product of thromboxane A_2 is thromboxane B_2. Thromboxane B_2 levels in normal plasma are probably extremely low and below the limit of detection for most assays. Measurements of plasma thromboxane B_2 may be useful, however, under specific conditions where levels are substantially elevated. The best metabolite to assay in human plasma is not yet established.

II. LEVELS OF URINARY METABOLITES

Measurement of the metabolites of prostaglandins and related chemical in the urine has been useful under some conditions, but these measurements also have their limitations. For example, prostaglandin production in the kidney may be overrepresented in assessing the primary prostaglandins and perhaps immediate metabolites. Production of one of the major body metabolites of thromboxane B_2 (2,3-dinor thromboxane B_2) and prostacyclin (2,3-dinor-6-keto-$PGF_{1\alpha}$) is more useful, but will reflect total body production, not necessarily just platelet and vascular production (4). Similar assays for 9-hydroxy-11,15-dioxo-2,3,4,5-tetranorprostane-1,16-dioic acid, 7_α-hydroxy-5,11-diketotetranorprostane-1,16-dioic acid, and 5_α,7_α-dihydroxy-11-keto-tetranorprostane-1,16-dioic acid, the principal urinary metabolites of PGD_2, PGE_2, and $PGF_{2\alpha}$, respectively, have been useful (1a,15-17). With each prostaglandin, the urinary metabolite mentioned is but one of a number of urinary metabolites which could be assessed. For a more detailed evaluation of urinary prostaglandin and thromboxane metabolites other references are available (3,18-20).

APPENDIX 15-1: VARIATION IN PLASMA $PGF_{2\alpha}$ METABOLITES IN VARIOUS SPECIES

Based on studies in several species, Granstrom (2,7a) has suggested using assays for 15-keto-13,14-dihydro $PGF_{2\alpha}$ in all species where prostaglandin release is slow and continuous, or where frequent samples can be taken. In the cow, this metabolite persists and can be used as a reasonable reliable index of all production for the previous several hours. In sheep, measurement of 5,7,11-dihydroxy-11-ketotetranorprostane-1,16-dioic acid and 5,7-trihydroxy-tetranorprostane-1,16-dioic acid is recommended, whereas in the rat assay of 5,7-dihydroxy-11-ketotetranorprostanoic acid is suggested. In the rabbit and guinea pig all metabolites are cleared from plasma so rapidly that assessment of urinary metabolites is probably best.

APPENDIX 15-2: SPECIES VARIATION IN $PGF_{2\alpha}$ and PGI_2 URINARY VERSUS FECAL METABOLISM

In rats, a considerable proportion of $PGF_{2\alpha}$ and PGI_2 is excreted in the feces, rather than in the urine as in humans (21,22).

REFERENCES

1a. M. Hamberg and B. Samuelsson. *J. Biol. Chem. 246*:6713 (1971).
1b. E. Granstrom, F. A. Fitzpatrick and H. Kindahl. *Methods Enzymol. 86*:306 (1982).
2. E. Granstrom, H. Kindahl, and M. L. Swahn. *Biochim. Biophys. Acta 713*:46 (1982).
3. C. K. Ellis, M. D. Smigel, J. A. Oates, O. Oelz, and B. J. Sweetman. *J. Biol. Chem. 254*:4152 1979).
4. L. J. Roberts, B. J. Sweetman, R. L. Maas, W. C. Hubbard, and J. A. Oates. *J. Lipid Res. 20*:117 (1982).
5. F. F. Sun, S. B. Armour, V. R. Bockstanz, and J. C. McGuire. *Adv. Prostaglandin Thromboxane Res. 1*:163 (1976).
6. M. F. Ruckrich, W. Schlegel, and A. Jung. *FEBS Lett. 68*:59 (1976).
7a. E. Granstrom and H. Kindahl. *Biochim. Biophys. Acta 713*:555 (1982).
7b. Y. Kikawa, S. Narumiya, M. Fukushima, H. Wakatsuka and O. Hayaishi. *Proc. Natl. Acad. Sci. USA 81*:1317 (1984).
8. I. A. Blair, S. E. Barrow, K. A. Waddell, P. J. Lewis, and C. T. Dollery. *Prostaglandins. 23*:579 (1982).
9. M. Greaves and F. E. Preston. *Thromb. Res. 26*:145 (1982).
10. E. Christ-Hazelhof and D. H. Nugteren. *Acta Therapeutic. 6*:33 (1980).
11. R. J. Haslam and M. D. McClenaghan. *Nature 292*:364 (1981).
12a. C. Patrono, F. Pugliese, G. Ciabattoni, P. Patrignani, A. Maseri, S. Chierchia, B. A. Peskar, B. M. Simonetti, and A. Pierucci. *J. Clin. Invest. 69*:231 (1982).
12b. J. C. Frolich and B. Rosenkranz. *Prostaglandins. 27*:355 (1984).
13. C. Williams, H. V. Stel, W. Van Aben, and J. A. VanMovrik. *Br. J. Haematol. 53*43 (1983).
14. B. Rosenkranz, C. Fischer, and J. C. Frolich. *Clin. Pharmacol. Ther. 29*:420 (1981).
15. L. J. Roberts, B. J. Sweetman, R. A. Lewis, K. F. Austen, and J. A. Oates. *N. Engl. J. Med. 303*:1400 (1980).
16. E. Granstrom and B. Samuelsson. *J. Biol. Chem. 241*:5254 (1971).
17. H. W. Seyberth, G. V. Segre, J. L. Morgan, B. J. Sweetman, J. T. Potts, and J. A. Oates. *N. Engl. J. Med. 293*:1278 (1975).
18. B. Samuelsson, E. Granstrom, K. Green, M. Hamberg, and S. Hammarstrom. *Ann. Rev. Biochem. 44*:669 (1975).
19. L. J. Roberts, II, B. J. Sweetman, and J. A. Oates. *J. Biol. Chem. 256*: 8384 (1981).
20. A. R. Brash, E. K. Jackson, C. A. Saggese, J. A. Lawson, J. A. Oates, and G. A. Fitzgerald. *J. Pharmacol. Exp. Ther. 226*:78 (1983).
21. K. Green. *Biochim. Biophys. Acta 231*:419 (1971).
22. F. F. Sun and B. M. Taylor. *Biochemistry 17*:4096 (1978).

16

Hemostasis, Thrombosis, and Atherosclerosis: The Response of Blood Cells to Vessel Wall Injury

The prevention of bleeding on injury to a blood vessel wall involves an interplay among the injured vessel site, platelets, and blood proteins. The rate of blood flow past the site, relatively fast in arteries and slower in veins, and the accompanying vasoconstriction also influence the process. In brief, injury to a vessel wall exposes subendothelial tissue. Collagen, a major component of this subendothelial layer, provides sites to which platelets can adhere. Platelets attach to collagen and spread over the injured surface. Von Willebrand factor appears to be important for platelet-collagen attachment at high shear rates. When the platelets spread, they secrete their granule contents. The release of tissue factor in the area of injury promotes blood protein coagulation and fibrin formation. The surface of the activated platelet accelerates this reaction. At the same time thromboxane A_2 and ADP secreted from activated platelets will act on other platelets in the vicinity and promote aggregation of these platelets at the site. Thromboxane A_2 produced by platelets and thromboxane A_2 and leukotrienes produced by the injured vessel wall will stimulate vasospasm.

As these events promoting clotting occur, other processes act to limit the extent of the platelet-fibrin clot and the degree of vasospasm. Endothelial cells, where these are left following the injury, will produce

PGI_2 in response to injury or as a result of stimulation by thrombin. PGI_2 will act to inhibit further platelet aggregation and to dilate the blood vessel to alleviate the vasospasm. Thrombin formed during the coagulation sequence will also bind to a receptor, thrombomodulin, on the endothelial cell surface. Thrombomodulin blocks the platelet-stimulating and fibrin-forming effects of thrombin and promotes thrombin activation of protein C. The activated protein C inhibits further fibrin formation, preventing the downstream propagation of the clot and, acting together with plasminogen activator released from the endothelial cells, it promotes plasmin formation and clot lysis.

During hemostasis, the balance of reactions is clearly critical. With a significant vessel injury, adequate platelet-fibrin plug formation and local vasospasm are essential to stop bleeding. Failure of these reactions will lead to a bleeding disorder. On the other hand, overactive clot formation, unnecessary vasospasm, or failure of clot lysis may lead to an unwanted vessel obstruction and ischemia to the region supplied by the blood vessel, a thrombotic disorder.

Secretion of a growth factor by platelets during the response to injury can lead to smooth muscle proliferation, one of the components of atherosclerosis. Healing platelet-fibrin thrombi may also be incorporated into and thus augment the atherosclerotic plaque.

I. BLEEDING AND THROMBOTIC TENDENCY

Some information on factors which predispose to bleeding and thrombotic tendencies is helpful to the later discussion of the effects of prostaglandins and related substances.

A. Bleeding Tendency

Bleeding difficulties are more likely with decreased platelet numbers, impaired platelet function, decreased or abnormal coagulation factors (including von Willebrand factor), accelerated fibrinolysis, and perhaps (this is less well defined) with an abnormal blood vessel site for stimulating coagulation or platelet adhesion.

B. Thrombotic Tendency

Circumstances predisposing to thrombosis include those associated with platelets which are hyperfunctional or activated in vivo, conditions of altered or decreased blood flow including venous stasis (i.e., varicose veins), and increased blood viscosity (i.e., dehydration, decreased red blood cell deformability, and increased fibrinogen), as well as altered coagulation factor levels (i.e., inherited high factor V or VIII, decreased antithrombin III or protein C, or, from large population studies, raised VII, VIII, or fibrinogen), and decreased fibrinolysis (i.e., decreased plasminogen activator). It is in these areas, platelet function, blood flow, coagulation, and fibrinolysis, that effects of arachidonic acid metabolites are important in terms of their regulation of hemostasis and thrombosis.

II. THE ROLE OF PROSTAGLANDINS AND RELATED CHEMICALS

A. The Balance of Thromboxane A_2 and Prostacyclin (PGI_2)

A widely studied hypothesis for the regulation of hemostasis and thrombosis is that the balance between the prothrombotic thromboxane A_2 and antithrombotic prostacyclin is critical to modulation of hemostasis (Fig. 16-1). According to this concept, a relative increase in production of thromboxane A_2 (primarily from platelets) with its action to promote platelet aggregation and stimulate vasoconstriction should be associated with an increased tendency to develop thromboses. In contrast, a relative increase in prostacyclin (primarily from endothelial cells) with its actions to inhibit platelet function and cause vasodilation should be associated with a decreased risk of thrombosis and an increased risk of bleeding. This hypothesis has been evaluated in several ways. Disease states associated with thrombotic or bleeding tendencies have been studied to look for alterations in the balance of thromboxane and prostacyclin. Drugs known to be antithrombotic, thrombogenic, or known to perturb the synthesis or effect of prostacyclin or thromboxane selectively have been evaluated. Prostacyclin, thromboxane A_2, or analogues of these compounds have been infused into animals or people to gain a more direct insight into their actions in vivo.

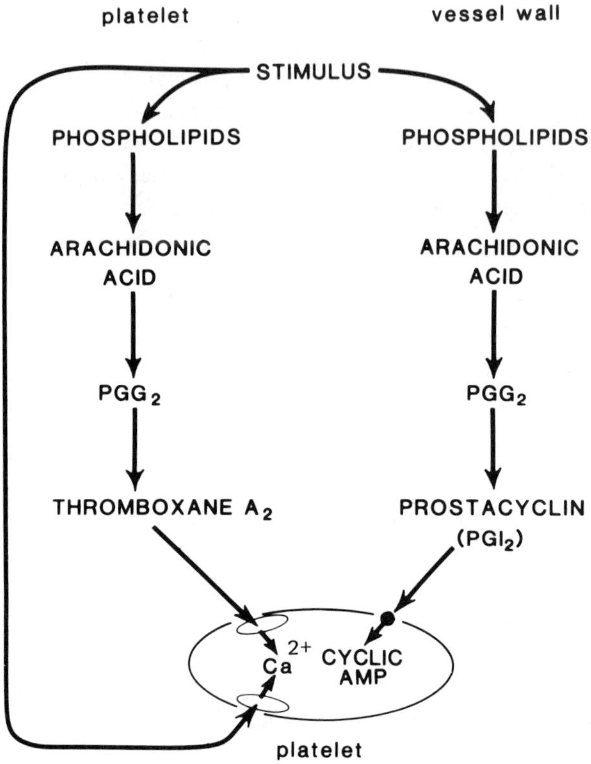

Fig. 16-1 A schematic outline of the balance of production and effects of PGI_2 (prostacyclin) and thromboxane A_2 on platelets. A thromboxane-independent pathway (left) is also shown as being important for platelet-activation. The effect of thromboxane A_2 to constrict (contract) blood vessels, while prostacyclin dilates (relaxes) such vessels may be as important (perhaps sometimes more important) as the effects shown on platelets.

1. Infusion of Arachidonic Acid, Thromboxane, or Prostacyclin In Vivo

Arachidonic acid. Intravenous injection of arachidonic acid, but not other fatty acids, into rabbits produces extensive platelet aggregates in the lung and sudden death (1). The effect is due to production of thromboxane A_2, as it is preventable by pretreating the rabbits with aspirin or imidazole (2).

Thromboxane A_2. Injection of thromboxane A_2, generated by incubation of PGH_2 with platelet microsomes, into coronary arteries or at the origin of the aortic arch in guinea pigs and rabbits produces myocardial ischemia, subendocardial necrosis, and sometimes ventricular fibrilation (3-6). Cholesterol feeding of rabbits renders them more likely to develop myocardial infarction when thromboxane A_2 is infused (6).

A major component of the effect of thromboxane A_2 is its ability to cause vasospasm. This is evident from studies of carbocyclic thromboxane A_2 (CTA_2), which constricts blood vessels but has no effect on platelets. Like thromboxane A_2, it causes sudden death in rabbits; however, with CTA_2 the effect is solely due to vasospasm for there is no platelet aggregation or thrombus formation (7).

Prostacyclin (PGI_2). In vitro prostacyclin acts to inhibit platelet adhesion to an injured vessel wall, platelet aggregation, and the platelet contribution to coagulation as well as relaxing most vascular smooth muscle cells—all actions which are antithrombotic.

Infusion of prostacyclin in humans produces vasodilating and antiplatelet effects, including a fall in diastolic blood pressure; facial, palmar, and pedal erythema; and a prolongation of the bleeding time (8,9). Prostacyclin has antithrombotic activity in a wide variety of animal models (5-8). Some evidence has been obtained for a beneficial effect of the infusion of prostacyclin in humans with arteriosclerosis obliterans and other forms of peripheral arterial disease (14,15). Such beneficial effects have not been found by all investigators, however, and it may be some time before a therapeutic role for prostacyclin in such disorders is clearly established.

2. Conditions Where Evidence Exists for a Thrombotic Tendency Associated with a Disturbance in Prostacyclin/Thromboxane Balance

Diabetes. Diabetes is associated with a tendency to thrombosis, particularly in small vessels and arteries. Platelets, in vitro, from diabetic animals and humans produce increased amounts of thromboxane A_2 in response to stimuli such as thrombin (16-21). Blood vessels from diabetic animals and humans also make less prostacyclin than normals (17,18,22-26). This is true in the umbilical cord vessels from infants of diabetic mothers as well as vessels from patients with diabetes (27). Both abnormal platelet thromboxane production and vascular prostacyclin production can be corrected by islet tissue transplantation in rats, showing the effects are specific to the diabetic state (18). Continuous insulin infusion given to humans to give improved diabetic control appears to normalize platelet thromboxane production (28).

The enhanced platelet thromboxane production appears primarily due to an increased agonist-stimulated release of arachidonic acid from platelet phospholipids (18). The decreased vascular prostacyclin formation is due to decreased prostacyclin synthetase activity (Fig. 16-2) (18).

A limitation of the studies in diabetes as in many other conditions is that data on in vivo production are lacking. The in vitro data suggest that the diabetic platelets and vessels will respond abnormally to stimuli in vivo, but measurements to prove this point are needed. Given the complexity of diabetes and other potentially thrombotic factors present in at least some diabetics (i.e., elevated factor VII, VIIIc, ristocetin cofactor, immune complexes, and decreased fibrinolytic activity) (19-21), the abnormal prostacyclin/thromboxane balance is probably only one component of the thrombotic tendency in this disorder.

Radiation. Radiation produces tissue damage which is associated with thrombosis of the vessels in the irradiated area. Radiation has been shown to cause an inhibition of endothelial cell prostacyclin synthetase (32). This probably results from free radical fatty acid or peroxide-induced enzyme inhibition, although the precise mechanism has not yet been clearly elucidated. No effect of radiation on platelet thromboxane production has been shown. However, in one study, local irradiation was associated with a decrease in platelet sensitivity to prostacyclin (33).

Studies of irradiation in vivo suggest that immediately after irradiation there may be a temporary increase in PGI_2 production (possibly due to cell damage), followed by a long-lasting decrease (34a,b). The balance of thromboxane to prostacyclin as assessed by measuring the urinary products appears to be shifted toward a relative increase in thromboxane production (35).

Smoking and Nicotine. Cigarette smoking is a risk factor for atherothrombotic disorders. Nicotine has been shown to inhibit vascular prostacyclin synthesis (36,37). Umbilical arteries of infants born to mothers who smoke produce much less prostacyclin than those born to nonsmoking mothers (38a). Acutely, smoking has been shown to be associated with hyperaggregable platelets without a significant change in arachidonic acid metabolism (38b). Individuals who smoke, however, have increased thromboxane-synthesizing capacity compared with those who do not (38c).

Hypercholesterolemia. Hypercholesterolemia, a risk factor for atherothrombotic disorders, is associated with hyperfunctional platelets which produce increased thromboxane A_2 in response to physiologic

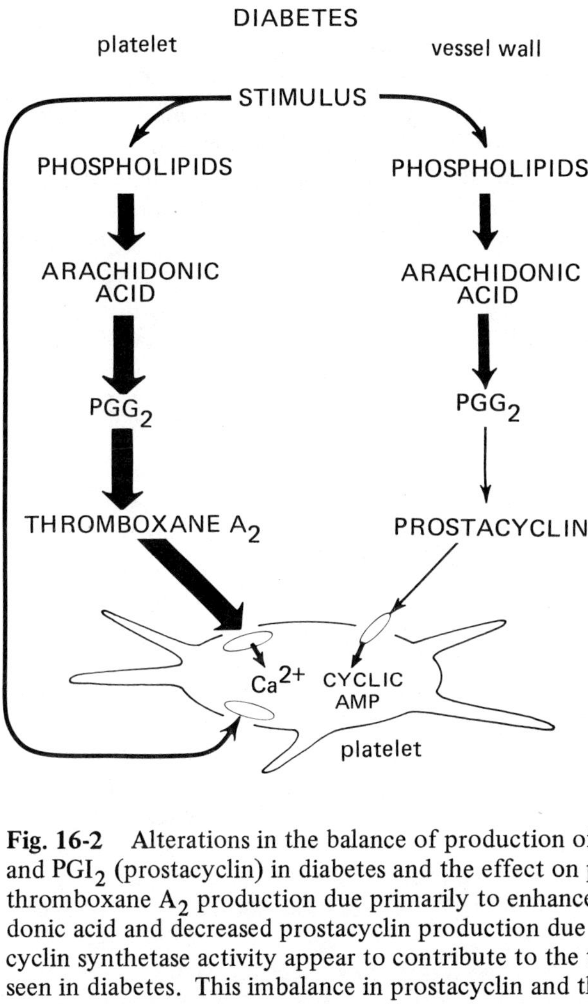

Fig. 16-2 Alterations in the balance of production of thromboxane A_2 and PGI_2 (prostacyclin) in diabetes and the effect on platelets. Enhanced thromboxane A_2 production due primarily to enhanced release of arachidonic acid and decreased prostacyclin production due to a lowered prostacyclin synthetase activity appear to contribute to the thrombotic tendency seen in diabetes. This imbalance in prostacyclin and thromboxane production leads to platelets which tend to aggregate more easily (as shown above), and vessels which tend to constrict (not shown).

agonists such as thrombin (39). The effect of the cholesterol is due to increased release of arachidonic acid from platelet phospholipids, and to increased conversion of released arachidonic acid to thromboxane A_2 (40). Effects of hypercholesterolemia on vascular prostacyclin synthesis are not well defined. However, recent studies suggest that platelets from hypercholesterolemic subjects are refractory to inhibition by prostacyclin (41,42), and that hypercholesterolemia delays the recovery of vascular prostacyclin production following vessel wall injury (43).

Vitamin E deficiency. A deficiency in vitamin E is associated in rats with fetal wastage due to thromboses in the placental vessels (55). Vitamin E deficiency is associated with increased platelet aggregability, increased platelet thromboxane A_2 production in response to physiologic agonists, and decreased vascular prostacyclin production (45-49b). The action of vitamin E is presumably to prevent formation of lipid peroxides. In the absence of vitamin E, lipid peroxides presumably build up and can then inhibit prostacyclin synthetase (Ch. 5). Deficient vitamin E in infants is associated with a defect in the ability of the infant plasma to regenerate PGI_2 production when added to "exhausted" blood vessels (49c). Such regeneration of PGI_2 production may be due to an action of vitamin E to "mop up" toxic radicals.

The reason for increased platelet thromboxane production in vitamin E deficiency may relate to enhanced phospholipase activity (48). Restoring vitamin E levels to normal in the diet in rats leads to a progressive normalization of vascular prostacyclin and platelet thromboxane production (48).

Chronic placental insufficiency and preeclampsia. Analysis of umbilical cord production of prostacyclin has shown decreased synthesis in vessels from infants with chronic placental insufficiency and intrauterine growth retardation (50a) and in infants of mothers with preeclampsia (50b, 50c). Adequate prostacyclin may be particularly critical to prevent thromboses in placental vessels. Decreased prostacyclin may be associated with high blood pressure in toxemia in pregnancy, and preliminary results from a recent study have shown benefit from prostacyclin treatment in toxemia, including a lowering of maternal blood pressure, increased placental perfusion, and a decrease in the number of occluded (thrombosed?) placental vessels (51,52).

Atherosclerosis. Atherosclerotic blood vessels have been found to have less capacity to produce prostacyclin than normal vessels (53-55), and the hypothesis has been put forward that a buildup of lipid peroxides in atherosclerotic vessels is responsible for this decrease in prostacyclin (56). However, evaluation of the urinary metabolites of individuals with diffuse atherosclerosis has shown an increased production of PGI_2 (57). This apparently contradictory finding may result from an increase in traumatic platelet-vascular interactions in patients with atherosclerosis. Thus, whereas less PGI_2 than normal may be produced in a given instance of vessel wall injury leading to a higher likelihood of thrombotic outcome, the increased incidence of vessel injury in atherosclerosis could lead to increased bodywide production of prostacyclin. In the later stages of atherosclerosis, there is increased platelet production of thromboxane A_2 (58-60).

Hyperoxia and Oxygen Toxicity. Exposure of umbilical arteries to higher than usual levels of oxygen inhibits the tissue synthesis of prostacyclin (61). This is probably a result of oxygen radical inhibition of prostacyclin synthase since the adverse effect on PGI_2 synthesis can be prevented by the antioxidant BHT (butylated hydroxytoluene). It is possible that some of the adverse effects of high oxygen levels in newborns undergoing treatment for respiratory difficulties are related to decreased PGI_2 synthesis.

Thrombotic thrombocytopenic purpura/hemolytic uremic syndrome. These two related disorders will be discussed together. In both, evidence for deficient production of prostacyclin has been presented, and in both cases this has been related to the deficiency of a plasma factor which normally stimulates prostacyclin production (62-67). Evidence for a shortened plasma half-life of prostacyclin in some patients and a familial tendency or an irreversible defect in some patients but not others suggest that the underlying basis for the decreased prostacyclin may be variable (68,69). Furthermore, none of these studies has assessed in vivo production of prostacyclin, and this would seem essential before it can be accepted unequivocally that defective prostacyclin production is a basic defect in this syndrome. Moreover, it is unknown at present whether the defective prostacyclin production is secondary (i.e., to a immune complex or other types of vessel wall injury) or primary. The presence of the defect in some patients with recurrent disease after full recovery suggests that it might be a primary defect in some instances.

Recent studies of patients with thrombotic thrombocytopenic purpura suggest the presence of von Willebrand factor multimers may be important in this disorder. The relationship between this finding and the prostacyclin deficiency is not yet celar.

Raynaud's phenomenon. The presence of high levels of thromboxane B_2 and PGE_2 in patients with Raynaud's syndrome has been reported (70). Patients with Raynaud's phenomenon have symptomatic improvement following intermittent prostacyclin infusion (71). Further studies of these patients are needed to better define the role of thromboxane and prostacyclin.

Angina. Although it has been suggested that the episodes of myocardial ischemia in patients with variant angina are due to altered PGI_2 and thromboxane A_2 (72), current evidence does not support this view. The increase in thromboxane B_2 seen is late, and no beneficial effect of cyclo-oxygenase inhibitors has been seen (73).

Hypertension. Diminished urinary 6-keto $PGF_{1\alpha}$ has been found in patients with essential hypertension (74). Decreased vascular PGI_2 production could potentially have a role in the development of hypertension. However, other studies have shown increased PGI_2 production by blood vessels from spontaneously hypertensive rats (75), and much more evidence is needed to link alterations in PGI_2 production in vivo to significant changes in blood pressure.

Homocysteinuria. Homocysteine, in vitro, appears to increase platelet thromboxane production in response to arachidonic acid, but has no effect on vascular prostacyclin synthesis (76a). The importance of these findings in vivo is uncertain as current evidence suggests vascular injury caused by homocysteine may be important to the thrombotic problems of individuals with homocysteinuria (76b).

Oral contraceptive use. Oral contraceptive use is associated with a thrombotic tendency. Platelets from individuals on oral contraceptives show increased production of thromboxane A_2 from arachidonic acid, increased aggregability to an endoperoxide analogue, and decreased sensitivity to prostacyclin (77,78).

Aging. Decreased PGI_2 production with advancing age has been reported (79). It is possible that this change in PGI_2 production with age may explain, in part, the decrease in the bleeding time with age.

Mental Stress. Endogenous opioid peptides, the enkephalins, increase endothelial cell PGI_2 production in response to either arachidonic acid or thrombin (80). Further studies are needed to evaluate a potential role for altered PGI_2 and thromboxane A_2 in stress, and the possible relationship of any such changes to the suggested role of type A (stressful) behavior in coronary artery disease.

Low-Density Lipoproteins. Increased serum low-density lipoproteins have been associated with increased vascular prostacyclin production (81).

Selenium Deficiency. Platelets from rats rendered selenium deficient show enhanced aggregation and increased thromboxane production in response to collagen (81b). It was suggested that the enhanced platelet thromboxane production may be due to increased cellular peroxide levels resulting from the low levels of glutathione peroxidase in the selenium deficient animals.

3. Conditions Where There is Evidence for a Bleeding Tendency Associated with an Altered Prostacyclin/ Thromboxane Balance

Diets Enriched in Eicosapentaenoic (Timnodonic) Acid. The diet of Greenland Eskimos in which the fat content of the diet comes largely from fish or fish-eating mammals such as seals, contains a high level of eicosapentaenoic acid and a low level of arachidonic acid. The platelets and blood vessels from these Greenland Eskimos contain much eicosapentaenoic acid and very little arachidonic acid (82). Greenland Eskimos have a mild bleeding tendency and a low incidence of atherosclerosis (83). The bleeding tendency appears to relate to the abnormal fatty acid and the difference in its metabolism compared with arachidonic acid. In human platelets, eicosapentaenoic acid can be metabolized by the platelet cyclooxygenase (84,85), but the thromboxane A_3 formed is only weakly active in promoting platelet aggregation (86,87). For this reason, and because eicosapentaenoic acid competes with arachidonic acid for incorporation into platelet phospholipids, inhibits the conversion of arachidonic acid to thromboxane A_2, and may itself be converted to PGD_3 (see Ch. 6), individuals on diets enriched in this fatty acid have platelets which function poorly (88,89).

Blood vessels incubated with eicosapentaenoic acid will produce a PGI_2-like substance which inhibits platelet aggregation (87). Initial controversy over whether PGI_3 was produced in vivo appears to be resolved as a species difference, with some species (i.e., rats) being unable to convert eicosapentaenoic acid to PGI_3 whereas others, including humans, will do so (Ch. 13). PGI_3 will, like PGI_2, inhibit platelet aggregation (Fig. 16-3).

Some recent data suggest other, as yet undefined, factors could be involved in the eicosapentaenoic acid-induced prolongation of the bleeding time (90).

Uremia. The bleeding tendency in uremia has been associated with increased vascular prostacyclin synthesis in vitro (91,92a). Until measurements are made in vivo and evidence provided that the defect can be corrected by PGI_2 synthetase inhibition, this concept must be viewed with caution.

Ethanol. Several studies have shown that moderate consumption of alcohol protects against cardiovascular disease (92b-g). Ethanol will inhibit platelet function and decrease platelet formation of thromboxane B_2 (92b,g). No effect of ethanol on aorta PGI_2 formation was found in studies of rats (92h).

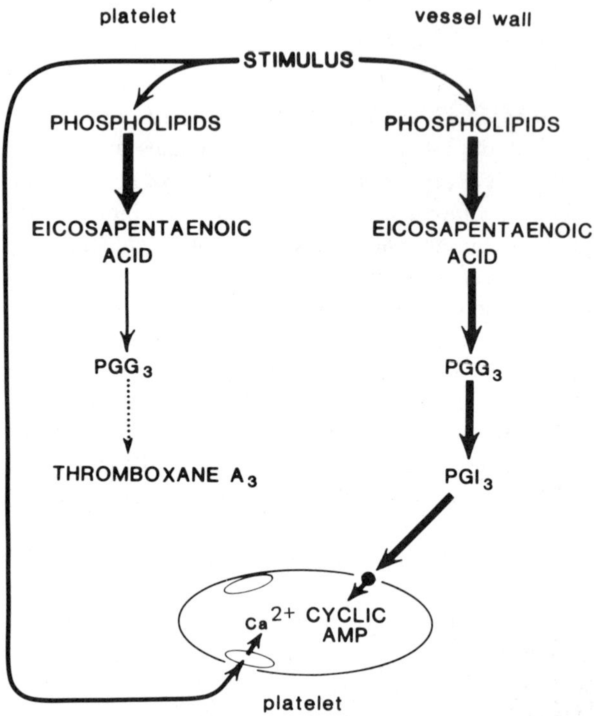

Fig. 16-3 In Greenland Eskimos, the arachidonic acid in the diet is largely replaced by eicosapentaenoic acid. The effect of this switch is to alter the pattern of prostacyclin and thromboxane production drastically to give a mild bleeding tendency. While platelets may produce small amounts of thromboxane A_3, this does not promote platelet aggregation. PGI_3, though produced by human blood vessels in lesser amounts than PGI_2 is produced from arachidonic acid, is nevertheless active in inhibiting platelets and relaxing vascular smooth muscle.

4. Selective Modulation of Thromboxane and Prostacyclin Production or Effects by Drugs

Cyclooxygenase inhibitors

Aspirin. Many studies have evaluated the clinical antithrombotic potential of aspirin. The results are still debated (93-96). Benefit of aspirin as an antithrombotic agent has been shown in animal models of thrombosis and in patients with hemodialysis shunts (160 mg p.o. daily) (97,98). However, trials of aspirin in myocardial infarction have shown, at best, a small and equivocal effect of aspirin, whereas trials of aspirin in stroke and postsurgical venous thromboses have ranged from showing some benefit in males but not females to equivocal results (93-96,99). An exception to the studies showing a small effect of aspirin is a recent study in patients with unstable angina which showed a 50% reduction in myocardial infarction and death. It is possible that a subset of patients at risk for myocardial infarction, those with unstable angina, may benefit significantly from aspirin at 325 mg/day (100a).

A tremendous amount of work using aspirin has been done to see if this drug can be used in humans to selectively inhibit the platelet cyclooxygenase while sparing the vascular enzyme. Early studies suggesting the vascular prostaglandin endoperoxide synthase was much less sensitive to aspirin have turned out to be mistaken (100b). Since endothelial cells can make new protein, whereas circulating platelets cannot, the possibility has been raised, using cultured endothelial cells, that the aspirin effect on endothelial cells might be of short duration compared with its effects on platelets. However, endothelial cells in vivo may be much less active than those in culture. Thus, whereas a discrepancy can be demonstrated in vitro, there may be less in vivo difference in the recovery of platelets and endothelial cells from exposure to aspirin. However, it remains possible that a schedule for administering aspirin can be found which will be relatively selective in its effects—inhibiting platelet thromboxane synthesis without significant effects on vascular prostacyclin.

Current work suggests that a single dose of 150 or 300 mg aspirin markedly inhibits both platelet thromboxane and vascular prostacyclin in vivo (101,102). A single dose of 40 mg aspirin appears to have a much greater effect on platelet thromboxane production than on vascular (total vessel or endothelial cell alone) prostacyclin production 12-16 h later (102-104). However, aspirin 20 mg daily for 7 days or more markedly suppressed both platelet thromboxane and endothelial cell PGI_2 (104), although total body PGI_2 was not affected (105), suggesting the deeper cell layers (i.e., smooth muscle) and their synthesis of PGI_2 are less affected. A regimen of 40 mg aspirin every other day may allow recovery of vascular prostacyclin production while maintaining inhibition of platelet thromboxane production (103a). Further studies are needed to confirm this.

In an alternate approach FitzGerald has used a dose of 1 mg aspirin over 30 mins. for 20 doses (103b). At this dose, aspirin appears to be fully metabolized to salicylate in its first passage through the liver. Platelets exposed to aspirin in the bloodstream (while in the venous or presystemic circulation) are inhibited while arterial PGI_2 production is not affected allowing a pronounced differential effect to inhibit platelet thromboxane while sparing vascular prostacyclin production.

Other cyclooxygenase inhibitors. A variety of cyclooxygenase inhibitors including sulfinpyrazone and ibuprofen have been shown to have antithrombotic effects in animal models.

Thromboxane synthetase inhibitors. Early enthusiasm for thromboxane synthetase inhibitors has been tempered somewhat with the realization that pure thromboxane synthetase inhibitors show very little inhibition of platelet function. The reason for this is that PGG_2 and PGH_2 synthesis are not blocked, and these two endoperoxides can function reasonably well to promote platelet aggregation in the absence of thromboxane A_2 (see Ch. 6). However, in the presence of thromboxane synthetase inhibition, PGH_2 produced by platelets can be converted to PGD_2 (a reaction promoted by albumin) and PGI_2 produced by endothelial cells), and some augmentation of production of platelet-inhibitory and vasodilator prostaglandins may therefore occur. Consistent with this, thromboxane synthetase inhibitors have been shown to have some antithrombotic effects in vivo (106). In other instances, no antithrombotic effects have been seen (107,108). The use of higher doses (109) or combination with very low-dose aspirin (110) could be explored further.

Thromboxane receptor antagonists. An antithrombotic effect of the thromboxane receptor antagonist 13-azaprostanoic acid has been demonstrated in an animal model (111). Further results are needed to assess the potential therapeutic role of this and other thromboxane receptor antagonists.

Agents which increase endothelial cell prostacyclin synthesis.

Nitroglycerin. Nitroglycerin has been used for many years because of its beneficial effects on pain and exercise tolerance in individuals with atherosclerotic heart disease. Nitroglycerin has been found to stimulate vascular prostacyclin synthesis (112,113), and part of the effect of nitroglycerin in angina may be due to its ability to stimulate vascular PGI_2 synthesis.

Others. Nafazatrom enhances vessel wall formation of prostacyclin (116), and bendrofluazide may do so (117). The antithrombotic potential of these drugs remains to be explored.

Vitamin E. As discussed previously, vitamin E deficiency is associated with a thrombotic tendency and abnormal prostacyclin balance. The possibility has been considered that therapy with vitamin E might be beneficial, particularly in circumstances where tissue vitamin E levels are low. This may be the case in diabetes (49c). Two separate trials of vitamin E therapy have recently shown that high doses of vitamin E can return the decreased vascular PGI_2 production and increased platelet production of diabetic rats toward normal (118,119). In spite of numerous trials of high-dose vitamin E as a potential antithrombotic agent, its use is not widely accepted. Most trials of vitamin E in atherosclerotic heart disease have been inconclusive, although double-blind trials of vitamin E for intermittent claudication have shown some benefit (120-122). It is possible that better understanding of the action of this vitamin may lead to a useful role for it in certain thrombotic disorders.

B. Other Fatty Acid, Prostaglandin, and Leukotriene Changes Which May Be Relevant to Hemostasis and Thrombosis

A study with eicosapentaenoic acid (90) and studies in patients with angina, showing reduction of thromboxane production using inhibitors without any effect on the ischemic threshold, suggest that mechanisms involving lipid mediators other than prostacyclin and thromboxane are important in some circumstances (123). A few comments will be made here on active lipids other than prostacyclin and thromboxane which may be important to hemostasis and thrombosis.

1. Dihomo-γ-Linolenic Acid and Prostaglandin E_1

Dihomo-γ-linolenic (DHGLA) acid can be converted by platelets to PGE_1. Since PGE_1 is a potent inhibitor of platelet aggregation, it seemed likely that a DHGLA-enriched diet might be antithrombotic. In spite of much work to evaluate this, the results have, in general, been disappointing. Perhaps, part of the problem is that DHGLA is also converted to PGH_1 which has some activity to stimulate platelet aggregation (124). In addition, DHGLA can be converted by many cells to arachidonic acid. Thus, the gain due to increased PGE_1 production may be relatively small.

2. Leukotrienes

Leukotrienes are vasoconstrictors in at least some circulatory beds. As such, they may promote thrombosis. In addition, the effect of leukotrienes to cause neutrophil aggregation could be prothrombotic. Much work remains to be done, but it is possible that lipoxygenase inhibitors or antagonists may be therapeutically useful under some circumstances.

3. Platelet-activating Factor

In circumstances of immune activation, release of platelet-activating factor can trigger intravascular platelet aggregation, and this may promote thromboses.

III. OVERVIEW

Much progress has been made in understanding the role of thromboxane and prostacyclin in hemostasis and thrombosis. It is probable that alterations in their balance contribute to thrombotic and bleeding tendencies in many circumstances. As research into these chemicals has increased rapidly in the last few years, so has the realization of the complex nature of the production and effects of these chemicals. Before prostacyclin was known, the therapeutic approach to thrombotic disorders seemed simple—take aspirin to inhibit thromboxane production. Now we realize it is much more complex. At the present time, a second generation of more specific drugs that may be useful in the treatment of thrombotic or vasospastic disorders is emerging—the thromboxane synthetase inhibitors and thromboxane antagonists, among others. These drugs, plus perhaps a more selective approach (a drug useful in one type of thrombotic or vasospastic disorder is not necessarily useful in another), are likely to considerably improve the therapy of these conditions over the next few years.

REFERENCES

1. M. J. Silver, W. Hoch, J. J. Kocsis, C. M. Ingerman, and J. B. Smith. *Science 183*:1085-1087 (1974).
2. P. Puig-Parellada and J. M. Planas. *Lancet 2*:40 (1977).
3. T. Shimamoto, M. Kobayashi, T. Takahashi, T. Motomiya, F. Numani, and S. Morooka. *Proc. Japan Acad. 53*:38 (1977).
4. Z. I. Terashita, H. Fukui, K. Nishikawa, M. Hirata, and S. Kikuchi. *Eur. J. Pharmacol. 53*:49 (1978).
5. S. Morooka, M. Kobayashi, T. Takahashi, Y. Takashima, M. Sakamoto, and T. Shimamoto. *Exp. Mol. Pathol. 30*:449 (1979).

6. F. Numano, M. Yajima, K. Nishiyama, K. Shimokado, F. Numano, S. Sasagawa, and K. Moriya. *Exp. Mol. Pathol. 37*:118 (1982).
7. A. M. Lefer, E. F. Smith, III, H. Araki, J. B Smith, D. Aharony, D. A. Claremon, R. L. Magolda, and K. C. Nicolaou. *Proc. Natl. Acad. Sci. USA 77*:1706 (1980).
8. R. J. Gryglewski, A. Szczeklik, and R. Nizankowski. *Thromb. Res. 13*: 153 (1978).
9. A. Szczeklik, R. J. Gryglewski, R. Nizankowski, J. Musial, R. Pieton, and J. Mruk. *Pharmacol. Res. Commun. 10*:545 (1978).
10. J. W. Aiken, R. R. Gorman, and J. J. Sheboski. *Prostaglandins 17*:483 (1979).
11. R. J. Gryglewski, R. Korbut, and A. Ocetkiewicz. *Prostaglandins 15*: 637 (1978).
12. E. A. Higgs, G. A. Higgs, S. Moncada, and J. R. Vane. *Br. J. Pharmacol. 63*:535 (1978).
13. F. B. Ubatuba, S. Moncada, and J. R. Vane. *Thromb. Haemostas. 41*: 425 (1979).
14. A. Szczeklik, R. Nizankowski, S. Skawinski, J. Szczeklik, P. Gluszko, and R. J. Gryglewski. *Lancet 1*:1111 (1979).
15. C. R. M. Prentice, J. J. F. Belch, A. McKay, B. McArdle, P. Leiberman, J. G. Pollock, G. D. O. Lowe, and C. D. Forbes. *Thromb. Haemostas. 50*:335 (1983).
16. V. A. Ziboh, H. Maruta, J. Lord, W. D. Cagle, and W. Lucky. *Eur. J. Clin. Invest. 9*:223 (1979).
17. M. T. R. Subbiah and D. Dietmeyer. *Biochem. Med. 23*:231 (1980).
18. J. M. Gerrard, M. J. Stuart, G. H. R. Rao, M. W. Steffes, S. M. Mauer, D. M. Brown, and J. G. White. *J. Lab. Clin. Med. 95*:950 (1980).
19. M. Johnson, A. H. Reece, and H. E. Harrison. *Adv. Prostaglandin Thromboxane Res. 8*:1283 (1980).
20. A. Butkus, V. A. Skrinska, and O. P. Schumacher. *Thromb. Res. 19*: 211 (1980).
21. P. V. Halushka, R. C. Rogers, C. B. Loadholt, and J. A. Colwell. *J. Lab. Clin. Med. 97*:87 (1981).
22. H. E. Harrison, A. H. Reece, and M. Johnson. *Life Sci. 23*:351 (1978).
23. K. Silberbauer, G. Schernthaner, H. Sinzinger, P. Clopath, H. Piza-Katzer, and M. Winter. *Thromb. Haemostas. 42*:334 (1979).
24. L. O. Carreras, D. A. F. Chamone, P. Klerckx, and J. Vermylen. *Thromb. Res. 19*:663 (1980).
25. K. Silberbauer, G. Schernthaner, H. Sinzinger, H. Piza-Katzer, and M. Winter. *N. Engl. J. Med. 300*:366 (1979).
26. M. Johnson, H. E. Harrison, A. T. Raftery, and J. B. Elder. *Lancet 1*: 325 (1979).
27. M. J. Stuart, S. G. Sunderji, and J. B. Allen. *J. Lab. Clin. Med. 98*:412 (1981).

28. J. W. McDonald, J. Dupre, N. W. Rodger, M. C. Champion, C. D. Webb, and M. Ali. *Thromb. Res. 28*:705 (1982).
29. J. A. Davis and G. P. McNicol. *Br. Med. Bull. 34*:113 (1978).
30. J. H. Fuller, H. Keen, R. J. Jarrett, T. Omer, T. W. Meade, R. Chakrabarti, W. R. S. North, and Y. Stirling. *Br. Med. J. 2*:964 (1979).
31. G. Davi, G. Triolo, E. Giardina, G. D. Bompiani, and A. Strano. *Thromb. Haemostas. 50*:397 (1983).
32. J. B. Allen, R. H. Sagerman, and M. J. Stuart. *Lancet 2*:1193 (1981).
33. D. G. Kieback, R. C. Briel, A. I. Schneider, R. G. A. Schmucker, and T. H. Lippert. *Thromb. Haemostas. 50*:455 (1983).
34a. H. Sinzinger, W.Firbas, and M. Cromwell. *Prostaglandins 24*:323 (1982).
34b. H. Sinzinger, M. Cromwell and W. Firbas. *Radiation Research. 97*:533 (1984).
35. M. J. Schneidkraut, P. A. Kot, P. W. Ramwell and J. C. Rose. *Adv. Prostaglandin Thrombox. Leukotriene Res. 12*:107 (1983).
36. A. Wennmalm. *Acta Physiol. Scand. 103*:107 (1978).
37. A. Wennmalm. *Br. J. Pharmacol. 64*:559 (1978).
38a. C. H. Dadak, C. Leithner, H. Sinzinger, and K. Silberbauer. *Lancet 1*: 94 (1981).
38b. D. Blache, E. Dumont, M. Ciavatte, and S. Renaud. *Thromb. Hemostas. 50*:274 (1983).
38c. D. J. Horns, J. M. Gerrard, G. H. R. Rao, W. Krivit, and J. G. White. *Thromb. Res. 9*:661 (1976).
39. E. Tremoli, G. Folco, E. Agradi, and C. Galli. *Lancet 1*:107 (1979).
40. M. J. Stuart, J. M. Gerrard, and J. G. White. *N. Engl. J. Med. 302*:6 (1980).
41. A. Strano, G. Davi, M. Averna, G. B. Rini, S. Novo, and A. Notarbartolo. *Thromb. Haemostas. 50*:138 (1983).
42. E. Tremoli, S. Colli, P. Maderna, A. Baraldi, G. Gianfranceschi, and S. Nicosia. *Thromb. Haemostas. 50*:286 (1983).
43. A. Eldor, D. J. Falcone, D. P. Hajjar, C. R. Minick, and B. B. Weksler. *Am. J. Pathol. 107*:186 (1982).
44. A. M. Evans and K. S. Bishop. *Science 56*:650 (1922).
45. A. M. Lake, M. J. Stuart, and F. A. Oski. *J. Peds. 90*:722 (1977).
46. L. J. Machlin, R. Filipski, A. L. Willis, D. C. Kuhn, and M. Brin. *Proc. Soc. Exp. Biol. Med. 149*:275 (1975).
47. C. W. Karpen, A. J. Merola, R. W. Trewyn, D. G. Cornwell, and R. V. Panganamala. *Prostaglandins 22*:651 (1981).
48. M. Okuma, H. Takayama, and H. Uchino. *Prostaglandins 19*:527 (1981).
49a. A. C. Chan and M. Leith. *Am. J. Clin. Nutr. 34*:2341 (1981).
49b. M. A. Valentovic, C. Gairola, and W. C. Lubawy. *Prostaglandins 24*: 215 (1982).

49c. M. J. Stuart. *Ann. N.Y. Acad. Sci. 393*:277 (1982).
50a. M. J. Stuart, D. A. Clark, S. G. Sunderji, J. B. Allen, T. Yambo, H. Elrad, and J. H. Slott. *Lancet 1*:1126 (1981).
50b. G. Remuzzi, D. Marchesi, G. Mecca, R. Misiani, E. Rossi, M. B. Donati, and G. de Gaetano. *Lancet 2*:310 (1980).
50c. U-M Makila, L. Viinikka and O. Ylikorkala. *Am. J. Obstet. Gynecol. 148*:772 (1984).
51. H. Sinzinger and C. Dadak. *Thromb. Haemostas. 50*:157 (1983).
52. H. Sinzinger, P. Husslein, S. Leodolter, K. Philip, N. Pateisky, and E. Gitsch. *Thromb. Haemostas. 50*:376 (1983).
53. V. Dangelo, S. Villa, M. Mysliwiec, M. B. Donati, and G. de Gaetano. *Thromb. Haemostas. 39*:535 (1978).
54. A. Dembinska-Kiec, T. Gryglewska, A. Zmuda, and R. J. Gryglewski. *Prostaglandins 14*:1025 (1977).
55. H. Sinzinger and A. Kefalides. *Thromb. Haemostas. 50*:240 (1983).
56. R. J. Gryglewski. In *Prostaglandins*, J. B. Lee (ed.). Elsevier, New York (1982).
57. G. A. FitzGerald, B. Smith, A. K. Pedersen, and A. R. Brash. *N. Engl. J. Med. 310*:1065 (1984).
58. A. Szczeklik and R. J. Gryglewski. In *International Conference of Atherosclerosis, Milan 1977*, L. A. Carlson, R. Paoletti, C. R. Siroti, and G. Weber (eds.). Raven Press, New York (1978).
59. A. Szczeklik, R. J. Gryglewski, J. Musial, L. Grodzinska, M. Serwonska, and E. Marcinkiewicz. *Thromb. Haemostas. 40*:66 (1978).
60. A. Zmuda, A. Dembinska-Kiec, A. Chytkowski, and R. J. Gryglewski. *Prostaglandins 14*:1035 (1977).
61. M. J. Stuart, Y. N. B. Setty, and R. W. Walenga. *Thromb. Haemostas. 50*:240 (1983).
62. G. Remuzzi, R. Misiani, D. Marchesi, M. Livio, G. Mecca, G. de Gaetano, and M. B. Donati. *Lancet 2*:871 (1978).
63. D. A. F. Chamone, W. G. Proesmans, C. A. Monnens, P. Binda ki Muaka, and J. Vermylen. *Int. J. Ped. Nephrol. 3*:13 (1982).
64. G. Defreyn, W. Proesmans, S. J. Machin, F. Lemmens, and J. Vermylen. *Clin. Nephrol. 18*:43 (1982).
65. G. Remuzzi, E. Rossi, R. Misiani, D. Marchesi, G. Mecca, G. de Gaetano, and M. B. Donati. *Semin. Thromb. Hemostas. 6*:391 (1980).
66. D. M. Coccheto, L. Cook, A. E. Cato, and J. E. Niedel. *Semin. Thromb. Hemostas. 7*:43 (1981).
67. H. Deckmyn, W. Proesmans, and J. Vermylen. *Thromb. Res. 30*:13 (1983).
68. G. Remuzzi, D. Marchesi, R. Misiani, G. Mecca, G. de Gaetano, and M. B. Donati. *Thromb. Res. 16*:517 (1979).
69. K. A. Jorgensen and R. S. Pedersen. *Thromb. Res. 21*:311 (1981).

70. D. F. Horrobin, K. Jenkins, and M. S. Manku. *Lancet 2*:747 (1983).
71. J. J. F. Belch, J. K. Drury, H. Capell, C. D. Forbes, P. Newman, F. McKenzie, P. Leiberman, and C. R. M. Prentice. *Lancet 1*:313 (1983).
72. M. Tada, T. Kuzuya, M. Inoue, K. Kodama, M. Mishima, M. Yamada, M. Inui, and H. Abe. *Circulation 64*:1107 (1981).
73. R. M. Robertson, D. Robertson, L. J. Roberts, R. L. Maas, G. A. Fitz-Gerald, G. C. Friesinger, and J. A. Oates. *N. Engl. J. Med. 304*:988 (1981).
74. J. H. Grose, M. Level, and F. M. Gbeassor. *Clin. Sci. 59*:121s (1981).
75. C. R. Pace-Asciak, M. C. Carrara, G. Rangaraj, and K. C. Nicolaou. *Prostaglandins 15*:1005 (1978).
76a. J. E. Graeber, J. H. Slott, R. E. Alane, J. D. Schulman, and M. J. Stuart. *Pediatr. Res. 16*:490 (1982).
76b. L. A. Harker, R. Ross, S. J. Slichter, and C. R. Scott. *J. Clin. Invest. 58*:731 (1976).
77. A. E. Schorer, J. M. Gerrard, J. G. White, and W. Krivit. *Prostaglandins Med. 1*:5 (1978).
78. J-Q. Pan, E. R. Hall, and K. K. Wu. *Blood 62*:308a (1983).
79. R. S. Kent, B. B. Kitchell, D. G. Shand, and A. R. Wharton. *Prostaglandins 21*:483 (1981).
80. M. A. Boogaerts, J. Vermylen, H. Deckmyn, C. Roelant, R. L. Verwilghen, H. S. Jacob, and C. F. Moidow. *Thromb. Haemostas. 50*:572 (1983).
81a. A. Szczeklik, R. J. Gryglewski, B. Domagala, A. Zmuda, J. Hartwich, E. Wozny, M. Grywacz, J. Modej, and T. Gryglewska. *Prostaglandins 22*:795 (1981).
81b. N. W. Schoene, V. C. Morris and O. A. levander. *Fed. Proc. 43*:477 (1984).
82. H. O. Bang, J. Dyerberg, and H. M. Sinclari. *Am. J. Clin. Nutr. 33*:2657 (1980).
83. J. Dyerberg, H. O. Bang, and E. Stoffersen. *Lancet 2*:117 (1978).
84. B. R. Culp, B. G. Titus, and W. E. M. Lands. *Prostaglandins Med. 3*:269 (1979).
85. G. Hornstra, E. Haddeman, G. A. A. Kivits, and J. A. Don. *Thromb. Haemostas. 50*:275 (1983).
86. A. Raz, M. S. Minkes, and P. Needleman. *Biochim. Biophys. Acta 488*:305 (1977).
87. R. J. Gryglewski, J. A. Salmon, F. B. Ubatuba, B. C. Weatherly, S. Moncada, and J. R. Vane. *Prostaglandins 18*:453 (1979).
88. J. Dyerberg and H. O. Bang. *Lancet 2*:433 (1979).
89. R. Lorenz, U. Spengler, S. Fischer, J. Duhm, and P. C. Weber. *Circulation 67*:504 (1983).
90. M. Thorngren, S. Shafi, and G. V. R. Bora. *Thromb. Haemostas. 50*:286 (1983).

91. G. Remuzzi, A. E. Cavenaghi, G. Mecca, M. B. Donati, and G. de Gaetano. *Thromb. Res. 11*:919 (1977).
92a. H. Deckmyn, W. Proesmans, and J. Vermylen. *Thromb. Res. 30*:13 (1983).
92b. M. G. Marmot, G. Rose, M. J. Shipley, and B. Thomas. *Lancet 1*:580 (1981).
92c. A. L. Klatsky, G. D. Friedman, and A. B. Siegelaub. *Ann. Intern. Med. 95*:139 (1981).
92d. H. W. Grochow, R. G. Hoffman, A. J. Anderson, and J. J. Barboviak. *Atherosclerosis 43*:393 (1982).
92e. D. J. Kozararevic, D. McGree, N. Vojvodic, Z. Racic, T. Dawber, T. Gordon, and W. Zukel. *Lancet 1*:613 (1980).
92f. K. Yano, G. G. Rhoads, A. Kagan, and J. Tillotson. *Am. J. Clin. Nutr. 31*:1270 (1978).
92g. D. H. Cowan. *Semin. Hematol. 17*:137 (1980).
92h. D. P. Mikhaildis, J. Y. Jeremy, M. A. Barradas, N. Green, and P. Dandona. *Br. Med. J. 287*:1495 (1983).
93. H. J. B. Barnett, J. Hirsch, and J. F. Mustard (eds.). *Acetylsalicyclic Acid: New Uses for an old Drug.* Raven Press, New York (1982).
94. L. Goldman and A. R. Feinstein. *Ann. Intern. Med. 90*:92 (1979).
95. J. Hirsch. *Progr. Pharmacol. 4*:21 (1982).
96. J. R. A. Mitchell. *Br. Med. Bull. 39*:289 (1983).
97. R. B. Philp. *Meth. Find. Exptl. Clin. Pharmacol. 1*:197 (1979).
98. H. R. Harter, J. W. Burch, P. W. Majerus, N. Stanford, J. A. Delmez, C. B. Anderson, and C. A. Weerts. *N. Engl. J. Med. 301*:577 (1979).
99. Canadian Cooperative Study Group. *N. Engl. J. Med. 299*:53 (1978).
100a. H. D. Lewis, J. W. Davis, D. G. Archibald, W. E. Steinke, T. M. Smitherman, J. H. Doherty, H. W. Schnaper, M. M. LeWinter, E. Linares, J. M. Pouget, S. C. Sabharwal, E. Chesler, and H. DeMats. *N. Engl. J. Med. 309*:396 (1978).
100b. E. A. Jaffe and B. B. Weksler. *J. Clin. Invest. 63*:532 (1979).
101. F. E. Preston, S. Whipps, C. A. Jackson, A. J. French, P. J. Wyld, and C. J. Stoddard. *N. Engl. J. Med. 304*:76 (1981).
102. B. B. Weksler, S. B. Pett, D. Alonso, R. C. Richter, P. Stelzer, V. Subramanian, K. Tack-Goldman, and W. A. Gay, Jr. *N. Engl. J. Med. 308*:800 (1983).
103a. S. P. Honley, J. Bevan, S. R. Cockbill, and S. Heptinstall. *Br. Med. J. 285*:1299 (1982).
103b. G. A. FitzGerald. Conference on Prostaglandins and Leukotrienes '84. May 8-11, Washington, D.C., Abstract 52 (1984).
104. E. F. Grabowski, B. B. Weksler, K. Tack-Goldman, P. Stelzer, V. Subramanian, and W. A. Gay, Jr. *Blood 62*:301a (1983).
105. C. Patrono. *Thromb. Haemostasis. 50*:413 (1983).
106. H. Tindall, J. E. Tooke, M. F. R. Martin, and J. A. Davies. *Thromb. Haemostas. 50*:281 (1983).

107. M. Goldman, C. Hall, R. J. Hawker, and C. N. McCollum. *Thromb. Haemostas. 50*:222 (1983).
108. G. P. Lewis, J. R. Smith, and I. H. M. Williamson. *Thromb. Haemostas. 50*:241 (1983).
109. G. A. FitzGerald, A. R. Brash, and A. K. Pederson. *Thromb. Haemostas. 50*:280 (1983).
110. V. Bertele, A. Falanga, M. Tomasiuk, E. Dejana, C. Cerletti, and G. de Gaetano. *Thromb. Haemostas. 50*:282 (1983).
111. S. E. Burke, O. M. Rith, and A. M. Lefer. *Thromb. Res. 29*:473 (1983).
112. R. I. Levin, A. E. Jaffe, B. B. Weksler, and K. Tack-Goldman. *J. Clin. Invest. 67*:762 (1981).
113. K. Schror, L. Grodzinska, and H. Darius. *Thromb. Res. 23*:59 (1981).
114. E. Morcillio, P. R. Reid, N. Dubin, R. Ghodgaonkar, and B. Pitt. *Am. J. Cardiol. 45*:53 (1980).
115. J. Van Dusen and S. J. Fischl. *Am. J. Cardiol. 47*:390 (1981).
116. J. Vermylen, D. A. F. Chamone, and M. Verstraete. *Lancet 1*:518 (1979).
117. J. Webster, C. T. Dollery, and C. N. Hensby. *Clin. Sci. 59*:125s (1980).
118. C. W. Karpen, K. A. Pritchard, Jr., J. H. Arnold, D. G. Cornwell, and R. V. Panganamala. *Diabetes 31*:947 (1982).
119. V. A. Gilbert, E. J. Zebrowski, and A. C. Chan. *Horm. Metab. Res. 15*:320 (1983).
120. P. D. Livingstone, and C. Jonas. *Lancet 2*:602 (1958).
121. A. M. Boyd and J. Marks. *Angiology 14*:198 (1963).
122. H. T. G. Williams, D. Fenna, and R. A. Macbeth. *Surg. Gynecol. Obstet. 132*:662 (1971).
123. M. Cortellaro, C. Boschetti, G. Moreo, V. Antoniazzi, S. Repetto, E. Verna, M. Boscarino, and G. Binaghi. *Thromb. Haemostas. 50*:374 (1983).
124. W. Siess and E. G. Lapentina. *Thromb. Haemostas. 50*:275 (1983).

BIBLIOGRAPHY

J. M. Gerrard and J. G. White. *Progr. Hemostas. Thromb. 4*:87 (1978).

S. Moncada and J. R. Vane. *Fed. Proc. 38*:66 (1979).

J. Mehta and P. Mehta (eds.) *Platelets and Prostaglandins in Cardiovascular Disease*. Futura Publishing Co., Mount Kisco, N.Y. (1981).

B. Pitt, M. J. Shea, J. L. Romson, and B. R. Lucchesi. *Ann. Intern. Med. 99*: 83 (1983).

A. L. Bloom and D. P. Thomas (eds.) *Haemostasis and Thrombosis*. Churchill Livingstone, Edinburgh (1981).

17

The Role of Prostaglandins in Host Defense Against Bacteria, Viruses, and Tumors and in Inflammation

Blood cells are involved in the body's reaction to infectious agents and to neoplastic transformation. Prostaglandin synthesis inhibitors such as aspirin are widely used by individuals with infections or malignancies. They are used primarily for their ability to abort secondary, unwanted reactions (fever, pain, and so on), yet the effects of this inhibition of prostaglandin synthesis has effects on host defense and immunity which are still poorly understood.

At the present time we can identify some of the specific effects of prostaglandins, but an adequate overall picture is still some distance away. Are there times during the process of some infections when host defense would be improved by having more or fewer prostaglandins and related chemicals? As with the role of these chemicals in hemostasis and thrombosis, it is likely that there is a critical balance and perhaps a critical sequence in their production. At present our knowledge is sketchy, but it would appear that for host defense the critical balance is not between thromboxane A_2 and prostacyclin, but perhaps between leukotriene B_4 and prostaglandin E_2. Indeed, the various positive and negative effects of these agents on white blood cell function suggest aspects of such a balance, if it exists, will be more complex than the balance of thromboxane A_2 and PGI_2 in hemostasis and thrombosis. Knowledge of this area will likely increase dramatically within the next few years. At the present time, it is only possible to provide an outline of the pieces as we are now aware of them.

I. DEFENSE AGAINST BACTERIA (Fig. 17-1)

A. Neutrophils

The initial response of the host to bacteria involves predominantly the polymorphonuclear leukocytes. Here, leukotriene B_4 and to a lesser extent various hydroxy fatty acids appear to be critical neutrophil activators, stimulating cell chemotaxis and secretion. In carrageenin-induced inflammation, at least, the early presence of LTB_4 derived primarily from neutrophils has been confirmed (1). Studies using selective lipoxygenase inhibitors in vivo to determine how critical the production of these compounds is in host defense have not so far been conducted. Perhaps the closest thing would be the use of steroids, which act at the phospholipase level to inhibit the release of arachidonic acid and formation of hydroxy fatty acids and leukotriene B_4 by neutrophils. Experience with steroids in vivo has shown that they can increase the severity of some bacterial infections consistent with an important role for leukotriene B_4 in host defense. However, whether the adverse effect of steroids is due solely to their effect to suppress leukotriene B_4 production is uncertain.

Thromboxane A_2 is also produced early on in the inflammatory response (1). No studies of the effect of thromboxane inhibitors on the inflammatory response are available. However, the use of the prostaglandin synthetase inhibitors aspirin, indomethacin, and phenylbutazone has not been associated with an increase in the severity of bacterial infections, unless these agents were used in very high doses (2).

B. Monocytes and Lymphocytes

In the initial stages of a bacterial infection the lymphocytes begin to mount an immune response. The effect of neutrophil-derived leukotriene B_4 on the early stages of the immune response is unknown, but may be important. The relative absence of PGE_2 (and perhaps also PGI_2) during the initial stage of the immune response may be important since these prostaglandins inhibit lymphocyte (particularly T cell and NK cell) function. Relatively little PGE_2 or PGI_2 would be expected at this time since neutrophils produce little of these prostaglandins; however, some tissue synthesis of PGE_2 may

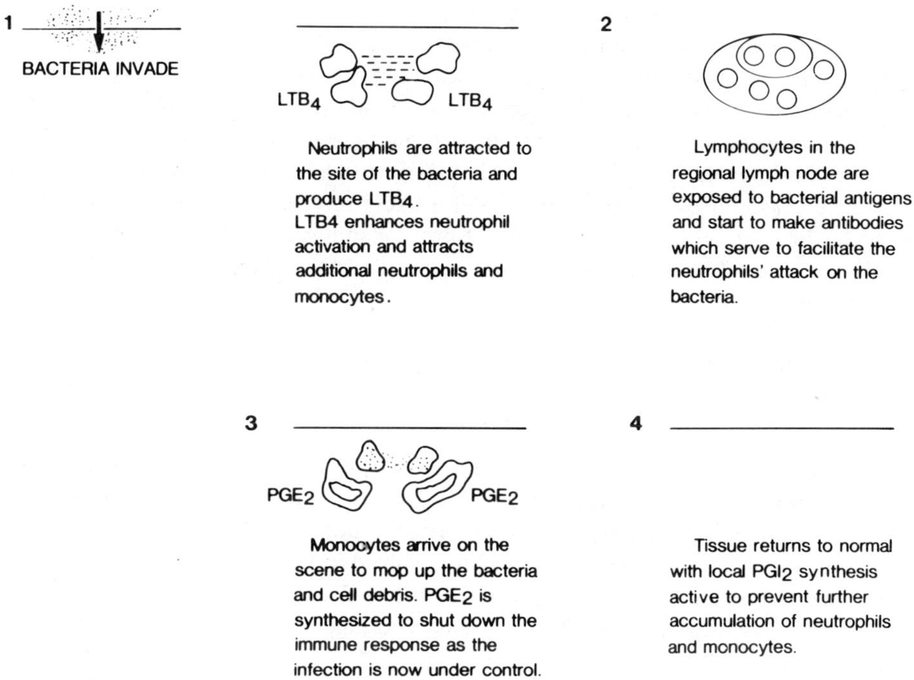

Fig. 17-1 A simplistic and speculative concept of the role of LTB_4 and PGE_2 at the site of an infection, based on our current knowledge.

occur (1). Monocytes/macrophages with a considerable ability to produce PGE_2 become more important only after the first few hours. However, Cahill and Hopper have shown that during the initial stages of infection with *Salmonella enteritidis* the ability of macrophages to produce PGE_2 in response to bacterial lipopolysaccharide is decreased (3). It is possible that initially macrophage PGE_2 production is depressed in order to allow the immune response to develop.

As the infection progresses, PGE_2 may be important in order to activate the macrophages (2). At the same time, PGE_2 inhibits most lymphocyte and granulocyte functions. At this stage of the infection, if the bacteria are under control, the macrophage activation would be important primarily for a cleanup operation to clear the site of cell debris, antigen-antibody and complement complexes, and so on, so that the recent battle scene between bacteria, neutrophils, antibody, and so forth can be cleared and the tissue returned to its preinfection status. PGI_2 and PGE_2 produced by the tissue may be important late in the process to shut down the macrophage activity and prevent further influxes of neutrophils, macrophages, or NK cells into the tissue. This short overview necessarily presents a simplistic and somewhat speculative view. As knowledge of prostaglandin involvement in these events improves, much more detail is likely to be added. Indeed it is likely that the pattern of production of prostaglandins and related chemicals will vary considerably, depending on the nature of the bacteria, the site of infection, and the host.

C. Clinical Relevance

1. Fever Associated with Infection

Fever associated with bacterial infection probably results from the action of pyrogens to stimulate hypothalamic prostaglandin production. Aspirin and acetaminophen reduce the fever by inhibiting hypothalamic synthesis of prostaglandins. Blood cells are probably involved in the generation of pyrogens. Prostaglandins synthesized by blood cells at the site of the infection probably do not ordinarily reach the hypothalamus in sufficient quantities to produce the fever directly.

2. Pain and Infection

Pain is one of the cardinal signs of an inflammatory reaction and usually develops at the site of a bacterial infection. Prostaglandins used alone do not produce pain, although prostaglandins, notably PGE_1, injected into human skin will induce an increased sensitivity to touch (i.e., hyperalgesia) (5,6). More important PGE_1, PGE_2, and PGI_2 will strongly potentiate pain responses to histamine and bradykinin (7-9). Inhibitors of prostaglandin synthesis such as aspirin are analgesic as a result of inhibition of the prostaglandin sensitization of pain receptors to other agonists.

3. Septicemia and Shock

In severe bacterial infection, there is an overproduction of prostaglandins and related lipid mediators (10). Production of these active chemicals appears to contribute in a variety of ways, including lung injury (see subsequent discussion), to the symptoms of shock. Prostaglandin and thromboxane synthetase inhibitors have been shown to have beneficial effects in shock, consistent with this concept (11-13).

4. Lung Injury

The infusion of complement-activated plasma, endotoxin, or live gram-negative organisms into sheep or goats causes thromboxane synthesis and produces pulmonary vasoconstriction (increased pulmonary artery and pulmonary wedge pressures) and an increase in pulmonary vascular permeability as shown by increased extravascular lung water (10,14-20). Associated with these changes in the lung is a significant fall in cardiac output. Treatment with cyclooxygenase or thromboxane synthetase inhibitors largely prevents the acute pulmonary vasoconstriction and fall in cardiac output but has a lesser effect on the change in pulmonary vascular permeability and the development of pulmonary edema. Some evidence suggests that lipoxygenase products derived from arachidonic acid may have an important role in the vascular permeability changes and in the mild late-appearing pulmonary hypertension seen in sheep (19). This production of thromboxane A_2 may be secondary to an initial synthesis of leukotriene C_4/D_4 and platelet activating factor. The application of these findings to man is not yet certain.

5. Hemostasis and Thrombosis

Secondary consequences of bacterial infections relating to hemostasis and thrombosis include effects of activated granulocytes to promote vessel wall injury and effects of platelet-activating factor and thromboxane A_2 produced by activated granulocytes and monocytes to stimulate platelets. The reader is referred to Ch. 16 for a more detailed discussion of this.

6. Hodgkin's Disease and Susceptibility to Infection

In Hodgkin's disease the T-lymphocyte response to phytohemagglutinin is reduced, associated with a higher risk of infections. Investigations have shown that the reason is abnormal (early on? or increased?) production of PGE_2 by monocytes (21). Incubation of the cells with indomethacin will normalize this response. Whether the use of indomethacin in patients with Hodgkin's disease can be used clinically to decrease the risk of infection has not been established. A similar situation may occur in some patients with melanoma who have a decreased lymphocyte response to concanavalin A as a result of increased monocyte production of PGE_2 (22a).

7. Aging

In a preliminary report the decline in immune responsiveness in old mice has been associated with an increase in splenic production of PGE_2 (22b). Vitamin E was shown to normalize both the enhanced PGE_2 production and the deficient cell-mediated immune response.

II. DEFENSE AGAINST VIRUSES

Viral infection in a number of host virus interactions has been shown to be associated with increased host PGE_2 and $PGF_{2\alpha}$ production in circumstances where interferon was also induced (23). However, it is likely that in vivo a variety of other arachidonic acid metabolites may be produced as well, depending on the particular circumstances. Our present knowledge in this area is very rudimentary and permits only a few observations.

A. Arachidonic Acid Metabolites Which May Inhibit Viral Infection

1. Direct Inhibition of Virus Replication and Infection

Santoro et al. have made the striking observation that prostaglandins A_1 and A_2 have potent antiviral activity when added to cell lines treated with Sendai virus, Vaccinia virus, or vesicular stomatitis virus (24-27). The effect is not due to inhibition or adsorption of virus to the cells or the first stages of viral replication. Rather, PGAs appear to act by inhibiting virus maturation or budding of the virus from the cells. The relevance of these observations to normal physiology is uncertain because PGAs are not known to be produced in vivo.

However, PGE_1, PGE_2, and $PGF_{2\alpha}$ have been shown to have antiviral activity against both parainfluenza and measle viruses in some studies (28,29).

2. Indirect Inhibition of Virus Infection via Altered Immunity

Enhancement of host immunity against viruses has been reported in vitro, but the effect of leukotriene B_4 to enhance natural killer cell cytotoxicity of herpes virus-infected target cells was small (30).

B. Enhancement of Virus Replication by Prostaglandins

1. Direct Enhancement

PGE_2 and $PGF_{2\alpha}$ have both been found to increase the size of herpes simplex virus plaques in Vero cells (31) and thromboxane B_2 and PGA_2 to enhance measles virus replication (29).

2. Enhancement Through Altered Immunity

Prostaglandins E_1 and E_2 have been shown to inhibit NK cell activity. Moreover, prostaglandins generated by monocytes/macrophages generally inhibit lymphocyte function (PGE_2 primarily), including natural killer cell activity (32,33), and indomethacin use has been associated with enhanced natural killer cell cytotoxicity toward herpes simplex virus-infected cells (34). Thus, a reasonable case can be put forward to support an effect of endogenous PGE_2 to indirectly accelerate a virus infection. Whether a significant effect ever occurs in vivo is not yet known.

C. Secondary Effects of Virus Infections

In general, pain, fever, and so on where they occur with viral infections may be related to production of prostaglandins in a similar fashion to that seen with bacterial infections.

1. Bronchiolitis and Respiratory Syncytial Virus Infection

Immune complexes resulting from an interaction of antibody with respiratory syncytial virus have been shown to activate neutrophils to produce superoxide, thromboxane A_2, and a smooth muscle-contracting activity (35,36). The experiments have been used to suggest that products of arachidonic acid metabolism could mediate the bronchoconstriction and tissue damage seen in respiratory syncytial virus infections.

III. HOST DEFENSE AGAINST PARASITES

Leukotriene B_4 has been shown to enhance neutrophil- and eosinophil-mediated, complement-dependent killing of the schistosomula of *Schistosoma mansoni* (37). LTC_4, LTD_4, 5-HETE, and 5-HPETE had no effect. No direct effect of any of these agents on schistosomular motility or viability was seen.

IV. DEFENSE AGAINST TUMORS

A. Direct Effects

PGD_2 has a direct cytotoxic action on mouse neuroblastoma cells in vitro (38). PGA_1 is also effective, but PGA_2, PGB_1, PGE_1, PGE_2, $PGF_{2\alpha}$, PGI_2, and thromboxane B_2 are not. The mechanism of the effect is unknown, but is not related to an elevation of cellular cAMP since PGE_2 is as effective in elevating cell cAMP as PGD_2. Used in vivo, PGD_2 significantly reduced tumor growth. PGD_2 has been found to inhibit DNA synthesis in human and murine leukemia, mouse melanoma, and mouse mastocytoma (39-41), but whether this is the mechanism of the effect of PGD_2 on neuroblastoma cells is not certain.

B. Indirect Effects

Natural killer (NK) lymphocytes have an important action to destroy tumor cells. Studies with phospholipase A_2 inhibitors suggest that an arachidonic acid metabolite might be involved in the stimulation of NK cell activity (42, 43). So far the arachidonic acid metabolite has not been identified, but studies with indomethacin suggest it is not a prostaglandin or thromboxane (33). If such an NK cell-stimulatory metabolite (perhaps leukotriene B_4?) does exist, it might be expected to promote the defense of the host against tumors.

PGE_1 and PGE_2 inhibit NK-cell lysis of tumor cells (32). PGE_2 produced by monocyte/macrophages may inhibit NK-cell activity. Some evidence to support such a macrophage/NK cell-interaction exists (33).

C. Clinical Relevance

Many tumor cell lines produce PGE_2, and such production may inhibit host NK-cell activity to facilitate tumor spread (Fig. 17-2). Indomethacin, or other prostaglandin synthetase inhibitors, have been used in some patients with various cancers, with occasional beneficial responses. This could eventually become standard adjunctive therapy for some cancers.

V. CHEMICAL INFLAMMATION

A. Effects of Prostaglandins to Promote Inflammation

Nonsteroidal anti-inflammatory drugs which inhibit prostaglandin synthesis, suppress the vasodilation, edema, and pain associated with most inflammatory processes, including the chemical carrageenin. As discussed previously, (Ch. 14 and Sec. I.C.2 of this chapter), while PGE_2 and PGI_2 are potent vasodilators, their role in edema and pain responses is to potentiate the effects of other agonists (i.e., histamine, bradykinin, and C5a). To date, the principal prostaglandins found in inflamed human skin have been PGD_2, PGE_2, $PGF_{2\alpha}$, and PGI_2 (44-47). Of these, PGE_2 and PGI_2 are much more potent than PGD_2 or $PGF_{2\alpha}$ in potentiating the vascular permeability increase of bradykinin (48).

The drug MK-447 facilitates conversion of PGG_2 to PGH_2 with a resultant increase in PGE_2 and $PGF_{2\alpha}$. Yet it is anti-inflammatory. This

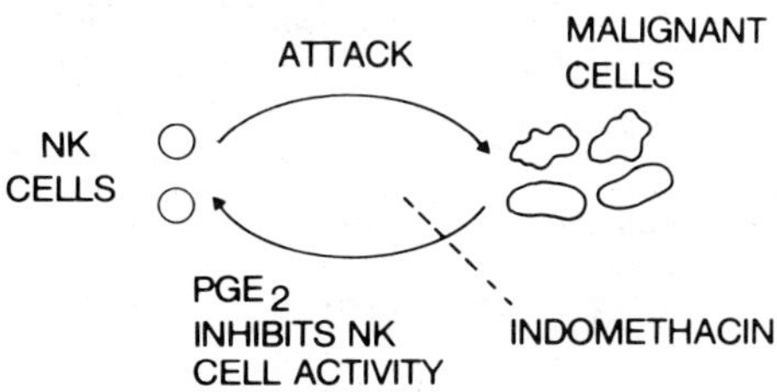

Fig. 17-2 The potential importance of PGE_2 synthesized by malignant cells to inhibit the action of natural killer (NK) cells in host defense against the tumor cells.

has been used to suggest that PGG_2 or a free radical usually formed in its metabolism is more important than PGE_2 (49). MK-447 is a reducing agent and a free radical scavenger. This is the mechanism by which it facilitates conversion of PGG_2 to prostaglandins. However, it has not been unequivocably established that the PGG_2 radical is the only or primary radical on which MK-447 acts. Nevertheless, the results suggest some caution in accepting the view that PGE_2 is the prostaglandin species principally responsible for inflammation.

Furthermore, indomethacin and other nonsteroidal anti-inflammatory drugs, while they suppress inflammation, do not completely inhibit it (50). It is probable that lipoxygenase products, especially the leukotrienes, are also important, and sometimes more important than the prostaglandins in the production of inflammation. In this regard the lipoxygenase inhibitors, benoxaprofen, eicosatetraynoic acid, and 13-cis-retinoic acid, have shown success in the treatment of acne, an inflammatory disease of human skin (51-53).

Preliminary reports of the effects of selective lipoxygenase inhibitors and combined cyclooxygenase and lipoxygenase inhibitors in a variety of models of inflammation suggest that in general lipoxygenase products may be more important for the cellular infiltrate (neutrophils particularly) while cyclooxygenase products are more important for the edema of inflammation (53b,53c). However, overlap is apparent and one pathway may be more critical in any given situation. Prostaglandins by promoting enhanced vascular permeability may facilitate egress of cells. LTB_4 primarily promotes neutrophil migration. However, it also increases vascular permeability, but only when neutrophils are present (i.e., not in neutrophil depleted animals) suggesting that edema produced by LTB_4 is secondary to its effects on neutrophils. Where LTC_4 and LTD_4 are significant lipoxygenase products more direct effects to increase vascular permeability occur. Additional studies with selective inhibitors are likely to be available in the near future to clarify the situation.

B. Effects of Prostaglandins to Inhibit Inflammation

There are a few conditions, including cotton pellet granulomas and adjuvant arthritis in rats, which can be suppressed by PGE_2 and/or PGE_1 (54-58). The effect of these agents could be due to their ability to inhibit leukocyte, lymphocyte, and monocyte function by stimulating cAMP synthesis in these cells. Prostaglandins may also help limit chronic inflammation by inhibiting fibroblast proliferation (59,60a).

C. Clinical Relevance

1. Gout

Monosodium urate crystals, important in the etiology of the arthritis in gout will stimulate the production of leukotriene B_4 by neutrophils (60b). Colchicine, widely used for the treatment of gout, inhibits LTB_4 synthesis in response to the crystals. Whether this is the reason that colchicine is efficacious in gout is not yet established. However, the finding of LTB_4 in the fluid from affected joints from patients with gout lends credence to this concept (60c).

VI. THE INVOLVEMENT OF PROSTAGLANDINS AND RELATED CHEMICALS IN DISEASES WITH AN ALTERED INFLAMMATORY RESPONSE

A. Psoriasis

Psoriasis is a skin disorder characterized by excessive proliferation of epidermal cells. Commonly, lesions develop at sites of trauma (surgical incisions, burns, scratches, and so on) consistent with an altered tissue response to injury. High concentrations of lipoxygenase products including 12-HETE and LTB_4 have been identified in affected skin (61,64). Also of interest, the response of psoriatic skin to PGE_1 (accumulation of cAMP) is much less than that of normal skin (65). It is tempting to speculate that psoriasis develops because of an imbalance in the production and/or effect of LTB_4 and PGE_2, resulting in excessive and prolonged neutrophil accumulation and epidermal proliferation. The finding of increased phospholipase A_2 (66) and lipoxygenase activities (67) in uninvolved skin from individuals with psoriasis has been used to suggest that one of these might be the basic defect in psoriasis, but more work is necessary before a firm conclusion can be reached.

However, better understanding of the therapy of psoriasis has already resulted. Benoxaprofen, a 5-lipoxygenase inhibitor, has been found to produce substantial improvement in psoriasis (68,69), whereas indomethacin which inhibits cyclooxygenase activity and diverts more arachidonic acid toward the lipoxygenase pathway appears to make the psoriasis worse (70,71).

B. Inflammatory Bowel Disease

Recent studies of the influence of sulfasalazine, a drug widely used to treat inflammatory bowel disease, on arachidonic acid metabolism may provide a new understanding of the mechanism of its effect, and a new view of the role of cyclooxygenase and lipoxygenase products in this disorder. Sulfasalazine has been found to inhibit the 5-lipoxygenase and thromboxane synthetase while sparing the 12-lipoxygenase and only partly affecting cyclooxygenase activity (72,73). The expected result of its action would be to decrease production of 5-HETE, LTB_4, and thromboxane A_2 while leaving relatively intact synthesis of PGE_2. Perhaps inflammatory bowel disease is associated with an overproduction or effect of 5-HETE, LTB_4, and thromboxane A_2 relative to PGE_2. Much more work needs to be done to assess this concept however.

C. Rheumatoid Arthritis

Rheumatoid arthritis is a chronic inflammatory disease of the joints. It is usually classified as autoimmune due to the frequent presence of autoantibodies. The presence of chronic inflammation and autoantibodies suggests that a mechanism for the "turn-off" of inflammation and antibody formation could be decreased or absent. Recent studies of B-cell proliferation induced by Epstein-Barr virus show individuals with rheumatoid arthritis have a deficiency in the normal control (turn-off) of this response (74-77). Under normal circumstances, T cells are activated to produce γ-interferon which down-regulates the virus-induced lymphoblast transformation by promoting the generation and/or activity of cytotoxic T cells (78-80). T-cell production of γ-interferon can be inhibited by monocyte-produced PGE_2. Studies of patients with rheumatoid arthritis show their monocytes may produce more PGE_2 (81), but this has not been confirmed (82). Rather, the most recent studies suggest that the interferon producing T lymphocytes from rheumatoid arthritis patients are much more sensitive to PGE_2 so that in the presence of minute quantities, they fail to generate the γ-interferon necessary for the turn-off of the B-cell lymphocyte response (82). For reasons which are not clear, the increased sensitivity to PGE could be reversed by indomethacin. It is too early to be sure that this mechanism is of major importance in rheumatoid arthritis. However, the potential for reversal of the defect by nonsteroidal anti-inflammatory drugs fits well with the widespread success with these agents in this disorder.

D. Autoimmune Disorders

As mentioned previously, the auto-antibody production seen in autoimmune disorders suggests that a component important for the normal down-regulation of the immune response might be decreased or missing. In this regard, Webb and Osheroff and co-workers have emphasized the rapid production of prostaglandins (PGE_2 and $PGF_{2\alpha}$) by the spleen of mice injected with sheep red blood cells (83,84). Within 2 min of the injection of the foreign red cells there was a 20-80-fold increase in splenic prostaglandins. In old NZB mice, widely used as a model for autoimmunity, there was no increase in splenic prostaglandin production although baseline levels were somewhat elevated. Indomethacin-treated and essential fatty acid-deficient animals (rats in this study) which do not show the splenic prostaglandin response have an enhanced plaque-forming cell response compared with the controls (85). These studies indicate that normal splenic prostaglandin production is important to dampen the overall extent of the immune response. The prostaglandin-deficient, immunostimulated state has been related to the accelerated development of the autoimmune disorder, experimental allergic encephalitis, as well as the autoimmunity of NZB mice (86,87). Furthermore, treatment of NZB mice with PGE_1 prevents the progression of their nephritis and increases their survival dramatically (88,89). Taken together, these studies support an important role for prostaglandins, particularly PGE_2, in the prevention of the excessive immune responses of autoimmunity and emphasize the potential role of drugs and diet in the prevention and treatment of these disorders.

VII. OVERVIEW

Recent advances have highlighted the important role of prostaglandins, thromboxanes, and leukotrienes in host defense and inflammation. However, this area of research is a complex one, and definitive understanding is still, for the most part, elusive. Nevertheless, present evidence suggests an important role for 5-lipoxygenase products, particulary LTB_4, in the initial granulocyte response, and an important role for PGE_2 to dampen the overall extent of the immune response. Excessive production of lipoxygenase products, and perhaps thromboxanes, may be important for the development of psoriasis and inflammatory bowel disease. Lack of normal PGE_2 production may be a factor in the development of autoimmune disorders. As an illustration of the potential complexity of the interactions of these chemicals, however, in rheumatoid arthritis, considered to be an autoimmune disorder, failure of suppressor cell activity has been linked to excessive PGE sensitivity of one subpopulation of T cells. Furthermore, while LTB_4 may usually act to enhance host defense, it can also stimulate suppressor cell activity (90). Thus, whereas LTB_4 may generally enhance and PGE_2 inhibit host granulocyte, monocyte, and lymphocyte responses, their ability to act similarly with regard to suppressor T lymphocytes means that their overall effect on immunity is not necessarily straightforward.

15-HETE, produced by eosinophils and some lymphocytes, is an inhibitor of the 5-lipoxygenase. 15-HETE production could be an important component in the effective balance of arachidonic acid metabolites in vivo, but to date, except for its production in nasal polyps (91), we know very little about it in vivo.

There may be significant therapeutic potential in the use of prostaglandins to treat immunologic disorders. Beneficial effects of PGE_1 in NZB mice were described above. PGE_2 and $PGF_{2\alpha}$ can markedly inhibit the myocardial damage and the nephritis produced in rats by injection of anti-rat serum, and PGI_2 has been shown to prolong the survival of cat and dog renal xenografts (92-94). Further exploration of the use of prostaglandins and analogues to ameliorate undesirable effects of immunologic reactions is clearly needed.

REFERENCES

1. P. M. Simmons, J. A. Salmon, and S. Moncada. *Biochem. Pharmacol. 32*:1353 (1983).
2. H. J. Robinson, H. F. Phares, and O. E. Grassele. In *Prostaglandin Synthetase Inhibitors*, H. J. Robinson and J. R. Vane (eds.). Raven Press, New York. (1974).
3. J. Cahill and K. E. Hopper. *Cell. Immunol. 67*:229 (1982).
4. M. E. Snider, R. H. Fertel, and B. S. Zwilling. *Cell. Immunol. 74*:234 (1982).
5. L. M. Solomon, L. Juhlin, and M. B. Kirschenbaum. *J. Invest. Dermatol. 51*:280 (1968).
6. L. Juhlin and G. Michaelsson. *Acta Derm. Venereol. 49*:251 (1969).
7. S. H. Ferreira. *Nature (New Biol.) 240*:200 (1972).
8. S. H. Ferreira, M. Nakamura, and M. S. de Abreu Castro. *Prostaglandins 16*:32 (1978).
9. E. A. Higgs, S. Moncada, and J. R. Vane. *Prostaglandins 16*:153 (1978).
10. J. Harlan, R. Winn, J. Weaver, J. Hildebrandt, and L. Harker. *Chest (Suppl) 83*:75S (1983).

11. R. Winn, J. Harlan, B. Nadir, L. Harker, and J. Hildebrandt. *J. Clin. Invest. 72*:911 (1983).
12. J. R. Fletcher and P. W. Ramwell. *Adv. Prostaglandins Thromboxane Res. 7*:821 (1980).
13. W. C. Wise, J. A. Cook, T. Eller, and P. V. Halushka. *J. Pharmacol. Exp. Ther. 215*:160 (1980).
14. J. D. Cooper, J. W. McDonald, M. Ali, E. Menkes, J. Masterson, and P. Klement. *Surgery 88*:215 (1980).
15. J. R. Snapper, M. L. Ogletrie, A. A. Hutchison, and K. L. Brigham. *Am. Rev. Resp. Dis. 123*:200 (1981).
16. W. D. Watkins, D. K. Huttemeier, and M. B. Peterson. *Prostaglandins 23*:273 (1982).
17. M. L. Ogletree and K. L. Brigham. *Am. Rev. Resp. Dis. 123*:247 (1981).
18. J. W. McDonald, M. Ali, E. Morgan, E. R. Townsend, and J. D. Cooper. *Circ. Res. 52*:1 (1983).
19. K. L. Brigham, M. Ogletree, J. Snapper, J. Hinson, and R. Parker *Chest (suppl.) 83*:70S (1983).
20. M. L. Ogletree, K. L. Brigham, J. A. Oates, and W. C. Hubbard. *Fed. Proc. 40*:767 (1981).
21. J. S. Goodwin, R. P.Messner, A. D. Bankhurst, G. T. Peake, J. H. Saiki, and R. C. Williams, Jr. *N. Engl. J. Med. 297*:963 (1977).
22a. J. L. Murray and G. M. Kollmorgen. *J. Clin. Immunol. 3*:268 (1983).
22b. S. N. Meydan, M. Meydan, C. P. Verdon, J. C. Blumberg, and K. C. Hayes. *Fed. Proc. 43*:478 (1984).
23. F. Fitzpatrick and D. Stringfellow. *J. Immunol. 125*:431 (1980).
24. M. G. Santoro, A. Benedetto, G. Carruba, E. Garaci, and B. M. Jaffe. *Science 209*:1032 (1980).
25. M. G. Santoro, G. Carruba, E. Garaci, B. M. Jaffe, and A. Benedetto. *J. Gen. Virol. 53*:75 (1981).
26. M. G. Santoro, A. Benedetto, S. Zaniratti, E. Garaci, and B. M. Jaffe. *Prostaglandins 25*:353 (1983).
27. M. G. Santoro, B. M. Jaffe, E. Garaci, and M. Esteban. *J. Gen. Virol. 63*:435 (1982).
28. M. Lucksak, W. Gumulka, S. Szmigielski, and M. Korbecki. *Arch. Virol. 49*:377 (1975).
29. P. Dore-Duggy. *Prostaglandins Leuk. Med. 8*:73 (1982).
30. M. Rola-Pleszczynski, L. Gagnon, and P. Sirois. *Biochem. Biophys. Res. Commun. 113*:531 (1983).
31. A. Benedetto, S. Zaniratti, P. Meo, and G. B. Rossi. *J. Gen. Virol. 45*:407 (1979).
32. J. C. Roder and M. Klein. *J. Immunol. 123*:2785 (1979).
33. H. S. Koren, S. J. Anderson, D. G. Fischer, C. S. Copeland, and P. J. Jensen. *J. Immunol. 127*:2007 (1981).

34. S. Kohl, P. M. Jansen, and L. S. Loo. *Prostaglandins Leuk. Med. 9*:159 (1982).
35. T. N. Kaul, H. S. Faden, E. Middleton, T. Figutani, and P. L. Ogra. *Pediatr. Res. 16*:224A (1982).
36. H. Faden, T. N. Kaul, and P. L. Ogra. *J. Infect. Dis. 148*:110 (1983).
37. R. Moqbel, S. P. Sass-Kuha, E. J. Goetzl, and A. B. Kay. *Clin. Exp. Immunol. 52*:519 (1983).
38. H. Higashida, K. Kano-Tanaka, S. Natsuume-Sakai, K. Sudo, H. Fukami, Y. Nakagawa, and N. Miki. *Int. J. Cancer 31*:797 (1983).
39. M. Fukushima, T. Kato, R. Cleda, K. Ota, S. Marumiya, and O. Hayaishi. *Biochem. Biophys. Res. Commun. 105*:956 (1982).
40. M. Kawamura and Y. Koshihara. *Prostaglandins Leuk. Med. 12*:85 (1983).
41. Y. Sasaki, C. Qwatani, and M. Tsuboshima. *Proc. Jap. Cancer Assoc. 41th Ann. Meeting*, p. 246 (1982).
42. T. Hoffman, F. Hirata, P. Bougnoux, B. A. Fraser, R. H. Goldfarb, R. B. Herberman, and J. Axelrod. *Proc. Natl. Acad. Sci. USA 78*:3839 (1981).
43. P-C. Quan, T. Ishizaka, and B. R. Bloom. *J. Immunol. 128*:1786 (1982).
44. M. W. Greaves, J. Sondergaard, and W. Gibson-McDonald. *Br. Med. J. 2*:258 (1971).
45. J. Sondergaard, M. W. Greaves, and H. P. Jorgensen. *Arch. Dermatol. 110*:556 (1974).
46. A. K. Black, N. Fincham, M. W. Greaves, and C. N. Hensby. *Br. J. Clin. Pharmacol. 10*:453 (1980).
47. W. Schalla, C. Hensby, A. Civier, J. Cambrou, L. Juhlin, and H. Schaefer. *J. Invest. Dermatol. 80*:345 (1983).
48. T. J. Williams. *Br. J. Pharmacol. 65*:517 (1979).
49. F. A. Kuehl, J. L. Humes, R. W. Egan, E. A. Ham, G. C. Beveridge, and C. G. Van Arman. *Nature (Lond.) 265*:170 (1977).
50. A. K. Black, M. W. Greaves, C. N. Hensby, N. A. Plummer, and A. P. Warin. *Br. J. Clin. Pharmacol. 6*:261 (1978).
51. C. Hindson, F. Lawlor, and H. Wacks. *Lancet 1*:1415 (1982).
52. J. S. Strauss, P. E. Pochi, and E. N. Whitman. *J. Invest. Dermatol. 48*:492 (1967).

53a. C. Fiedler-Nagy, C. Hamilton, C. Batula-Bernardo, and J. W. Coffey. *Fed. Proc. 42*:949 (1983).

53b. R. F. Meyers, J. C. Anthes, C. J. Casmer and M. I. Siegel. *Fed. Proc. 43*:955 (1984).

53c. J. M. Young, A. J. Tomolonis, J. B. Kheifets, J. A. Rovito, D. J. Henricksen, A. C. Allison, D. V. Krishnamurthy, M. Kruseman-Aretz and D. K. Kosai. Conference on Prostaglandins and Leukotrienes '84, May 8-11, Washington, D.C. Abstract 138 (1984).

54. I. L. Bonta and M. J. Parnham. *Biochem. Pharmacol. 27*:1611 (1978).
55. R. L. Aspinall and P. S. Cammarata. *Nature (Lond.) 224*:304 (1969).
56. I. L. Bonta, M. J. Parnham, and L. Van Vliet. *Ann. Rheum. Dis. 37*: 212 (1978).
57. E. M. Glenn and N. Rohloff. *Proc. Soc. Exp. Biol. Med. 139*:290 (1972).
58. R. B. Zarier and M. Ballas. *Arthritis Rheum. 16*:251 (1973).
59. H. D. Peters, B. A. Peskar, and P. S. Schonhofer. *Naungn-Schmiedebergs Arch. Pharmacol. 297*:589 (1977).
60a. P. S. Schonhofer, H. D. Peters, A. Wasmus, B. A. Peskar, K. Von Figura, and I. Klappstein. *Pol. J. Pharmacol. Pharm. 30*:183 (1978).
60b. C. N. Serhan, U. Lundberg, G. Weissman and B. Samuelsson. *Prostaglandins 27*:563 (1984).
60c. S. A. Rae, E. M. Davidson, and M. J. M. Smith. *Lancet 2*:1122 (1982).
61. S. Hammarstrom, M. Hamberg, B. Samuelsson, E. A. Duell, M. Stawiski, and J. J. Voorhees. *Proc. Natl. Acad. Sci. USA 72*:5130 (1975).
62. S. D. Brain, R. D. Camp, P. M. Dowd, A. K. Black, P. M. Woollard, A. I. Mallet, and M. W. Greaves. *Lancet 2*:762 (1982).
63. R. D. Camp, A. Mallet, P. Wollard, S. Brain, A. K. Black, and M. W. Greaves. *J. Invest. Dermatol. 80*:359 (1983).
64. S. Brain, R. D. Camp, A. K. Black, P. M. Dowd, and M. W. Creaves. *J. Invest. Dermatol. 80*:360 (1983).
65. J. J. Voorhees. *Ann. Rev. Med. 28*:467 (1977).
66. S. Forster, E. Ilderton, R. Summerly, and H. J. Yardley. *Br. J. Dermatol. 108*:103 (1983).
67. S. Hammarstrom, J. A. Lingren, C. Marcelo, E. A. Duell, T. F. Anderson, and J. J. Voorhees. *J. Invest. Dermatol. 73*:180 (1979).
68. B. R. Allen and S. M. Littlewood. *Br. Med. J. 285*:1241 (1982).
69. K. Kragballe and T. Herlin. *Arch. Dermatol. 119*:548 (1983).
70. H.Katayama and A. Kawada. *J. Dermatol. (Tokyo) 8*:323 (1981).
71. C. N. Ellis, J. D. Fallen, J. L. Heezen, and J. J. Voorhees. *J. Invest. Dermatol. 80*:362 (1983).
72. W. F. Stenson and E. Lobos. *J. Clin. Invest. 69*:494 (1982).
73. W. F. Stenson and E. Lobos. *Biochem. Pharm. 32*:2205 (1983).
74. P. A. Bardwick, H. G. Bluestein, N. J. Zvaifler, J. M. Depper, and J. E. Seegmiller. *Arth. Rheum. 23*:626 (1980).
75. G. Tosato, A. D. Steinberg, and R. M. Blaese. *N. Engl. J. Med. 305*: 1238 (1981).
76. J. M. Depper, H. G. Bluestein, and N. J. Zvaifler. *J. Immunol. 127*: 1899 (1981).
77. F. Hasler, H. G. Bluestein, N. J. Zvaifler, and L. B. Epstein. *J. Exp. Med. 157*:173 (1983).
78. D. J. Moss, A. B. Rickinson, and J. H. Pope. *Int. J. Cancer 23*:618 (1979).

79. A. B. Rickinson, L. E. Wallace, and M. A. Epstein. *Nature 283*:865 (1980).
80. C. D. Tsoukas, R. I. Fox, S. F. Slovin, D. A. Carson, M. Pellegrino, S. Fong, J-L. Pasquali, S. Ferrone, P. Kung, and J. H. Vaughan. *J. Immunol. 126*:1742 (1981).
81. G. S. Panayi, V. Covrigall, and L. I. F. Youlten. *Scand. J. Rheumatol (Suppl.) 38*:9 (1981).
82. F. Hasler, H. G. Bluestein, N. J. Zvaifler, and L. B. Epstein. *J. Immunol. 131*:768 (1983).
83. D. R. Webb and P. L. Osheroff. *Proc. Natl. Acad. Sci. USA 73*:1300 (1976).
84. D. R. Webb, T. J. Roger, and I. Nowowiejski. *Ann. N.Y. Acad. Sci. 332*:262 (1979).
85. G. A. Boissonneault and P. V. Johnston. *J. Nutr. 113*:1187 (1983).
86. P. G. Weston and P. V. Johnston. *Lipids 13*:408 (1978).
87. P. G. Weston and P. V. Johnson. *Lipids 13*:876 (1978).
88. R. B. Zurier, I. Damjanov, D. M. Sayadoff, and N. F. Rothfield. *Arthritis Rheum. 20*:1449 (1977).
89. R. B. Zurier, I. Damjanov, P. L. Miller, and B. F. Biewar. *J. Clin. Lab. Immunol. 2*:95 (1979).
90. M. Rola-Pleszczynski, P. Borgeat, and P. Sirois. *Biochem. Biophys. Res. Commun. 108*:1531 (1982).
91. D. M. Smith, J. M. Gerrard, S. K. Juhn, and J. G. White. *Minn. Med. 64*:605 (1981).
92. A. R. Mundy. *Transplantation 30*:226 (1980).
93. E. Pausescu, D. Laky, M. V. Popescu and D. Chiper. *Biomed. Biochim. Acta 42*:235 (1983).
94. E. Pausescu, D. Laky, M. V. Popescu and D. Chiper-Stancu. *Clin. Nephrol. 21*:169 (1984).

BIBLIOGRAPHY

R. B. Zurier. In *Prostaglandins*, J. B. Lee (ed.). Elsevier, New York (1982).
T. J. Williams. *Br. Med. Bull. 39*:239 (1983).
K. Kragballe and J. J. Voorhees. *J. Invest. Dermatol. 81*:293 (1983).

18

The Role of Blood Cells in Allergic or Hypersensitive Disorders

The cell which appears to be of central importance in allergy and hypersensitivity is the tissue mast cell. As discussed in Ch. 9, mast cells exposed to antigen-IgE complexes produce several lipid mediators including prostaglandin D_2, leukotrienes C_4 and D_4 (slow-reacting substance of anaphlaxis), and platelet-activating factor. Mast cells also secrete significant amounts of the important mediator histamine. Much of this chapter will be devoted to a consideration of immediate hypersensitivity reactions and the various components of these reactions, with some discussion of other allergic disorders. Because of the central role of the mast cell, systemic mastocytosis will be considered first as an example of excessive numbers of mast cells and the resultant systemic effects.

I. SYSTEMIC MASTOCYTOSIS

This disorder is characterized by abnormal proliferation of tissue mast cells. Symptoms include skin lesions (urticaria pigmentosa), episodes of flushing, tachycardia, and hypotension, and sometimes diarrhea. The disorder is associated with increased amounts of circulating histamine and increased production of prostaglandin D_2 (1,2). Therapy with H_1 and H_2 histamine receptor blockers only partially improves symptoms (2-4). A significant decrease in the episodes of flushing, tachycardia, and hypotension has been observed in one patient treated with prostaglandin synthetase inhibitors (2) and in the diarrhea of a second patient so treated (5). These findings implicate both histamine and prostaglandin D_2 as important mediators of the symptoms of systemic mastocytosis. It is possible that the relative importance of these two compounds may vary from patient to patient.

II. IMMEDIATE HYPERSENSITIVITY AND ANAPHYLAXIS

Components of immediate hypersensitivity and anaphylaxis include the following: (a) bronchospasm; (b) localized edema and/or vasodilation as manifested by urticaria or with edema of the hypopharynx and larynx; (c) hypotension, pulmonary edema, and vascular collapse; (d) platelet activation and thrombocytopenia; and (e) neutrophil activation and neutropenia. In a given anaphylactic reaction one or more of these components may be particularly prominent. Each will be discussed individually.

A. Bronchospasm

At least some asthma is an immediate hypersensitivity reaction (IgE-antigen mediated) in which bronchospasm is the principal component. In systemic IgE anaphylaxis, a similar bronchospastic component is often present, but is accompanied by and often overshadowed by other aspects of the response (i.e., laryngeal edema and/or systemic vascular collapse). Mast cell-derived products with bronchoconstrictor activity include leukotrienes C_4, D_4, and E_4 (slow-reacting substance of anaphylaxis), histamine, platelet-activating factor, and PGD_2 (6-8). In addition, thromboxane A_2 and $PGF_{2\alpha}$, both with bronchoconstrictor activity, could be produced from nonmast cell sources in the lung.

In allergic asthma, considerations of the relative potencies of these agents, their relative production by lung tissue, and studies with inhibitors lead to the high probability that the leukotrienes (C_4, D_4, and E_4) are major mediators of allergic bronchoconstriction in man (9,10). In systemic anaphylaxis, significant quantities of other mediators including thromboxane A_2 and platelet-activating factor are likely produced as well (see Sec. II.C) and could be important. Studies in guinea pigs show that the lipoxygenase inhibitor BW755C gives only partial protection from the respiratory distress of anaphylaxis (11).

B. Localized Edema and/or Vasodilation

The general use of antihistamines as the first agent for the treatment of urticaria suggests that histamine secretion plays an important role in this reaction. The effect of histamine may be potentiated (and perhaps sometimes superceded) by production of other mediators, including leukotrienes, platelet-activating factor, and prostaglandins.

C. Pulmonary Hypertension and Systemic Hypotension

Leukotrienes (C_4, D_4, and E_4), prostaglandin D_2, thromboxane A_2, and platelet-activating factor are all potential mediators of the pulmonary hypertension and systemic hypotension seen in IgE anaphylaxis. Recent evidence implicates thromboxane A_2 production, perhaps secondary to leukotriene or platelet-activating factor action, as being important in a number of shock states (see Chs. 14 and 17), including that resulting from transfusion of heterologous blood. For example, cyclooxygenase and thromboxane synthetase inhibitors largely suppressed the development of pulmonary hypertension and systemic hypotension when rabbit blood was infused into cats without affecting the thrombocytopenia and neutropenia (12). Leukotrienes (C_4 and D_4) and platelet-activating factor may be more important for the development of the cardiovascular changes of IgE anaphylaxis (13a,b).

D. Thrombocytopenia and Neutropenia

Studies of rabbit and baboon models of IgE anaphylaxis have been used to suggest that platelet-activating factor is critical to the development of thrombocytopenia and neutropenia, as well as some of the other changes in anaphylaxis. In the rabbit model, intraperitoneal antigen (bovine serum albumin) administration to rabbits within the first 24 hr after birth results in the preferential, long-term expression of specific IgE antibody in response to this antigen (14,15). This IgE rabbit subsequently will respond to intravenous antigen challenge with the rapid development of systemic anaphylactic shock accompanied by a profound thrombocytopenia and neutropenia (14,16,17). As discussed in the chapter on basophils, challenging of these cells with appropriate antigen-IgE results in the production or secretion of various active chemicals, a principal one being platelet-activating factor (18). Intravenous antigen challenge of IgE rabbits has shown significant in vivo production of platelet-activating factor (19,20), coincident with the thrombocytopenia and neutropenia. Intravenous injection of purified acetyl glyceryl ether phosphorycholine (AGEPC) (platelet-activating factor) produced a similar thrombocytopenia and neutropenia (21). In this circumstance, AGEPC caused the platelets and neutrophils to aggregate in vivo as it does in vitro. Accompanying thrombocytopenia and neutropenia, there were severe cardiovascular and pulmonary alterations (22) indistinguishable from those seen in IgE-induced systemic anaphylactic shock (23). These findings implicate platelet-activating factor as the principal mediator of anaphylaxis in the IgE rabbit.

It should be mentioned that during intravenous infusion of AGEPC into rabbits there is a rise in plasma thromboxane B_2 (13), similar to that seen in IgE-induced anaphylaxis (24). The role of such thromboxane production (due principally to AGEPC stimulation of platelets) is not clear, but is probably relatively minor, representing a secondary effect in this circumstance.

Intravenous infusion of AGEPC into baboons produces thrombocytopenia and neutropenia accompanied by cardiovascular and pulmonary alterations similar to those seen in human anaphylaxis (25,26). Compared with the rabbits, however, the thrombocytopenia is very transient. It would clearly be desirable to have a specific inhibitor of the production or effect of platelet-activating factor which could be used to test the role of this mediator in human anaphylaxis and possibly to provide a new specific therapeutic approach.

Platelet activation, not necessarily associated with thrombocytopenia, is a feature of antigen challenge in several hypersensitivity disorders including asthma (27) and patients with rheumatoid arthritis with specific food intolerance (28). Whether this represents a lesser production of a mediator such as platelet-activating factor or whether this might represent a direct effect of immune complexes on platelets is not certain.

III. OTHER ALLERGIC DISORDERS

A. Eczema

Evening primrose oil, which is rich in dihomo-γ-linolenic acid, the precursor of PGE_1, has been used to treat eczema on the hypothesis that the disease is due to a disordered production of prostaglandins. Some success has been achieved with this therapy (29), although the biochemical evidence for altered prostaglandin production is not yet convincing.

IV. RESULTS OF STUDIES OF DRUGS AFFECTING ARACHIDONIC ACID METABOLISM

A. Steroids

The successful use of steroids, which can inhibit the release of arachidonic acid from phospholipids (see Ch. 4), to treat allergic conditions such as asthma and eczema suggests arachidonic acid metabolites may be important in these disorders. Steroids are not helpful in identifying the particular metabolite involved, and indeed effects of steroids on other processes besides their action to promote the synthesis of phospholipase-inhibitory proteins may be important.

B. Cyclooxygenase Inhibitors

1. Adverse reactions

Aspirin intolerance (acute urticaria-angioedema, bronchospasm, severe rhinitis, or rarely shock occurring within 3 hr of aspirin ingestion) is a significant problem in up to 20-30% of patients with chronic urticaria, nasal polyps, or nasal asthma (30). Although the pathophysiology of aspirin intolerance is still a matter of debate, several observations suggest strongly that it results from inhibition of prostaglandin synthesis (31,32). Patients with aspirin intolerance react similarly to other cyclooxygenase inhibitors. Clinical desensitization is associated with cross-desensitization to other cyclooxygenase inhibitors and can be achieved so rapidly that an immunological process is unlikely. The reaction to aspirin could result either from blocking synthesis of an inhibitory prostaglandin (i.e., PGI_2 or PGE_2 in the bronchospasm reaction), or from the diversion of an increased proportion of arachidonic acid toward production of bronchoconstrictor lipoxygenase products such as LTD_4. It is also possible that some aspirin-sensitive people may be allergic to the drug itself.

2. Beneficial Effects of Aspirin

A very small proportion of patients with asthma (about 1% of adult asthmatics) show striking clinical improvement after taking aspirin (33). This observation implies that in a small subset of asthmatics the bronchoconstriction results primarily from the production of a cyclooxygenase product with bronchoconstrictor activity (i.e., PGD_2, $PGF_{2\alpha}$, or thromboxane A_2). In some individuals PGE_2 is also a bronchoconstrictor. A possible relationship between the reaction to PGE_2 and the response to aspirin could be tested, but has not been so far.

A study of six patients with urticaria, four of whom were aspirin intolerant, showed that during treatment with aspirin (following desensitization in the aspirin-intolerant individuals) the subjects no longer reacted to foods which had previously caused moderate or severe reactions (32). Confirmation of this finding in a double-blind study is needed.

C. Thromboxane Synthetase Inhibition

Beneficial effects of thromboxane synthetase inhibitors on bronchospasm have been reported in animal experiments (34,35), but no human experience has been reported.

Dazoxiben, a thromboxane synthetase inhibitor, has been reported to decrease the extent of local edema produced late (1-8 hr), following intradermal injection of antihuman IgE or compound 48/80 even though the size of the immediate wheal was slightly increased (36). The basis for the differential effect of this drug on early and late reactions is not clear. Thromboxanes, as prostaglandins and leukotrienes, have to be synthesized since they are not stored in cells. However, ordinarily such synthesis occurs very rapidly, and the necessity for such de novo synthesis does not by itself explain the possible role of thromboxane in delayed but not in immediate responses.

VI. POTENTIAL EFFECTS OF CHANGES IN DIET

A. Eicosapentaenoic Acid

Mastocytoma cells from mice grown in the peritoneal cavities of mice fed a diet enriched in eicosapentaenoic acid produce proportionately much less LTC_4 and LTC_5 and more LTB_4 and LTB_5 (37). If this happens with human cells, fish-based diets might have beneficial effects in patients with asthma by decreasing production of LTCs.

VII. OVERVIEW

The role of arachidonic acid metabolites in hypersensitivity reactions appears complex. Perhaps the most interesting recent development is evidence that

LTC_4, LTD_4, and LTE_4 may have a major role in asthmatic reactions. An important role for platelet-activating factor in anaphylaxis also appears possible. With evidence that eosinophils and monocytes/macrophages, as well as mast cells, can produce LTC_4, the possible role of these cells in some allergic disorders may need to be reevaluated. The development and clinical testing of specific inhibitors of the synthesis or actions of these compounds are eagerly awaited.

REFERENCES

1. D. J. Demis. *Ann. Intern. Med. 59*:195 (1963).
2. L. J. Roberts, II, B. J. Sweetman, R. A. Lewis, K. F. Austen, and J. A. Oates. *N. Engl. J. Med. 303*:1400 (1980).
3. J. W. Gerrard and C. Ko. *J. Pediatr. 94*:843 (1979).
4. B. I. Hirschowitz and J. F. Groarke. *Ann. Intern. Med. 90*:769 (1979).
5. T. Poynard, C. Nataf, B. Messing, R. Modigliani, T. Lecompte, P. Nicolas, F. Dray, and C. Ferme. *N. Engl. J. Med. 307*:186 (1982).
6. J. M. Drazen, K. F. Austen, R. A. Lewis, D. A. Clark, G. Goto, A. Marfat, and E. J. Corey. *Proc. Natl. Acad. Sci. USA 77*:4354 (1980).
7. S. M. M. Karim, P. G. Adaikan, and S. R. Kottegoda. *Adv. Prostaglandin Thromboxane Res. 7*:969 (1980).
8. B. B. Vargaftig, J. Lefort, M. Chignard, and J. Benveniste. *Eur. J. Pharmacol. 65*:185 (1980).
9. S-E. Dahlen, G. Hansson, P. Hedqvist, T. Bjorck, E. Granstrom, and B. Dahlen. *Proc. Natl. Acad. Sci. USA 80*:1712 (1983).
10. M. Griffin, J. W. Weiss, A. G. Leitch, E. R. McFadden, Jr., E. J. Corey, K. F. Austen, and J. M. Drazen. *N. Engl. J. Med. 308*:436 (1983).
11. B. J. Everitt and W. D. Spiegel. *Fed. Proc. 42*:443 (1983).
12. S. Bunting, S. Castro, J. A. Salmon, and S. Moncada. *Thromb. Res. 30*:609 (1983).

13a. R. N. Pinckard, L. M. McManus, and D. J. Hanahan. *Adv. Inflammation Res. 4*:147 (1982).

13b. R. J. Gordon, J. Travis, H. R. Godfrey, D. Sweeney, P. S. Wolf, P. T. Pruss, E. Neiss, J. Musser, U. Chakraborty, H. Jones, and M. Liebowitz. Conference on Prostaglandins and Leukotrienes '84, May 8-11, Washington, D.C. Abstract 266 (1984).

14. R. N. Pinckard, M. Halonen, and A. L. Meng. *J. Allergy Clin. Immunol. 49*:301 (1972).
15. M. Halonen, H. K. Fisher, C. Blair, C. Butler, and R. N. Pinckard. *Am. Rev. Resp. Dis. 114*:961 (1976).
16. M. Halonen, R. N. Pinckard, and A. L. Meng. *J. Immunol. 111*:331 (1973).

17. M. Halonen and R. N. Pinckard. *J. Immunol. 115*:519 (1975).
18. J. Benveniste, P. M. Henson, and C. G. Cochrane. *J. Exp. Med. 136*: 1356 (1972).
19. P. M. Henson. *J. Exp. Med. 143*:937 (1976).
20. R. N. Pinckard, R. S. Farr, and D. J. Hanahan. *J. Immunol. 123*:1847 (1979).
21. L. M. McManus, D. J. Hanahan, C. A. Demopoulos, and R. N. Pinckard. *J. Immunol. 124*:2919 (1980).
22. M. Halonen, J. D. Palmer, I. C. Lohman, L. M. McManus, and R. N. Pinckard. *Am. Rev. Resp. Dis. 122*:915 (1980).
23. M. Halonen, H. K. Fisher, C. Blair, C. Butler, and R. N. Pinckard. *Am. Rev. Resp. Dis. 114*:961 (1976).
24. L. M. McManus, J. O. Shaw, and R. N. Pinckard. *J. Immunol. 125*: 1950 (1980).
25. R. N. Pinckard, L. M. McManus, R. A. O'Rourke, M. H. Crawford, and D. J. Hanahan. *Clin. Res. 28*:358 (1980).
26. L. M. McManus, R. N. Pinckard, F. F. Fitzpatrick, R. A. O'Rourke, W. G. Johnson, and D. J. Hanahan. *Lab. Invest. 45*:303 (1981).
27. K. A. Knauer, L. M. Lichtenstein, N. F. Adkinson, Jr., and J. E. Fish. *N. Engl. J. Med. 304*:1404 (1981).
28. C. H. Little, A. G. Stewart, and M. R. Fennessy. *Lancet 2*:297 (1983).
29. C. R. Lovell, J. L. Burton, and D. F. Horrobin. *Lancet 1*:278 (1981).
30. G. A. Settipane. *Am. J. Med. 64(6A)*:102 (1983).
31. A. Szczeklik and R. J. Gryglewski. *Am. Rev. Respir. Dis. 118*:799 (1978).
32. S. I. Asad, L. J. F. Youlten, and M. H. Lessof. *Clin. Allergy 13*:459 (1983).
33. A. Szczeklik, R. J. Gryglewski, G. Czerniawska-Mysik, and E. Nizankowska. *Adv. Prostaglandin Thromboxane Res. 7*:993 (1980).
34. D. N. Harris, R. Greenberg, M. B. Philips, G. H. Osman, and M. J. Antonaccio. *Adv. Prostaglandin Thromboxane Res. 6*:437 (1980).
35. W. Dorsch, L. Frey, and J. Neuhauser. *Allergologie 6*:94 (1983).
36. W. Dorsch, J. Ring, and H. Melzer. *J. Allergy Clin. Immunol. 72*:168 (1983).
37. R. C. Murphy, W. C. Pickett, B. R. Culp, and W. E. M. Lands. *Prostaglandins 22*:613 (1981).

BIBLIOGRAPHY

M. K. Bach. *Ann. Rev. Microbiol. 36*:371 (1982).

19

The Regulation of Blood Cell Production

The regulation of the synthesis of blood cells in the bone marrow is complex. There are numerous cell lines involved, and each line undergoes a sequential maturation, each step involving biochemical changes which are not always associated with major morphological changes. As one example, addition of prostaglandin E_2 to a human promyelocytic leukemia cell line has been found to induce biochemical evidence of maturation (induction of chemotactic receptors, NBT reduction, and glass adherence) without morphological evidence of maturation (1).

Hampering our present understanding of the effect of various arachidonic acid metabolites on the bone marrow is the lack of studies using lipoxygenase-derived products, the hydroxy fatty acids, and leukotrienes. Thus, whereas the effects of prostaglandins (especially prostaglandin E) and inhibitors such as indomethacin have been studied, the lack of knowledge relating to other metabolites of arachidonic acid likely gives us a very incomplete picture. The recent demonstration that immature red blood cells synthesize the lipoxygenase product 15-HETE makes such studies all the more relevant (2).

I. THE HEMOPOIETIC STEM CELL

The multipotential hemopoietic stem cells present in marrow and spleen represent for the most part a dormant or noncycling population. Utilizing the ability of these cells to form spleen colonies when injected into lethally irradiated mice, prostaglandin E_1 and E_2 have been shown to activate mice stem cells into DNA synthesis (3-5), increasing the proportion of stem cells in S phase from 5 to 30%, and producing a transient increase (6-24 hr later) in colony-forming units in culture. Evidence of Pelus that addition of PGE_1 or PGE_2 to human bone marrow cells produces an increase in Ia-positive CFU-GM (the granulocyte-macrophage committed stem cell) (6) could be the result of stimulation of an earlier (perhaps the multipotential) stem cell.

A. Clinical Relevance

Cases of aplastic anemia following prolonged use of the prostaglandin synthetase inhibitor indomethacin have been reported (7). It is possible that the effect of indomethacin was secondary to prostaglandin synthesis inhibition by the drug, but another mechanism (antibody or hypersensitivity or other) cannot be excluded.

II. THE ERYTHROCYTE SERIES

A. Stimulation of Erythropoiesis

Injection of various prostaglandins, alone or together with low doses of erythropoietin, into polycythemic mice results in a stimulation of erythropoiesis as assessed by the incorporation of ^{59}Fe into erythrocytes (8). Prostaglandins were effective in the following order: $PGA_2 > PGE_2 > PGE_1 > PGA_1$. PGI_2 is also effective (9). $PGF_{2\alpha}$ and $PGF_{2\beta}$ had no effect.

Evaluation of the *site of action of prostaglandins* has shown that prostaglandins stimulate the presumed early erythrocyte progenitor cells [burst-forming units (BFU-E)], the presumed late erythrocyte progenitor cells [colony-forming units (CFU-E)], and stimulate the production of erythropoietin. Using human bone marrow and a methylcellulose culture system, prostaglandins stimulated BFU-E in the following order of potency: $PGB_1 > PGA_2 > PGE_1 > PGA_1 > PGE_2 > PGF_{2\beta} > PGF_{1\alpha} > PGB_2$ (10). In a separate study, PGI_2 was also found to be stimulatory (11). CFU-E growth in vitro was similarly stimulated by various prostaglandins, although to a lesser extent than BFU-E. The order of potency was $PGE_1 > PGA_2 > PGF_{2\beta} > PGF_{1\alpha} > PGE_2 > PGB_1 > PGB_2$ (10).

The mechanism of the stimulatory action of prostaglandins may result from stimulation of adenylate cyclase to raise cellular cAMP. However, the only evidence for this presented to date has been an effect of lithium to inhibit the stimulation due to prostaglandins. In other systems lithium has been shown to block cAMP-mediated effects (acting after the generation of cAMP (12).

PGE_1 and PGE_2 stimulate renal production of erythropoietin (13, 14). PGE_2 produced in the kidney appears to be important for endogenous erythropoietin production since indomethacin will block erythropoietin production in response to renal artery constriction and to hypoxia (15-17).

B. Clinical Relevance

A trial of PGE_2 in patients with anemia due to end-stage renal disease has been reported (18). PGE_2 given three times a week for 4-8 weeks increased circulating BFU-E in three patients and produced a slight increase in plasma erythropoietin in two. In mice, two PGE_2 derivatives which are resistant to degradation by the prostaglandin dehydrogenase because of protected 15-hydroxy [15(S)-methyl and 16,16-dimethyl PGE_2-methyl ester] were 100 times more potent than PGE_2 in stimulating erythropoiesis in vivo (19). Thus, it may be possible in the future to use PGE_2, or more likely a stable derivative, to treat some forms of anemia.

C. Inhibition of Erythropoiesis

$PGF_{2\alpha}$ (used as the free acid) inhibits both BFU-E and CFU-E growth in culture (10,20). Since prostaglandins which stimulate erythropoiesis inhibit granulopoiesis and $PGF_{2\alpha}$ which inhibits erythropoiesis enhances granulopoiesis (10,21), it is possible that prostaglandins produced in the bone marrow regulate the balance between erythropoiesis and granulopoiesis (Fig. 19-1). However, whether $PGF_{2\alpha}$ is made by bone marrow cells is not known at present. Since $PGF_{2\alpha}$ has been shown to interact with the thromboxane receptor in other cell systems (22a), it is possible that prostaglandin endoperoxides or thromboxanes are involved here as well.

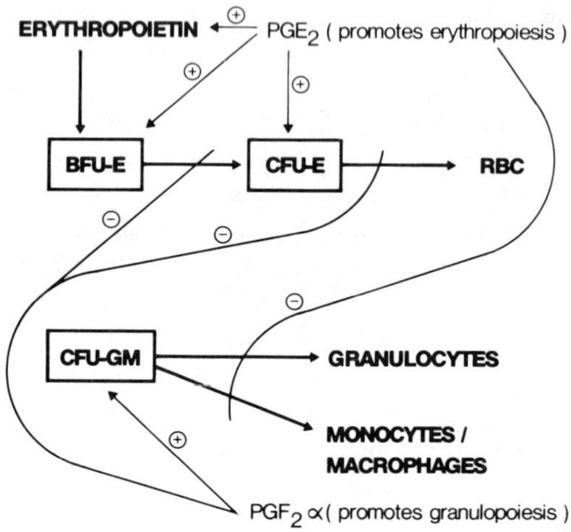

Fig. 19-1 Experiments to date suggest opposite effects of PGE_2 and $PGF_{2\alpha}$ on erythropoiesis and granulopoiesis. (BFU-E - burst-forming unit-erythrocyte; CFU-E = colony-forming unit-erythrocyte; CFU-GM = colony forming unit-granulocyte/macrophate.)

III. GRANULOCYTE-MACROPHAGE FORMATION

A. Stimulation of Granulopoiesis

The proliferative ability of the granulocyte-macrophage progenitor cell (CFU-GM) is augmented by low concentrations of prostaglandin $F_{2\alpha}$ (21). cGMP has been implicated as a second messenger in this effect of $PGF_{2\alpha}$ (21), however, the evidence for such a role for cGMP is far from conclusive. However, lipoxygenase inhibitors but not indomethacin inhibited the growth of granulocyte-macrophage colonies stimulated by colony stimulating factor suggesting leukotrienes rather than $PGF_{2\alpha}$ (22b) might be important endogenous activators. Studies evaluating the direct effect of leukotrienes are needed.

B. Inhibition of Granulopoiesis

Prostaglandins E_1 and E_2 can both inhibit the in vitro proliferation of the committed granulocyte-macrophage progenitor cell (CFU-GM) when used at concentrations as low as 10^{-10} M (23). $PGF_{1\alpha}$ and $PGF_{2\alpha}$ are ineffective.

The effect of PGE_1 is dose dependent, with complete inhibition of proliferation seen at 10^{-5} M.

Studies on the human leukemia cell line (HL60) from a patient with acute promyelocytic leukemia show that PGE_1 not only inhibits cellular proliferation but also stimulates biochemical maturation as evidenced by increased chemotactic receptor expression, increased NBT reduction, and increased glass adherence (1). Morphologic maturation was not seen concomitantly, suggesting that the effect of PGE_1 is selective. Recent studies have provided evidence that the granulocyte-macrophage progenitor cell is sensitive to prostaglandins only when the Ia-antigen is expressed on the cell surface (24).

Since macrophages (see Ch. 10) can synthesize significant quantities of PGE_2, these cells have been implicated in the provision of PGE_2 to regulate granulocyte-macrophage formation and differentiation (23). A fibroblastoid cell line has been shown to produce an unidentified prostaglandin (PGE_2 or possibly PGI_2) which can similarly inhibit CFU-GM formation (25). Thus, marrow fibroblasts as well as macrophages may be involved.

Colony-stimulating factor (CSF) required for proliferation of the granulocyte-macrophage precusor cell (CFU-GM) is also a stimulus for macrophage PGE synthesis (26). Synthesis of CSF and PGE_2 may occur in separate macrophage subpopulations. CSF-stimulated PGE_2 synthesis could provide a negative feedback message to prevent overpopulation of granulocytes and macrophages under conditions of high levels of CSF.

C. Clinical Relevance

Abnormal prostaglandin regulation of granulocyte-macrophage production has been implicated in two disease states—cyclic neutropenia and chronic myelogenous leukemia.

1. Cyclic Neutropenia

In canine cyclic hematopoiesis, dogs show an intermittent neutropenia. In vitro studies have shown that the adherent cells (probably predominantly macrophages and fibroblasts) from the bone marrow of these dogs show an intermittent inhibition of normal marrow granulocyte colony-forming units. Synthesis of the inhibitory stimulus by these adherent cells can be prevented by indomethacin, suggesting it is a prostaglandin (27).

2. Chronic Myelogenous Leukemia

Whereas PGE_2 is effective in suppressing normal granulocyte-macrophage colony formation (CFU-GM), it is ineffective in suppressing CFU-GM growth in chronic myelogenous leukemia (28). The absence of prostaglandin-mediated inhibition could be the reason for the unregulated granulocyte-macrophage proliferation in chronic myelogenous leukemia.

IV. THE MACROPHAGE-COMMITTED PROGENITOR CELL

The granulocyte-macrophage progenitor cell can give rise to a purely macrophage progenitor. This cell and its growth can be assessed using thioglycollate-stimulated peritoneal exudate cells. The growth of these cells is inhibited by PGE_1 at concentrations of 10^{-6}-10^{-10} M (21).

V. MEGAKARYOCYTOPOIESIS

Isolated megakaryocytes (guinea pigs), like platelets, will convert arachidonic acid to thromboxane B_2 and the hydroxy fatty acids HHT and 12-HETE, with one megakaryocyte, synthesizing as much as 2,500-4,000 platelets (29).

The growth and maturation of megakaryocytes appear to require a megakaryocyte colony-stimulating activity, which promotes proliferation of the progenitor cells, and thrombopoietin, which promotes megakaryocyte development. To date, the effects of prostaglandins and other arachidonic acid metabolites on megakaryocytopoiesis are unknown.

VI. LYMPHOCYTE PRODUCTION AND DIFFERENTIATION

Knowledge of the influence of prostaglandins and other arachidonic acid metabolites on lymphocyte development is presently at a very primitive level. Prostaglandin E_1 is a potent inhibitor of colony formation by mouse splenic B lymphocytes (21). PGE_2 has been shown to increase the percentage of T cells which act as suppressor cells in the humoral response induced by antigens such as pokeweed mitogen (T cells capable of binding the Fc fragment of IgG) and to decrease the percentage of T cells which help B-cell differentiation (IgM-Fc receptor-bearing cells) (30). However, since PGE_2 can inhibit the activity of a suppressor T-cell population which modulates immunoglobin production by B lymphocytes, its overall effect may be to enhance polyclonal immunoglobin production (31). The effects of PGE_2 may be important as this is a major prostaglandin produced by macrophages, and could be involved in macrophage regulation of lymphocyte production and function. However, there are many other arachidonic acid metabolites which may also be important.

VI. PROSTAGLANDIN PRODUCTION BY WHOLE BONE MARROW

One study of rat bone marrow homogenates suggests PGD_2 is the primary prostaglandin produced (32). A second, using rat bone marrow microsomes, suggests PGE_2 and $PGF_{2\alpha}$ are the major metabolites (33). Clearly, much more work needs to be done in this area.

VIII. SUMMARY

At the present time studies of the production and effects of prostaglandins, thromboxanes and leukotrienes on blood cell production are at an early stage. Perhaps the best studied finding is the enhancement of erythropoiesis and depression of myelopoiesis by PGE_2. Abnormalities in prostaglandin mediated regulation of myelopoiesis have been implicated in cyclic neutropenia and chronic myelogenous leukemia, but further studies are needed to fully establish these possibilities. With the many leukotrienes still to be tested for their effects and specific inhibitors of thromboxane and leukotriene synthesis to be studied it is likely there will be some exciting new developments in this field in the near future.

REFERENCES

1. T. J. Chaplinski and J. E. Niedel. *J. Clin. Invest. 70*:953 (1982).
2. R. W. Bryant, J. M. Bailey, T. Schewe, and S. M. Rapoport. *J. Biol. Chem. 257*:6050 (1982).
3. I. Feher and J. Gidali. *Nature (Lond.) 247*:550 (1974).
4. J. W. Byron. *Exp. Hematol. 3*:44 (1975).
5. J. Gidali and I. Feher. *Cell Tissue Kinet. 10*:365 (1977).
6. L. M. Pelus. *J. Clin. Invest. 70*:568 (1982).

7. A. Kornberg, and E. A. Rachmilewitz. *Acta Hematol. 67*:136 (1982).
8. P. P. Dukes, N. A. Shore, D. Hammond, J. A. Ortega, and M. C. Datta. *J. Lab. Clin. Med. 82*:704 (1973).
9. P. K. Nelson and J. W. Fisher. *Fed. Proc. 37*:607 (1978).
10. H. S. L. Chan, E. F. Saunders, and M. H. Freedman. *J. Lab. Clin. Med. 95*:125 (1980).
11. P. P. Dukes. In *Prostaglandins: Organ and Tissue Specific Actions*, S. Greenberg, P. J. Kadowitz, T. F. Burks (eds). Marcel Dekker, Inc., New York (1982), pp. 283.
12. J. N. Forrest, Jr. *N. Engl. J. Med. 292*:423 (1975).
13. L. G. Paulo, R. D. Wilkerson, B. L. Roh, W. J. George, and J. W. Fisher. *Proc. Soc. Exp. Biol. Med. 142*:771 (1973).
14. D. M. Gross, J. Brookins, G. D. Fink, and J. W. Fisher. *J. Pharmacol. Exp. Ther. 198*:489 (1976).
15. V. M. Mujovic and J. W. Fisher. *J. Pharmacol. Exp. Ther. 191*:575 (1974).
16. D. M. Gross, V. M. Mujovic, W. Jubiz, and J. W. Fisher. *Proc. Soc. Exp. Biol. Ther. 15*:498 (1976).
17. V. M. Mujovic and J. W. Fisher. *Life Sci. 16*:463 (1975).
18. J. A. Ortega, M. H. Malekzadeh, P. P. Dukes, a. Ma, and N. A. Shore. *Clin. Res. 30*:123A (1982).
19. P. P. Dukes, N. A. Shore, D. Hammond, and J. A. Ortega. In *Erythropoiesis*, K. Nakae, J. W. Fisher, and F. Takaker (eds.). University of Tokyo Press, Tokyo (1975), p. 3.
20. H. S. L. Chan, M. H. Freedman, and E. F. Saunders. *Exp. Hematol. (Suppl. 3) 6*:35 (1978).
21. J. I. Kurland, J. W. Hadden, and M. A. S. Moore. *Cancer Res. 37*:4534 (1977).
22a. S. C. Hung, N. I. Galli, D. L. Venton, and G. C. LeBreton. *Prostaglandins 24*:195 (1982).
22b. D. S. Snyder and J. F. Desforges. Conference on Prostaglandins and Leukotrienes '84. May 8-11, Washington, D.C., Abstract 255 (1984).
23. J. Kurland and M. A. S. Moore. *Exp. Hematol. 5*:357 (1977).
24. L. M. Pelus. *J. Clin. Invest. 70*:568 (1982).
25. H. M. Garnett, E. P. Cronkite, and K. Harigaya. *Proc. Natl. Acad. Sci. USA 79*:1545 (1982).
26. J. I. Kurland, L. M. Pelus, P. Ralph, R. S. Bockman, and M. A. S. Moore. *Proc. Natl. Acad. Sci. USA 76*:2326 (1979).
27. J. B. Jones and J. D. Jolly. *Br. J. Hematol. 50*:607 (1982).
28. L. M. Pelus, H. E. Broxmeyer, B. D. Clarkson, and M. A. S. Moore. *Cancer Res. 40*:2512 (1980).
29. J. L. Moller, M. J. Stuart, and R. W. Walenga. *Biochem. Biophys. Res. Commun. 107*:752 (1982).
30. P. A. Kaszubowski and J. S. Goodwin. *Cell Immunol. 68*:343 (1982).

31. J. L. Ceuppens and J. S. Goodwin. *Cell Immunol.* *70*:41 (1982).
32. A. Kojima, M. Shiraki, R. Takahashi, H. Orimo, I. Morita, and S. Murota. *Prostaglandins 20*:171 (1980).
33. V. A. Ziboh, J. Lord, G. Blick, I. Kursunoglu, J. Poitier, and A. A. Yunis. *Cancer Res. 37*:3974 (1977).

20
An Overall Perspective

This book has been written from my own point of view, that of an inquiring physician who has some clinical involvement, but who spends most of the time in a laboratory searching for an understanding of basic and fundamental mechanisms of cellular function. I have sought to provide an up to date evaluation of the role of prostaglandins, thromboxanes, and leukotrienes in the general scheme of things, and in the function of blood and vascular cells in particular. Out of the expanding research effort in this area, there is emerging a vast array of new drugs as well as new insights into the mechanisms and uses of old drugs. The potential benefits in the prevention and treatment of disease are enormous. At present we have barely scratched the surface.

I. WHY SHOULD MANIPULATION OF THE PRODUCTION AND EFFECTS OF PROSTAGLANDINS AND RELATED LIPID MEDIATORS HAVE SUCH EXTRAORDINARY THERAPEUTIC POTENTIAL?

The answer to this question is, in essence, simple. There is a wide variety of prostaglandins, and an even greater number of closely related chemicals–

thromboxanes, leukotrienes, hydroxy fatty acids, and so forth. Each of these compounds has a unique spectrum of activity, often promoting or inhibiting cell function at very low concentrations. Furthermore, the effects of these compounds on cells—their modulating function (promoting or inhibiting cellular activities depending on the compound and the circumstance)—are often desirable for the treatment of patients with specific diseases, but in some cases are undesirable. For example, manipulation of platelet function so that the platelets are more responsive as desirable in a patient with a bleeding disorder, but undesirable in a patient with a tendency to develop thromboses. Conversely, inhibition of platelet function is inappropriate for the former patient, but desirable for the second. Last, it is now becoming clear that through changes in diet or drugs we can modify the production and effects of prostaglandins and related chemicals in a bewildering variety of ways.

If each prostaglandin (PG), thromboxane, or leukotriene (LT) exerted its specific effects only on one particular cell type, and if drugs that affected a given aspect of the production or effect were entirely specific, designing and using chemicals that modify this system might be simplified. In reality, overlapping (sometimes complementary, sometimes antagonistic), actions of prostaglandins and related chemicals on the functions of different cells frequently make rather complex the manipulation of these pathways to achieve desirable goals. For example aspirin inhibition of platelet synthesis of the proaggregatory and vasoconstrictor thromboxane would be much more antithrombotic if it were not counterbalanced by aspirin usually also inhibiting endothelial cell synthesis of the antiaggregatory and vasodilator prostacyclin. An additional order of complexity may be operative in lymphocytes where the overall effects of prostaglandin E_2 (PGE_2) may depend on its relative inhibition of lymphocyte subtypes (helper cells, suppressor cells, etc.), and the overall effect of leukotriene B_4 may similarly depend on its ability to promote activation of suppressive versus other cells. Such complexity means that therapeutic intervention will not always be easy. Sophisticated approaches may often be essential for optimum results.

II. ARE THERE GENERAL PRINCIPLES THAT CAN FACILITATE THE UNDERSTANDING OF THESE COMPLEX CHEMICALS?

I believe that there are several concepts that can provide a framework on which to build the finer details of prostaglandin-cell interaction. These have been discussed in earlier chapters but will be reviewed here as part of this overall synthesis.

A. Response to Injury

Blood cells, in general, respond to injurious or noxious stimuli (platelets to an injured vessel wall; neutrophils to bacteria; lymphocytes and mast cells to foreign antigens; natural killer cells to malignant cells etc.). There are strong reasons for believing that the present specific response of a given blood cell type to a specific stimulus has evolved from a nonspecific cellular response to damage to its cell membrane (Fig. 20-1). Blood cells will still respond to nonspecific injury by breakdown of their membrane, release of fatty acids, and synthesis of prostaglandins. The rate-limiting step in stimulus-specific formation of prostaglandins is the release of arachidonic acid from membrane phospholipids—a process involving enzymes that hydrolyze or break down specific arachidonic acid-enriched membrane phospholipids.

B. The Synthesis of Prostaglandins and Leukotrienes Are Just Specific Forms of Fatty Acid Oxidation

Polyunsaturated fatty acids with their double bonds are very susceptible to oxidation. In the presence of a transition metal such as Fe^{2+} and oxygen, the oxidation of polyunsaturated fatty acids occurs rapidly but nonspecifically. I suspect that current blood cells have evolved from the situation in more primitive cells where nonspecific oxidation occurred, to their present specific mechanisms. Blood cells have probably, in essence, harnessed the innate potential for oxidation of fatty acids by channeling it in specific directions. Rather than nonspecific oxidation of fatty acids by transition metals, we now have specific patterns of oxidation induced by iron- or heme-containing enzymes. There are two major pathways—a cyclooxygenase (prostaglandin endoperoxide synthetase) pathway giving rise to prostaglandins and thromboxanes and a lipoxygenase pathway giving rise to hydroxy fatty acids such as hydroxyeicosatetraenoic acids (HETEs) or DiHETES derived from arachidonic acid or leukotrienes (Fig. 20-2). Certain leukotrienes (C_4, D_4, and E_4) have the added complexity of having one or more amino acids linked to their basic structure, whereas others (A_4, B_4) do not.

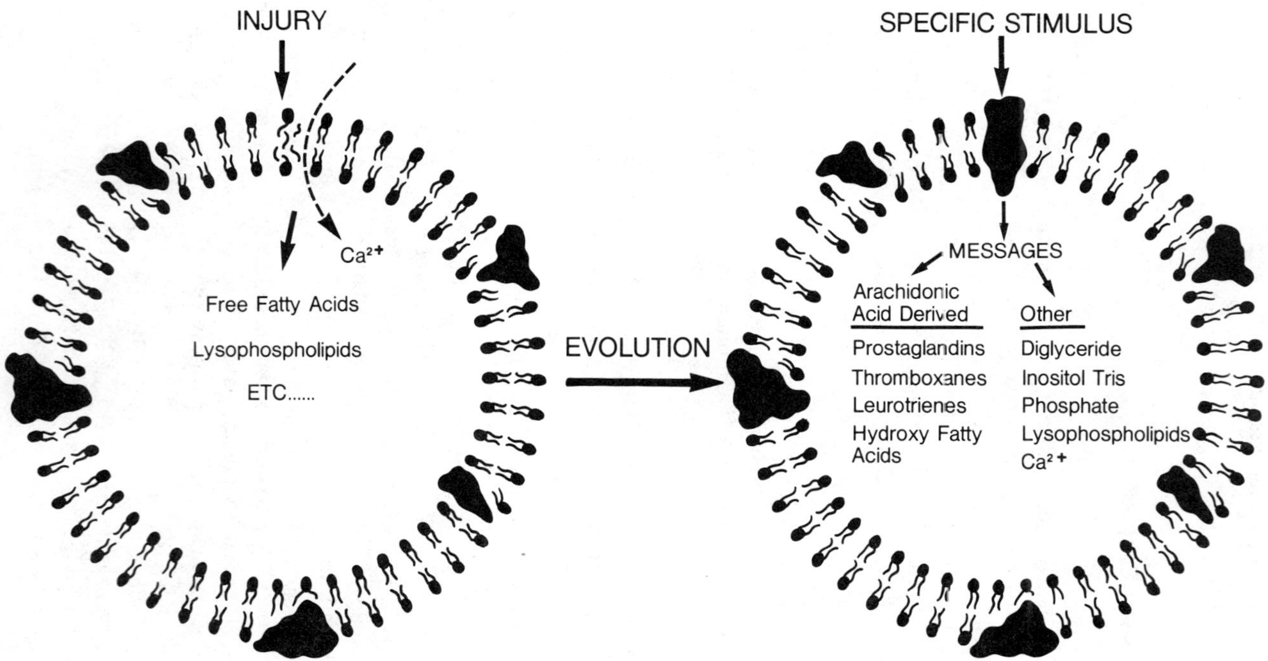

Fig. 20-1 It is very likely that the present production of prostaglandins and other messengers in response to specific stimuli (right) has evolved from a more general response to injury and nonspecific membrane damage by a more primordial cell type (left).

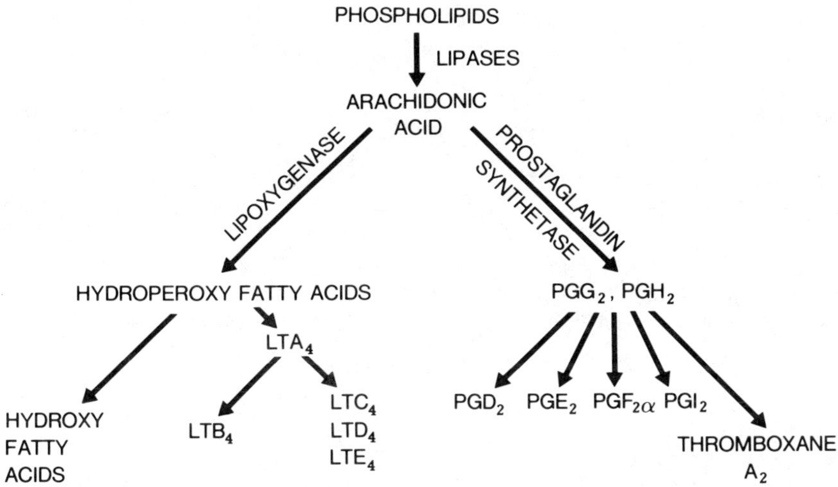

Fig. 20-2 Following the release of unsaturated fatty acids such as arachidonic acid from cellular phospholipids, it is metabolized primarily through either the prostaglandin synthetase (fatty acid cyclooxygenase) or lipoxygenase pathway. A considerable variety of further metabolites is then produced from the initial products of these pathways (i.e., PGG_2 and PGH_2 from the prostaglandin synthetase pathway, and hydroperoxy fatty acids from the lipoxygenase pathway). Additional products not shown including lipoxans and prostaglandin cyclic inositol have recently been described, but it is not yet certain whether these are produced in vivo.

C. Autocoids or Local Acting Messengers

Prostaglandins and related chemicals may act as intracellular messengers, having effects inside the cell where they were produced, or as extracellular messengers, having effects on cells other than the one in which they were produced. In either case, the site of action is almost always relatively close to the site of synthesis. Prostaglandins and related chemicals are short-lived in vivo, either because the native chemical is unstable or because it is rapidly degraded by enzymes such as the prostaglandin dehydrogenase present in the lung. PGE_2, for example, is more than 90% degraded in a single passage through the lung. Prostaglandins are therefore not hormones in the usual sense of this word but rather autocoids—short-lived, local-acting messengers (Fig. 20-3).

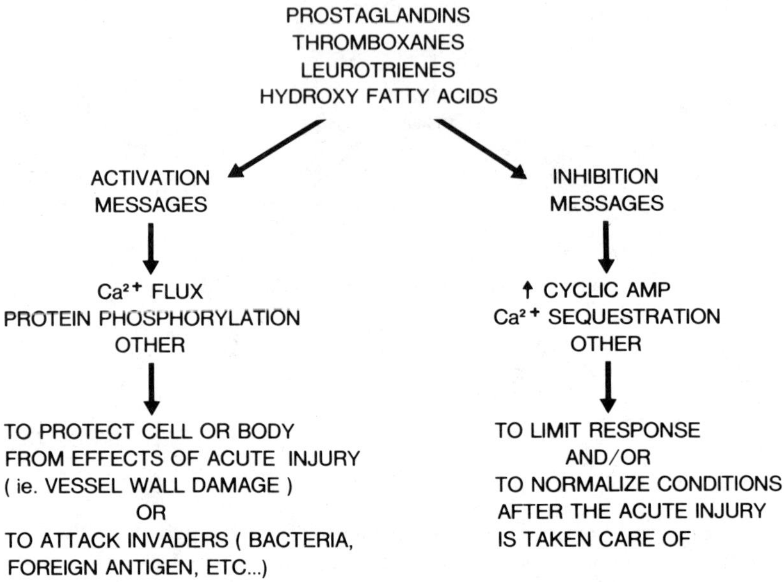

Fig. 20-3 Effects of prostaglandins, thromboxanes, leukotrienes, and hydroxy fatty acids on blood cells can be generally divided into those which promote cellular activation and those which inhibit cell function.

1. Positive or Agonist Messengers: Calcium and Calcium-Interactive Processes

A rise in the level of cytoplasmic calcium is an important component in the activation of blood cells (platelet aggregation, neutrophil chemotaxis, mast cell secretion, lymphocyte transformation, endothelial and smooth muscle cell contraction, etc.). Evidence has been provided that the following prostaglandins and related chemicals promote cellular activation by stimulating a flux of calcium into the cytoplasm (prostaglandin endoperoxides and thromboxane A_2, platelets; LTB_4, neutrophils; LTD_4, smooth muscle cells; $PGF_{2\alpha}$, smooth muscle cells). Of these, thromboxane A_2 and LTB_4 have been shown to have some properties of calcium ionophores. The cell-specific nature of their actions and inhibition of their effects by structurally related chemicals argues against a purely calcium-ionophore mechanism of action. However, it is possible that blood cells may have evolved from responding nonspecifically to these chemicals, which may under defined conditions act as calcium ionophores to more specific and controlled receptor-coupled calcium flux-promoting mechanisms.

In the last few years, it has become apparent that cells have mechanisms for activation which, although requiring calcium, are not calcium controlled in the sense that activation occurs primarily as a result of a change in the cytosol level of calcium. At present, diglyceride and phorbol myristate acetate activation of cells through stimulation of protein kinase C clearly fits in this category. It is probably only a matter of time before effects of prostaglandin or related chemical to promote activation of this kinase, or some other process which is not calcium driven, is described. Already in platelets, arachidonic acid and prostaglandin endoperoxides are known to actively promote phosphorylation of a 47,000-dalton protein phosphorylated by protein kinase C. In neutrophils, 5-HETE and LTB_4 are synergistic in promoting cell responsiveness, suggesting they act slightly differently. Thus, while the promotion of calcium flux by prostaglandins and related chemicals appears to be an important mechanism of their stimulatory actions, other processes will undoubtedly be important to an overall view of their agonist effects.

2. Negative or Inhibitory Messengers and Cyclic Adenosine Monophosphate

For each blood cell type studied, there are prostaglandins that convey inhibitory messengers. There is a greater consistency in the prostaglandins responsible for such inhibition, with PGI_2, PGE_2, PGD_2, and PGE_1 being the most important. However, cell-specific differences do exist (i.e., PGE_2 is inactive as an inhibitor of platelet function, although it is effective on most other blood cell types). In each case where it has been well studied, cellular inhibition by these prostaglandins results from an action to stimulate cell adenylate cyclase to raise the intracellular level of cyclic adenosine monophosphate (cAMP). With the possible exception of a non-cAMP-mediated effect of PGE_1 described by Sinha and Colman in platelets (1a), there has been no clear demonstration of alternate mechanisms for inhibition.

D. Pathways for Cell Stimulation Independent of Prostaglandins, Thromboxanes, and Leukotrienes

It is quite clear that the platelet response to the critical in vivo agonist thrombin, is largely independent of platelet thromboxane production except at low thrombin concentrations. Platelets thus have mechanisms for bypassing the requirement for thromboxane A_2, an important concept, in view of the potential untoward effects if platelet function were completely inhibited by aspirin. Thrombin appears to bypass a requirement for thromboxane production through an effect to break down phosphatidylinositols and produce mediators such as diglyceride, inositol trisphosphate, phosphatidic acid, and lysophosphatidic acid, which can act independent of thromboxane production. Other blood cells are almost certain to be similar (i.e., neutrophil stimulation by C5a or FMLP may be largely independent of LTB_4, etc.). Indeed the initial breakdown of phosphoinositides is emerging as important in most and perhaps all blood cell types. For the present overview, the important concept is that although prostaglandins, thromboxanes, and leukotrienes are important modulators of cell function, they may not be essential in the sense that without them the cell can still respond even if it requires a slightly larger stimulus.

E. The Balance of Production and Effect May be More Critical Than the Level of Any Individual Substance

In situations where there is a stimulus (vessel wall injury, bacteria, immune complexes, etc.) there is likely to be more than one prostaglandin, thromboxane, or leukotriene produced. In such circumstances, the end result may be significantly influenced by the sequence of their production or the specific balance of products present at a given time. In many circumstances in vivo, we are still hampered by limitations in our ability to measure the full array of potentially important products, and sometimes even in clearly knowing which products should be measured. In the evaluation of thrombotic problems, thromboxane A_2 and PGI_2 are clearly important, but in some instances (i.e., coronary vasospasm) leukotriene D_4 may also be critical. In the evaluation of disorders involving neutrophil infiltration of tissues, measurement of LTB_4 and the HETEs would appear to be most valuable. With hypersensitivity disorders and anaphylaxis, the mast cell products LTC_4, LTD_4, PGD_2 and platelet-activating factor appear to be most involved, but secondary thromboxane A_2 production clearly occurs and may be important. With disorders of immunological function, levels of PGE_2, LTB_4, and 15-HETE may be most important, but given our current state of knowledge this is less certain than in other areas.

Measurement of prostaglandins and related substances is easiest with a single cell type and a defined stimulus. The more complex the situation, the greater the difficulties in assessing the production of these substances as discussed in Chapter 15. Gradually, improved understanding of how best to approach a given situation and how to interpret the results is emerging.

III. DIRECTIONS FOR THE FUTURE

We are presently nearing the point where we have an understanding of the major metabolites of arachidonic acid in each blood cell type and the amount of each produced (Table 20-1). It is apparent, however, that a number of discrepancies between different investigators need to be resolved. Less well understood are variations in the amounts of each product with the type of stimulus, the influence, if any, of the nature of the resuspending medium, and the products produced by combinations of different cells. Understanding the relative amounts of each product produced under various conditions in vivo is clearly the next step, and this process has hardly begun.

There is a tremendous potential to alter the pattern of production and effect of prostaglandins and related metabolites by dietary changes. Diets enriched in eicosapentaenoic acid, a fatty acid found in fish from northern waters, is one example. Benefit may occur in individuals prone to develop thrombotic disorders as described in Chapter 16. Benefit is also possible in inflammatory disorders involving neutrophils, since LTB_5 derived from eicosapentaenoic acid is only about one-tenth as potent in stimulating the chemotaxis and aggregation of neutrophils as LTB_4 derived from arachidonic acid (1). Furthermore, mast cells enriched in eicosapentaenoic acid produced LTB_4 and LTB_5 in preference to LTC_4 and LTC_5. This switch away from a normal preponderance of LTC_4 might be of significant benefit in disorders such as asthma where LTC_4 and LTD_4 derived from mast cells may be the cause of bronchospasm.

Alternate dietary approaches using dihomo-γ-linolenic acid and other fatty acid-enriched diets may have benefit under particular circumstances either through direct modulation of the production of metabolites or through effects as diverse as changing the availability of prostaglandin receptors as has been shown with corn oil diets and PGE_2 receptors on monocytes (2). A particular example of an effect of diet is the production of 12-hydroxy 20:3ω9, a hydroxy fatty acid produced by the platelet lipoxygenase from 20:3ω9, a fatty acid found in higher than usual levels in individuals on a high saturated fatty acid diet. 12-Hydroxy 20:3ω9 promotes platelet aggregation, and its production may account for the enhanced platelet aggregation seen in individuals on such diets. Better understanding

Table 20-1 Representative Production of Prostaglandins and Related Chemicals by Human Blood and Vascular Cells

Cell type	Stimulus	Production (ng/10^6 cells except platelets where ng/10^8 cells is used)[a]									Reference
		Thromboxane B_2	PGD_2	PGE_2	$PGF_{2\alpha}$	PGI_2	5-HETE	15-HETE	LTB_4	LTC_4/D_4	
Platelet	Thrombin (1 Um)			2	0.7						3
	Thrombin (5 Um1)		3								4
	AA[b] (1.6 mM)	340									5
	collagen (1 μg/m1)	18									5
Neutrophil	A23187 (20 μM)						50	0	17		6
	AA + A23187 (20 μM)						280	15	33		6
	A23187 (5 μM)								50	7	7
	Serum-treated zymosan	0.07									8
Eosinophil	(normal donors)										
	A23187 (10 μM)						0.5	2.5	2.1	3.5	9
	A23187 (5 μM)								6.0	38	7
	AA (100 μM) + A23187 (10 μM)							47			9
Basophil	Anti-IgE	0.04								4	10

Mast cell	Anti-IgE	4.60	58	0.33	3.1	0.3		110	10
	IgE/antigen						<4	25	1
Monocyte	PHA[b]			109					1
	PHA	17		2.5					12
	PHA + T cells	44		8					12
	A23187						70	30	1
	Zymosan						10	2	1
Alveolar macrophage:	A23187						190	10	7,13
Endothelial cells:	AA (20 μM)					20			14
	AA (10 μM)	35				200			15
Vascular (aorta) smooth muscle cell	AA (10 μM)	0				50			15

[a]Values given are means from the published references.
[b]AA = arachidonic acid; PHA = phytohemagglutinin.

of this and other changes with diet should allow an improved knowledge of the effects of diets on disease and how diets might be altered in a beneficial fashion.

The prostaglandin synthetase inhibitors, aspirin, indomethacin and so on, are presently in widespread use. Many new drugs are rapidly being synthesized and tested. These include specific thromboxane synthetase and lipoxygenase inhibitors and receptor antagonists for the thromboxanes and leukotrienes, as well as other drugs which modify pathways involved in the release of arachidonic acid. These new agents are likely to revolutionize the treatment of a broad spectrum of human ailments. The years ahead will be exciting ones.

REFERENCES

1a. A. K. Sinha and R. W. Colman. *Thromb. Res. 30*:533 (1983).
1b. R. A. Lewis and K. F. Austen. *J. Clin. Invest. 73*:889 (1984).
2. F. A. Opmeer, M. J. P. Adolfs, and I. L. Bonta. *J. Lipid Res. 25*:262 (1984).
3. J. B. Smith, C. Ingerman, J. J. Kocsis, and M. J. Silver. *J. Clin. Invest. 52*:965 (1973).
4. O. Oelz, R. Olez, H. R. Knapp, B. J. Sweetman, and J. A. Oates. *Prostaglandins 13*:225 (1977).
5. J. Docherty, E. Israels, and J. M. Gerrard. Unpublished manuscript.
6. P. Borgeat and B. Samuelsson. *Proc. Natl. Acad. Sci. USA 76*:2148 (1979).
7. P. F. Weller, C. W. Lee, D. W. Foster, E. J. Corey, K. F. Austen, and R. A. Lewis. *Proc. Natl. Acad. Sci. USA 80*:7626 (1983).
8. I. M. Goldstein, C. L. Malmsten, H. Kindahl, H. B. Kaplan, O. Radmark, B. Samuelsson, and G. Weissmann. *J. Exp. Med. 148*:787 (1978).
9. W. R. Henderson, J. B. Harley, and A. S. Fauci. *Immunology 51*:679 (1984).
10. D. W. MacGlashan, Jr., R. P. Schleimer, S. P. Peters, E. S. Schulman, G. K. Adams, A. K. Sobotka, H. H. Newball, and L. M. Lichtenstein. *Fed. Proc. 42*:2504 (1983).
11. A. D. Bankhurst, E.Hastain, J. S. Goodwin, and G. T. Peake. *J. Lab. Clin. Med. 97*:179 (1981).
12. M. E. Goldyne and J. D. Stobo. *Prostaglandins 24*:623 (1982).
13. P. M. Godard, F. B. Damon, F. B. Michel, E. J. Corey, K. F. Austen, and R. A. Lewis. *Clin. Res. 31*:548A (1983).
14. E. A. Jaffe and B. B. Weksler. *J. Clin. Invest. 63*:532 (1979).
15. C. Ingerman-Wojenski, M. J. Silver, J. B. Smith, and E. Macarak. *J. Clin. Invest. 67*:1292 (1981).

Glossary

47P: A 47,000-dalton protein found in platelets and perhaps in other blood cells which is phosphorylated by protein kinase C and may be involved in granule secretion.

A23187: A calcium ionophore widely used in the study of blood cell function because of its ability to transport calcium across biological membranes to stimulate cells. Because of its ability to stimulate calcium flux directly, A23187 can bypass certain receptor-coupled steps involved in signal transmission.

Arachidonic Acid: (20:4ω6) A polyunsaturated fatty acid with 20 carbons and 4 double bonds. The double bond closest to the CH_3-terminal end is 6 carbons (ω6) away. Arachidonic acid is widely distributed in mammalian tissues and is the principal fatty acid substrate for prostaglandins and related chemicals. Its structure is shown in Fig. 1-1.

Aspirin: Acetylsalicyclic acid is a widely used inhibitor of the prostaglandin synthetase enzyme (see Chapter 5).

B Cells: Lymphocytes which are involved in humoral immunity and immunoglobulin production. For further details see Chapter 12.

C5a: The activated (a) form of the fifth component of complement. This protein has potent chemotactic activity for neutrophils.

Calmodulin: A 17,000-dalton protein present in blood cells which serves as an intracellular receptor for calcium. When the cytoplasmic calcium level rises on cell stimulation, the calcium-calmodulin complex can activate a variety of intracellular proteins to promote the cellular response to the stimulus.

Concanavalin A: A vegetable protein which stimulates proliferation of B lymphocytes.

CCF: An 8,400-dalton neutrophil granule glycoprotein with chemotactic activity.

CFU-GM: The bone marrow precursor cell for granulocytes and macrophages (see Chapter 19).

CSF: Colony-stimulating factor, a factor important for the proliferation of the granulocyte-macrophage precursor cell (see Chapter 19).

cAMP: Adenosine 3′,5′-cyclic phosphate, an intracellular messenger which exerts its effects by activating protein kinases and causing phosphorylation of certain intracellular proteins. In blood cells many, but not all, of the actions of cAMP are inhibitory to cell function (see Chapter 3).

cGMP: Guanosine 3′,5′-cyclic phosphate, a high-energy phosphate species found in many blood cells in association with cellular activation events. In most circumstances its role is still uncertain (see Chapters 3 and 12).

Diglyceride: A neutral lipid with two fatty acids esterified to a glycerol backbone (see Fig. 2-16 for structure). One of the immediate products of the receptor-coupled phospholipase C hydrolysis of phosphoinositides in blood cells is a diglyceride, primarily stearoyl-arachidonyl diglyceride (see Fig. 4-2). Diglycerides can activate blood cells through stimulation of protein kinase C (see Chapter 3).

Diglyceride Lipase: An enzyme which removes one and perhaps both fatty acids from diglycerides.

DiHETE: Dihydroxyeicosatetraenoic acid refers to any one of several derivatives of arachidonic acid with two hydroxy substituents. One of the most important biologically appears to be LTB_4 (see Fig. 8-3 for structure).

Dihomo-γ-linolenic Acid: (20:3ω6) A polyunsaturated fatty acid with 20 carbons and 3 double bonds. The double bond closest to the CH_3-terminal end is 6 carbons (ω6) away. Dihomo-γ-linolenic acid is a precursor for 1-

series prostaglandins (i.e., PGE_1, PGD_1, $PGF_{1\alpha}$) and 3-series leukotrienes (i.e., LTB_3). In most mammalian tissues dihomo-γ-linolenic acid is present in much lower quantities than arachidonic acid, in part because of the rapid conversion of dihomo-γ-linolenic acid to arachidonic acid by most tissues.

Eicosapentaenoic Acid: (20:5ω6) (also called timnodonic acid): A polyunsaturated fatty acid with 20 carbons and 5 double bonds. The double bond closest to the CH_3-terminal end is 6 carbons (ω6) away. Eicosapentaenoic acid is the precursor for 3-series prostaglandins (i.e., PGE_3, PGD_3, $PGF_{3\alpha}$, PGI_3) and 5-series leukotrienes (i.e., LTB_5, LTC_5). Eicosapentaenoic acid is plentiful in fish from cold waters and in human populations such as the Greenland Eskimos whose diet is largely fish or fish-eating mammals such as seals.

Fatty Acid Cyclooxygenase: See prostaglandin synthetase.

FMLP: Formyl-methionyl-leucine-phenylalanine, a chemotactic peptide used in studies of leukocyte function.

HETE: Hydroxyeicosatetraenoic acid, a hydroxy derivative of arachidonic acid. There are a considerable number of HETEs formed biologically with 5-HETE (Fig. 8-3), 12-HETE (Fig. 2-10), and 15-HETE (Fig. 8-3) being the most common mono-HETEs. DiHETEs are derivaties with two hydroxy substituents. At present the most important of these appears to be LTB_4 but other DiHETEs also have biological activity.

HHT: 12-Hydroxy heptadecatrienoic acid, a hydroxy fatty acid formed in platelets during the conversion of PGH_2 to thromboxane A_2. It has some activity to stimulate neutrophil chemotaxis.

HPETE: Hydroperoxyeicosatetraenoic acid, a hydroperoxy derivative of arachidonic acid formed by the lipoxygenase enzymes which are intermediates in the synthesis of HETEs (see Fig. 2-10 for the structure of 12-HPETE).

Leukotrienes: Chemicals derived from polyunsaturated fatty acids which possess a conjugated triene (C=C–C=C–C=C) structure. The name was given as the first of these was found from leukocytes. The structures of several leukotrienes are shown in Figs. 2-14 and 8-3.

LTA_4: Leukotriene A_4, a leukotriene with a $C_{5,6}$ epoxide. LTA_4 is a labile intermediate in the synthesis of LTB_4 and LTC_4.

LTB_4: Leukotriene B_4, a leukotriene derived predomonantly from neutrophils and monocytes which has important biological activities on inflammatory cells (see Fig. 8-3 for structure).

LTC_4: Leukotriene C_4, a leukotriene derived from LTA_4 as a result of the addition of glutathione by the enzyme glutathione-S-transferase. LTC_4 has important actions on smooth muscle cells (see Fig. 2-14 for its structure and Chapter 14 for a description of its activity).

LTD_4: Leukotriene D_4, a leukotriene derived from LTC_4 through the loss of a glutamine residue as a result of the action of the enzyme glutamyl transpeptidase. It has important biological activities on smooth muscle cells (see Chapter 14; its structure is shown in Fig. 2-14).

LTE_4: Leukotriene E_4, a leukotriene derived from LTD_4 through the loss of a glycine residue. In general LTE_4 has considerably less biological activity than LTD_4 (see Fig. 2-14 for structure).

Lysophosphatidic Acid: A lysophospholipid present in very small amounts in unstimulated blood cells. In platelets, and perhaps in other cells, there is an increase in the amount of lysophosphatidic acid on stimulation. Lysophosphatidic acid has activity to stimulate platelet aggregation, enhance neutrophil chemotaxis, and to cause smooth muscle contraction. The structure of lysophosphatidic acid is shown in Fig. 2-16.

Myosin Light Chain: In platelets and smooth muscle cells calcium regulation of contractile activity is regulated through calcium-calmodulin activation of a protein kinase which phosphorylates myosin light chain. With its light chain phosphorylated, myosin can then interact with actin to generate tension (i.e., contract).

NK Cells: Natural killer cells, large granular lymphocytes with an important role in the destruction of tumor cells (see Chapter 12).

Oleoyl-acetyl-diglyceride: Most diglycerides do not penetrate readily into cells. This diglyceride was synthesized because it can penetrate into cells (as a result of the short acetyl group in the 2-position of the diglyceride) and, like the natural diglyceride, it stimulates the activity of protein kinase C.

PG: Prostaglandin.

PGA_2: Prostaglandin A_2, see Appendix 2-1 for structure.

PGB_2: Prostaglandin B_2, see Appendix 2-1 for structure.

PGC_2: Prostaglandin C_2, see Appendix 2-1 for structure.

PGD_2: Prostaglandin D_2, see Appendix 2-1 for structure.

PGE_2: Prostaglandin E_2, see Appendix 1-1 for structure.

$PGF_{2\alpha}$: Prostaglandin $F_{2\alpha}$, see Appendix 2-1 for structure.

PGG_2: Prostaglandin G_2, a prostaglandin endoperoxide (see Appendix 2-1 for structure).

PGI_2: Prostaglandin I_2, see Appendix 2-1 for structure.

PHA: Phytohemagglutinin.

Phorbol Myristate Acetate: A tumor promoter isolated from croton oil which promotes secretion in several blood cell types. Phorbol myristate acetate has been found to act by stimulating a protein kinase C.

Phosphatidylcholine: A phospholipid widely distributed in mammalian tissues. In red cells, platelets, and perhaps in other blood cells, it is found in considerable quantities in both halves of the plasma membrane. It is an important source of arachidonic acid for the synthesis of prostaglandins, thromboxanes, and leukotrienes in several blood cells (see Fig. 2-2 for its structure).

Phosphatidylethanolamine: A negatively charged phospholipid widely distributed in mammalian tissues. In red blood cells, platelets, and perhaps other blood cells, it is found primarily on the inner half of the plasma membrane (see Fig. 2-2 for structure).

Phosphatidylinositol: A negatively charged phospholipid found in biological membranes. In red blood cell and platelet plasma membranes phosphatidylinositol is located primarily on the inner leaflet of the bilayer (see Fig. 2-2 for structure). Phosphatidylinositol phospholipids in mammalian cells often have a high content of arachidonic acid and are important in that they frequently provide this fatty acid substrate for the synthesis of prostaglandins and leukotrienes.

Phosphatidylinositol-4-phosphate (PIP): A phospholipid found in small quantities in the membranes of cells which may be important for stimulus-transmission coupling (see Fig. 4-2).

Phosphatidylinositol-4,5-phosphate (PIP_2): A phospholipid found in small quantities in cells. The phosphate group in the 5 position turns over rapidly in resting cells. It is believed to be very important for stimulus-activation coupling (see Fig. 4-2). The structure of this phospholipid is shown in Fig. 4-1.

Phosphatidic Acid: A negatively charged phospholipid present in very small amounts in resting blood cells. When cells are stimulated frequently a significant increase in phosphatidic acid is seen. This increase in phosphatidic acid is related to the receptor-coupled breakdown of phosphoinositides (Fig. 4-2). The structure of phosphatidic acid is shown in Fig. 2-16.

Phospholamban: A protein found in cardiac muscle. When phosphorylated by cAMP, phospholambin promotes sequestration of calcium.

Phospholipase: An enzyme which cleaves one or more phospholipids. Four types, phospholipase A_1, phospholipase A_2, phospholipase C, and phospholipase D, are present in blood cells (see Chapter 4 for more details).

Phytohemagglutinin: A mucoprotein obtained from the red kidney bean which stimulates the proliferation of T lymphocytes.

PIP: See phosphatidylinositol-4-phosphate.

PIP$_2$: See phospatidylinositol-4,5-phosphate.

Platelet-Activating Factor: Acetyl glyceryl ether-phosphoryl choline (AGEPC). A phospholipid synthesized primarily in stimulated mast cells, monocytes, and neutrophils with potent activity to stimulate platelet and neutrophil aggregation.

Prostacyclin: See PGI_2.

Prostaglandin: Biologically active chemicals derived from polyunsaturated fatty acids with a 5-carbon ring as shown in the basic prostanoic acid skeleton in Fig. 2-11. The structure of prostaglandin E_2 (PGE_2) is shown in Fig. 1-1. The structures of additional prostaglandins are outlined in Appendix 2-1. The name prostaglandin was used initially as the compounds were first found in semen, and they were thought to be derived from the prostate gland. The name has been retained even though prostaglandins in semen are now known to be derived primarily from the seminal vesicles.

Prostaglandin Synthetase: The enzyme responsible for the formation of the prostaglandin endoperoxides PGG_2 and PGH_2 from arachidonic acid. Also known as the prostaglandin endoperoxide synthetase or fatty acid cyclo-oxygenase enzyme (see Chapter 5).

Protein Kinase C: A protein kinase which can phosphorylate certain intracellular proteins in platelets and probably in other blood cells, in association with cell stimulation.

Sphingomyelin: A sphingolipid which is an important constituent of the outer bilayer of the plasma membrane in red blood cells, platelets, and probably also in other blood cells.

Thromboxane A_2: An unstable lipid produced from PGH_2, through the action of a thromboxane synthetase enzyme, with potent activity to cause platelet aggregation and vasoconstriction in many vascular beds. The basic thrombanoic acid structure is shown in Fig. 2-13. Thromboxane A_2 has two substituent groups added on this basic skeleton C_9-O-C_{11} and an OH attached to C_{15}.

Thromboxane B_2: The stable metabolite of thromboxane A_2. Thromboxane B_2 has three hydroxyl groups attached to the basic thrombanoic acid skeleton (Fig. 2-13) at C_9, C_{11}, and C_{15}.

T Cells: Lymphocytes with an important role in cell-mediated immunity (for further details see Chapter 12).

Zymosan: A carbohydrate obtained from the walls of yeast cells. When added to serum, complement is activated and the chemotactic peptide C5a is produced.

Index